I0447077

The ULTIMATE
Supermarket Handbook

Your guide to what's *really* healthy

By Kylie Floate
BSc.(Nutrition).Grad.Dip.Edu.(ECS)

Contents

Overview

Supermarkets have become our lifelines. The average person is so consumed by a myriad of society constraints that we have become reliant on supermarket produce. The consumer is now at the mercy of clever marketing and the multi-nationals who appear to have a reckless disregard for our health. That is of course, if you discount the claims of 97% fat free and other so-called 'guilt-free' delights.

The bottom line is that much of our food supply is toxic and void of any nutrients. The food we are filling our trolleys with is making us unhealthy. Even consumers who try to choose healthy varieties are routinely sabotaged by clever marketing and deceptive labelling. In fact one really requires a science degree to make sense of a food label. Fortunately I have one!

I thought it was time to level the playing field and give the consumer the opportunity to make an informed choice. Each of the thousands of supermarket items were reviewed and rated according to the nutrient content; the presence of food additives and given a nutritious rating.

The nutrients that I assessed were total fat, sugar and salt. Generous allowances were given to each and are well above the legal labelling laws that deem a product as low in fat, sugar or salt.

To receive a tick, a product needed to have less than 8g of total fat per 100g; less than 10g of sugar per 100g and less than 500mg of salt per 100g. Please note that sugar doesn't necessarily need to be sucrose (conventional white sugar) to be listed as high in sugar. Many products have fruit syrups or concentrates added as a sweetener that doesn't make them any healthier. There are many forms of sugar. The most common ones used as sweetening agents are maltose, fructose and sucrose. While maltose is probably the healthiest of the three, they are all still sugar. Receiving a tick for nutrition does not mean that the food is necessarily 'nutritious'. It simply is low in fat, sugar and salt. Cardboard satisfies all of these criteria, yet could hardly be described as nutritious. Nutritious foods contain a variety of vitamins and minerals and are mostly found in minimally processed foods. However, the fat, sugar and salt content have been highlighted, as these seem to be what is of most concern to consumers.

Some items, like ice-cream, chips and chocolate, have obviously high amounts of fat, sugar or salt. Rather than discount them all, I have highlighted the best of the worst. There is still room for treats, the body is amazingly resilient, but some are much better than others.

This guide also assesses a grocery item according to the presence of food additives. After reviewing the research into the harmful effects of some food additives, I have highlighted those I believe should be avoided and included a summary of the associated effects. Many of these food additives have been banned in other countries, yet currently are still permitted in Australia and New Zealand. In addition, I have contacted each of the manufacturers to explore any hidden additives. In Australia and New Zealand if an ingredient contained is less than 5% of the overall product, it does not require labelling. A manufacturer can also use a pre-preserved ingredient such as vinegar and omit the preservative from the label. In fact they can also label the product as "No added preservatives", because technically they didn't add the preservative, someone else did!

I have also included some interesting research into food packaging and chemical migration to help to raise awareness to this issue.

Please note that I am not endorsing certain brands or suggesting that you eat those foods. Nor am I saying that you should never eat the foods that were awarded zero ticks. I am merely trying to help you make informed choices. I have found that food labels are very cryptic, with very small print. Research has also shown that the average person is time poor and heavily reliant on the information presented on the front of the label rather than the nutrition information panel on the back. The food industry is aware of this and uses it to their full advantage.

Most people I talk to, want to choose good food for their family, but they also just want to get in an out of the supermarket as quickly as possible. Now you can look up your family favourites at your leisure and take some of the headache out of grocery shopping.

Disclaimer

While every effort has been made to ensure that all information contained within is accurate and current, I am human and will not be held libel for any errors.

Introduction to Food Additives

A food additive is an ingredient that has been added to a food to perform one or more technical functions. Common functions of food additives include preservation, bulking, thickening, anti-separation, colouring, mould retardant, moisture retention, flavour enhancement and fermentation prevention. Many of these functions can be performed safely, such as with the use of tocopherols (vitamin E) and ascorbic acid (vitamin C).

However, many food manufacturers favour the cheaper and often toxic options. Avoiding food additives is not is an easy task, as they do seem to be in everything. However, there are usually one or two brands on the market that are mostly doing the right thing. My ultimate goal is to assert change in food manufacturing procedures. Many countries have banned the use of these harmful food additives and I am hoping that Australia and New Zealand can follow suit. For example, currently there are 877 colouring agents approved for use; Norway has just 34. It begs the question, why do we need 877 colouring agents?

The effects of tartrazine (102) and Sunset yellow (110) are well founded. Studies have shown that they cause hyperactivity, aggression, confusion, interference with mental computation and exacerbation of neurological disorders, such as depression. These colorants go hand in hand as additives to fruit juice, breakfast cereals, soft drinks, confectionary, biscuits and ice-cream. It is important to note that I am hoping these items will be re-formulated, not banned. With saying that, the body is very resilient and can cope with the occasional indulgence.

Colours

Colouring agents are used purely for aesthetic purposes; they serve no other function than looking good. There are three types of colours: naturally derived colours, like beetroot and paprika; chemically identical colours that are produced in a laboratory and are much cheaper than the natural counterpart; and the synthetic 'coal tar' colours, which are made from petro-chemicals. In Australia, there are thirteen coal tar colours still in use. It is important to note that natural colourings are still used in doses that exceed what they would in nature. 'Natural' colours or chemically identical colours are not consumed in 'natural' quantities and can still cause adverse reactions. All of the listed colouring agents are linked to hyperactivity, aggression, neurological disorders, migraines, skin rashes, asthma and eczema.

There are many colours that are shrouded in suspicion, however these are the colours where the evidence against their use is strong and have been banned elsewhere in the world. The Acceptable Daily Intake (A.D.I.) in Australia and New Zealand is 290g/kg in food or 70mg/L.

102	Tartrazine
104	Quinoline Yellow
110	Sunset Yellow
122	Carmoisine
123	Amaranth
124	Ponceau 4R
127	Erythrosine
129	Allura red
132	Indigotine
133	Brilliant blue
142	Green S
153	Carbon Black
154	Brown HT
160b	Annatto extract*
174	Silver
175	Gold

*<u>Annatto extract</u> has not been banned in other countries; however, double-blind studies have shown it can cause hyperactivity (head-banging, oppositional defiance etc) and skin rashes in sensitive people. Annatto is used extensively throughout our food supply. The A.D.I. varies with different food groups. The highest A.D.I. for annatto extract is 100mg/kg in breakfast cereals. Annatto can be found in cheese, butter, vegetable oil, ice-cream, yoghurt, biscuits, frozen chips and meat products.

<u>Cochineal or carmines (120)</u> are produced from scale insects. It is the colouring that produces the pretty candy pink and various shades of red. It is used in icings, confectionary, ice-cream, cooking sauces, canned fruit, jelly, cakes, biscuits and marinades. The use of additive 120 is very widespread and is produced by crushing the eggs or boiling the beetles (sometimes just their wings or eggs) in acid and forming a concentrated powder. The powder is either used as is, or dissolved in alcohol and sold as 'natural' food colouring. I am certainly not against eating insects, most are highly nutritious; but I hardly see what is 'natural' about this process.

<u>Sorbates</u>

Sorbates are used to keep food moist and prevent mould forming. This type of preservative is linked to the trigger of asthma attacks and behavioural problems.

The highest A.D.I. for sorbates is 1000mg/kg and are commonly found in confectionary, particularly fudge, ice confectionary, cream cheese, dips, yoghurt, cheese rennet, sausages and fruit juice.

200	Sorbic acid
201	Sodium sorbate
202	Potassium sorbate
203	Calcium sorbate

Benzoates

Benzoates are commonly used to prevent fruit products from fermenting or losing their flavour. They are also used with rennet enzymes in cheese-making. When benzoates combines with vitamin C, benzene is formed, a known carcinogen. Studies show that the various forms of benzoate can cause hyperactivity, aggression, skin rashes and can trigger asthma attack. The JENCFA database shows that test animals displayed hyper-excitability, incontinence, convulsions and all of the animals died within two-weeks. Benzoates have an A.D.I. of up to 2500mg/kg and are commonly found in soft drinks, fruit juices, fruit tubs, fruit pies, yoghurt and cheese products. Many products are free of benzoates; it is just a matter of reading the label.

210   Benzoic acid

211   Sodium benzoate

212   Potassium benzoate

213   Calcium benzoate

Sulphites

Sulphites are mostly used to stop ingredients going brown or losing their colour. Mostly, they are associated with asthma attacks. Research has shown that sulphite exposure irritates the airways, which exacerbates the effects of other known triggers. Sulphites are also linked to behavioural problems and stomach   upset. JENCFA research indicated that doses between 250mg-6g caused vomiting and severe stomach and intestinal irritation in most of the human test subjects. In addition, sulphite intake caused increased calcium excretion, thiamin inactivation and the gradual depletion of vitamin A in the liver.

A small handful of dried fruit may contain 80mg of sulphite, yet the A.D.I. is 0.7mg per kg of body weight. One sausage may contain 50mg. If you start adding up highly probable food sources that a small child might eat in any one-day, it greatly exceeds the A.D.I. Sulphites are found in fruit juice, dried fruit, nuts, instant noodles, soup, muesli bars, breakfast cereal, fresh prawns, canned vegetables, cheese and wine, just to mention a few. Manufacturers can use sulphites up to a level of 3000 mg/kg, depending on the type of food. It is possible to find food that is processed without the use of sulphites.

220	Sulphur dioxide
221	Sodium sulphite
222	Sodium bisulphite
223	Sodium metasulphite
224	Potassium metabisulphite
225	Potassium sulphite
228	Potassium bisulphite

Nitrates

Nitrates serve the function of a preservative but technically aren't classified as one and can legally be labelled as 'No Preservatives'. It is mostly used in fresh and cured meat products to prevent the growth of harmful micro-organisms. JENFCA strongly discourages the use of sodium nitrate in baby food or foods intended for small children. For this reason it is prohibited in baby foods. Unfortunately, sodium nitrate is used extensively in sausages, bacon, most crumbed or marinated meat, ham and other processed meats that are commonly eaten by small children, even babies. It would be appropriate to alert parents, so that they are able to make informed choices when feeding their children. Sodium nitrate consumption is associated with decreased growth, skin irritations, abdominal pain, headaches, confusion, nauseas and behavioural problems. The nitrites are more toxic than the nitrates, but unfortunately nitrate can be converted to nitrite in the gut. Nitrate can also react with amines and form nitrosamine, which is a poison.

The maximum A.D.I. for nitrate or nitrite is 125mg/kg.

249	Potassium nitrite
250	Sodium nitrite
251	Sodium nitrate
252	Potassium nitrate

Propionates

Propionates are mould retardants; the most notable is calcium propionate (282), which was famously exposed by Sue Dengate's double-blind study. Results revealed that additive 282 could cause irritability, inattention; sleep disturbance, irritable bowel syndrome, heart palpitations, speech delay and lethargy. It was also found that the effects built up slowly and seemed to accumulate in the body. Propionates can be used at a level of up to 4000mg/kg and can be found in cakes, bread and pastries. Many bakeries have removed the use of 282 in light of Sue Dengate's work, but commercial bread-makers have become savvier. They use preserved vinegar and vegetable oil.

280	Propionic acid
281	Sodium propionate

| 282 | Calcium propionate |
| 283 | Potassium propionate |

Antioxidants

Antioxidants sound healthy, but really aren't. These synthetic compounds prevent foods from going rancid from oxidation (exposure to oxygen causing micro-organisms to thrive). Antioxidants such as B.H.A. (320), B.H.T. (321) and T.B.H. (319) do not provide any health benefits. It has been found that B.H.A. and B.H.T. are readily absorbed in the fat tissue and takes three to four days to work its way through the system. This means that a regular consumption of foods containing B.H.A. or B.H.T. can result in an accumulation in the body, with higher levels than the recommended A.D.I. B.H.T. was found in animal studies to elevate serum cholesterol. B.H.T. also interacted with vitamin A to cause abnormalities in pregnancy and demonstrated a carcinogenic effect. B.H.T. and B.H.A. are prohibited for use in baby food or those intended for young children. It seems there is a need to inform pregnant women and parents of the dangers of B.H.T. and B.H.A. Particularly, as these two additives often go undeclared in vegetable oil used in commercial bread. These antioxidants are found wherever there is vegetable oil or animal fat and may be used at a level of up to 200mg/kg. The use of antioxidants can easily be avoided with the help of vitamin C, vitamin E, vacuum packaging, low temperature storage and storage away from light.

319	Tertiary butylated hydroquinone
320	Butylated hydroxyanisole
321	Butylated hydroxytoluene

Flavour Enhancers

Flavour enhancers, particularly MSG are associated with 'Chinese Food Syndrome'. Due to the bad publicity, most Chinese food eateries proudly display a 'No MSG' sign. Of course, this means that they're not sprinkling it into their dishes, but there has been several cases where ingredients have been used that already contain a flavour enhancer and have caused adverse reactions. Flavour enhancers are rarely labelled clearly and are often disguised as 'hydrolysed vegetable protein (HVP)', 'yeast extract (YE)', 'vegetable protein extract (VPE)' or 'natural flavouring'. All are linked to headaches, insomnia, asthma, allergic reactions, hyperactivity and nausea.

627 and 631 are prohibited for use in baby food. The additive 635 has been banned elsewhere in the world. They are likely to be found in potato chips, sauces, marinades, sushi, burgers, fried chicken, spreads, instant noodles and frozen foods. There is no A.D.I. set, which means that its use is unrestricted.

| 620 | L-Glutamic acid |
| 621 | Monosodium L-glutamate (MSG) |

622	Monopotassium L-glutamate
623	Calcium glutamate
624	Monoammonium L-glutamate
625	Magnesium glutamate
627	Disodium 5'-guaylate
635	Disodium 5'-ribonucleotides
641	L-Leucine

Artificial Sweeteners

Artificial sweeteners are used to reduce the kilojoule content of food. Until recently, the evidence against artificial sweeteners was weak. The studies were poorly designed and not reasonably translatable to humans. Compelling evidence has emerged in recent years, resulting in serious doubts of the continued use of artificial sweeteners.

The research has focused on aspartame, which has been found that it can over stimulate the brain causing or exacerbating neurological disorders. In addition, in animal studies aspartame exposure caused tumours. They also tend to have a laxative effect.

The current A.D.I varies according to its use, but the highest levels have been approved for confectionary at a concentration of 10000mg/kg. Almost every product has a 'diet' option that has been artificially sweetened.

951	Aspartame
952	Calcium cyclamate or sodium cyclamate
954	Saccharin
955	Sucralose
956	Alitame
957	Thaumatin
965	Maltitol
966	Lactitol
967	Xylitol

<u>Carrageenan (407)</u> is an emulsifier that is used in food to improve texture, as a thickening agent or to stop separation. It is currently allowed at a level of 2g/kg and often found in confectionary, dairy products and infant formula. Studies on test animals show that carrageenan interferes with pepsin activity during the digestion process. This results in the interference of nutrient absorption, kidney damage and deformities. I recommend exercising caution with this additive. However, products such as ice-cream are almost impossible to buy without a dose

of carrageenan. I am not suggesting that you never eat ice-cream again; the body is resilient and can handle the occasional indulgence. Awareness is the key.

Humectants comprise of a variety of substances used for moisture and texture retention. Dried fruits, muesli bars, biscuits and desserts are the most likely products to contain humectants. 420 and 421 are banned in baby foods or those intended for children. All cause a laxative effect and can interfere with nutrition absorption and hydration. The nastiest of the humectants is 1520. It is mostly used in baby wipes to stop them drying out and is used extensively on fresh fruit and vegetables. 1520 is a toxic chemical that is linked to neurological disorders, as well as kidney and liver damage. There are four main types.

420	Sorbitol
421	Mannitol
422	Glycerol
1520	Propylene glycol

Introduction to Food Packaging

Plastic has literally invaded our planet. Its use in food packaging commenced in the 1960's and has become progressively more widespread. By the 1990's, most of the waxed paper and glass packaging had been replaced by plastic.

Today, there are only a handful of lines that are produced exclusively in glass. The most notable is coffee. The reason for the glass packaging is simple; plastic chemicals migrate from the packaging to food/drinks. Irrespective of the type of plastic, or whether the packaged item is liquid, solid or aqueous – plastic will leach toxic chemicals. This is a fact. Coffee producers opt for glass, not because they are concerned with the consumers' health; but because they are ensuring the flavour integrity is maintained and not contaminated by the plastic.

There are six types of plastic used in food packaging.

Polyethylene Terephthalate (P.E.T.) – used to package soft-drink, water, fruit juice, salad dressing, jams and spreads. This type of plastic is known for being transparent and flexible.

High-Density Polyethylene (H.D.P.E) – used to package milk, fruit juice, sauces and breakfast cereals. This type of plastic is usually translucent and is available is various thickness. It can also be thin enough to make a plastic insert to package dry materials such as breakfast cereal.

<u>Low-Density Polyethylene (L.D.P.E)</u> – used to package frozen foods, bread, milk carton coatings, lids, squeeze bottles and disposable cups.

<u>Polyvinyl Chloride (P.V.C.)</u> – used to manufacture shrink-wrap, cling-film and vacuum packaging.

<u>Polypropylene</u> – used to manufacture containers for packaging margarine, yoghurt, cottage cheese, ice-cream and 'take-aways'. Consumers quite often reuse these containers, despite the fact that they are not suitable for multiple use or at all heat stable.

<u>Polycarbonate</u> – these are much sturdier plastics that are used to manufacture re-usable drink bottles, buckets of honey and canisters of rice or flour.

<u>Polystyrene</u> – often called 'foam' products, which are used to package instant noodles, meat trays and take-away containers.

Numerous studies, worldwide have been conducted into global chemical migration. Each reveals that that various components of food packaging contaminate the contents and usually at much higher rates than the regulations allow. The current legislation allows up to 60mg/kg of chemical migration.

The most common chemicals found to migrate from food packaging are: methylbenzene, ethylbenzene, 1-octene, zylene, styrene, 1,4 dichlobenzene, toluene, benzophenone (printing ink), bisphenol A (B.P.A.), phthalates and benzene. They are classified as volatiles, additives, monomers and oligomers.

The factors that have been found to have the most influence over chemical migration are temperature, pH, time, molecular size and weight, chemical structure, fat content and degrees of crystallinity.

Most of the studies have recommended a re-evaluation of the current legislation and in many cases, a complete ban of a plastic for use in food packaging. Researchers have noted that the safety of plastics is generally based on the individual chemicals and not the overall synergistic effects.

This is a three-fold issue. Firstly, there is often a lack of evidence that an individual chemical is appropriate for the use of food packaging. Secondly, there are many chemicals used to manufacture a type of plastic and there is limited data to support the safety of those chemical interactions. The area that is most lacking, is how these plastic compounds are affected by the unique chemical composition of the food or beverage. The food industry is not required to complete testing of their products and provide evidence that the packagings of their products are safe. Plastic manufacturers can only give a general guideline for the applications of their products and how they are actually used, is not really their responsibility.

The Government has set a limit of 60mg/kg or 10mg/dm2 of allowable chemical migration from food packaging. This might be fine for an isolated occurrence, as the body is very resilient. However, the ingestion of these toxic substances is not an isolated occurrence, they are happening on a daily basis and the long-term effects are unknown and not reflected in the current regulation. To take this one step further, on any given day the average person is consuming food from various plastic packaging, the various chemicals have unknown synergistic effects. Couple that with the multiple food additives contained within each food, also with unknown synergistic effects.

A study of British school children found that 67% of their daily consumption of food came from those packaged in plastic. They were also more likely to have kids-sized little packets of snacks. These smaller packets contain higher concentrations of plastic chemicals than the full sized varieties. Overall, the daily intake of plastic chemicals were higher per kilogram of body weight that that of adults. Infants under one year were found to consume 0.65dm2/kg of body weight of chemicals associated with plastic packaging. Children aged between one and four years consumed 0.81dm2/kg of body weight and four to six year-olds consumed 0.66dm2/kg of bodyweight. The current regulations assume that the average person would not exceed 0.1dm2/kg of bodyweight.

In fact most of the studies conducted show that the migration levels far exceed what is deemed to be safe.

P.E.T packaging has found to leach various forms of benzene and phythlates. The level of benzene was found in cooking oil was 73.9mg/L and 4.1mg/L in bottled water. Benzene has strong links to animal and human birth defects. Long-term exposure can affect normal blood production, damage the immune system and cause a range of cancers, particularly leukaemia.

Phythlates migration is particularly influenced by the presence of fat and heat. There are different types of phythlates, all differing in toxicity and ability to migrate. The worst is believed to be di-2, etheylhexl phythlate. Test animals show teratogenic effects, liver damage, kidney damage, weight gain, retarded growth and longevity, with none surviving beyond fifty-five weeks.

Humans have higher fat stores than test animals and it have been proposed, that we may actually have a greater capacity for absorbing plastic chemicals and have a higher level of risk.

L.D.P.E packaging has been found to contain high levels of benzoic anhydride and 4-hydroxybenzoic acid; 30-40% and 10-20% respectively, were found to migrate into the foods and liquids tested. Most of the migrating substances seem to reach a plateau where migration ceases due to saturation.

H.D.P.E packaging has been found to have high levels of nonyphenol migration. Researchers predict that the average person consumes 7.5µg per day of nonylphenol. Levels from H.D.E.P bottles were 180µg/L and 300µg in P.V.C bottles.

P.V.C. packaging has been found to contaminate cheese, poultry, cooked and uncooked meats, fruit and vegetables and baked goods. Uncooked meat and poultry contained up to 72.8mg/kg, depending on the fat content. Skinless chicken and trimmed meats had less contamination. Cooked chicken had up to 48.6mg/kg. Cheese contained up to 135mg/kg. Fruit and vegetables contained up to 2mg/kg and baked goods, including wrapped sandwiches had up to 212mg/kg depending on the fat content.

77% of the P.V.C films tested were deemed unsuitable for food packaging. Levels of di-(2-ethylhexl) adipate (D.E.H.A) were detected at levels ranging from 20-30mg/dm2 from films that are classified as "low migration". In a study of cheese wrapped in P.V.C cling-film, a level of 45mg/kg of D.E.H.A. was found after two hours at 5°C. After ten days, the level had increased to 150mg/kg. The maximum tolerable allowance (M.T.A.) of D.E.H.A. is 0.3mg/kg of body weight. The researchers concluded that the average person's exposure would easily exceed the current M.T.A. They also recommended the discontinuation of P.V.C as a food packaging material.

Polypropylene has been found to be one of the least stable food packaging materials. Migration occurs with all types of substances and between the temperature range of 20°C and 60°C. Various toxic chemicals contaminate the food, but migration has been shown to decrease with an increased thickness of the polypropylene used.

Polystyrene has been shown to leach the highly toxic substance styrene. Migration occurs at all temperatures, but is at their highest at room temperature and in the presence of oil. Researchers found that the concentration of styrene increased when a product was nearer the used-by-date and estimated that the average person consumes 12μg of styrene per day.

Other sources of chemical contamination come from paperboard, cellophane, aluminium cans, steel cans and foil.

Paperboard leaches benzophone, a printing ink, which is highly toxic and completely unregulated. Recycling has caused levels to increase further.

Cellophane has many applications in food packaging. It is currently manufactured by combining two layers. The outer layer is plant cellulose and the inner food-contact layer is made from a phythlate ester and a sulphuric acid mist. Both are human carcinogens. In addition to the harmful properties of phythlates already mentioned, the chemical has oestrogen-mimicing potential and has been implicated in the early on-set of puberty and cancers of the reproductive organs, including breast cancer.

Aluminium and steel cans are lined with the epoxy resin bisphenol-A (B.P.A.). Polycarbonate plastic also contains B.P.A. B.P.A. has been found in numerous studies to be an endocrine system disruptor. In other words it can interfere with hormone function, in particular, oestrogen. It has also been found to cause neurotoxicity. Animal studies revealed damage to the brain and reproductive organs, with changes in hormone levels and observed behaviour when fed low levels of B.P.A. in utero.

B.P.A. migrates into water at 0.79mg per hour at room temperature. The rate increases by 55% when exposed to heat. Most canned goods are either cooked in the can or packed when hot. Some baby food producers are now planning to phase out their use of B.P.A in canned goods, but to date, all canned goods contain B.P.A

Europe seems to be the most aware and active in making reforms to food packaging regulations. Recently we have seen the removal of B.P.A from baby bottles but until there is a public outcry for changes to food packaging, I believe the industry or the government will never instigate reform.

Guide to selecting staples

Bread

I strongly recommend buying bread from a bakery or baking your own. Bakery bread is baked fresh daily and without the use of preservatives. Preservatives can come in the form of intentionally added chemicals, such as calcium propionate (282); or pre-preserved ingredients, such as vegetable oil or vinegar. Typically, vegetable oil is preserved with T.B.H. (319), B.H.A. (320) or B.H.A. (321) and vinegar is preserved with a benzoic acid (210 - 212) or sulphites (220-228).

Supermarket bread tends to be packaged in plastic, often while still warm. Most bakeries offer the option of a paper bag.

White bread will usually have less energy (kilojoules) and nutrients than a multigrain wholemeal variety, but has a high glycaemic index. Subsequently, multigrain bread will help you to feel fuller for longer. It also contains a lot of fibre that assists with the digestion process, keeping you healthy and regular.

Butter and Margarine

Butter can be made easily at home in less than five minutes. A carton of cream that costs less than two dollars could easily supply the family with butter for a week. Commercial butter has a cocktail of additives in order to preserve its taste, texture and colour for at least a year. Why does butter need a use by date that far in the future? Not many of us would make our own butter and then consider storing it for up to a year, it would be rancid. Why does the dairy industry attempt to do that? Supermarkets have an exceptionally high stock turnover and I would love to a meet a consumer that is looking for that kind of shelf-life.

If it really is inconceivable to make your own butter, opt for the no-name brands as they tend to be lower in the additives and packaged in waxed paper. Margarine by nature is an artificial product and is always packaged in plastic. Don't get me wrong, I grew up on the stuff and have always preferred to taste of margarine to butter. If you really can't live without it, brands like Nuttelex, Meadow Lee and Black & Gold or Homebrand butter are the best options.

Cheese

Cheddar cheese is almost always packaged in plastic. Chemical migration is high due to the fat content. Cheese usually has a host of undeclared additives, including colours, annatto extracts, sulphites and sorbates. Research also shows that cheese is highly susceptible to chemical migration from plastic cling wrap that almost every household uses to maintain freshness.

If you are going to eat cheese, regard it as a treat. Cheese is not healthy. Never buy cheese pre-grated, as sorbates and sulphites are usually added to stop the cheese drying out and losing its colour. When storing the cheese after opening, wrap the block in paper towel and then place in a zip lock bag.

Speciality cheeses, such as Brie and Camembert are usually packaged in a waxed paper or foil. In terms of packaging, these chesses are a better option. However, in terms of fat content, they are usually worse and the additive risk remains the same.

Soft cheeses, such as cottage or ricotta are fairly low in fat, but high in salt. At present, I cannot find a brand that does not use food additives. I have a cheese-making book that shows how easy it is to make ricotta and cottage cheese........it might be an avenue to explore.

Coffee and Tea

Have you ever noticed that coffee and tea never comes packaged in plastic? No they aren't concerned with your health. The manufacturers just aren't willing to risk the plastic chemical migration altering the flavour of their product. Try to buy organic fair trade coffee. Most of the coffee is grown in third world countries that are poorly compensated for their efforts. I recommend the 'plunger' or coffee machine varieties as it is a better product and there are many brands offering organic fair trade.

I love herbal teas and get a kick out of sampling new varieties. I have found that there are many brands on the market that artificially flavour their tea. Read the label. There is hardly any price difference between the real deal and the synthetic varieties. It is like comparing fruit juice to cordial. While both can be satisfying, there is a clear difference in quality.

Make sure coffee and/ or black tea is restricted to one or two cups per day and are consumed two hours before or after eating as they interfere with nutrient absorption.

Confectionary

Confectionary refers to lollies, sweets, and candy – whatever it is you like to call them! Obviously, they are not a healthy food source. Generally they contain a lot of sugar and food additives. Contrary to the 99% fat free claim that many packets advertise, lollies WILL contribute to weight gain! When I was working in an office a colleague said to me quite seriously "but they are 99% fat free, lollies won't make you fat just rot your teeth" So for those that who are still labouring under a misapprehension, ALL food contributes to over all energy. The energy that is not used, is stored as fat.

This isn't to say that confectionary should be avoided all together, but I would

advise their consumption be kept to a minimum. All varieties of confectionary are void of nutrients and are basically empty kilojoules. In light of that, pick your favourites, as there really isn't much difference. Of course, I lean toward the 'natural' coloured varieties rather than those containing 102, 110, 127, 129, 133......
Nothing will possess me to feed anything with those colouring agents to my kids, the effects are just too obvious.

Deli Meats

Deli meats on the whole are preserved with sodium nitrate/nitrite (250/251), plumped with water (on average 30%) and packaged in plastic. Some contain propyl glycerol (1520), potassium sorbate (202), sodium benzoate (211) and flavour enhancers (621-635).

It worries me that deli meat is a common sandwich filling, particularly for school lunches.

I am aware that some butchers and speciality stores are selling preservative free ham and bacon. Alternatively, roast some meat and keep it sliced in the freezer; or consider having a vegetarian lunch – it is much healthier and cheaper.

Eggs

ALWAYS BUY FREE RANGE EGGS!!! There is no excuse for buying cage eggs. If you are oblivious to the cruelty that caged battery hens face –WAKE UP! As long as people continue to buy cage eggs, the cruelty will continue. Once the cage eggs business is debunked, the price of free range eggs will decrease. Make a stand. Remember the use by date on the carton is just a guide. Place the eggs in a container of water; if the eggs sink they are fresh, if they float, they need to be thrown away.

Flour

Flour is usually packaged is paper, although there are a few plastic canister varieties on the market. When storing flour in the pantry, either leave the contents inside the paper bag and seal in an air-tight container, or store the flour in a glass canister.

Always buy unbleached organic flour. Buying organic baked goods can be expensive. With the help of organic flour, sugar and eggs; a family can eat organically very cheaply. Where possible, buy wholemeal. Wholemeal flour provides more fibre, making it easier to reduce portion size and feel fuller for longer.

Fruit and Vegetables

Unfortunately the current practice in agriculture is to use dozens of pesticide chemicals during the growing period and then to wash the produce in bleach. Fruit is routinely harvested before the produce has had a chance to mature, then placed in 'cold storage' for months and finally artificially ripened with toxic chemicals. Vegetables are grown to maturation, but constantly doused in toxic chemicals after harvest to prevent deterioration.

Most of the chemicals used are carcinogenic. I suggest avoiding fruit and vegetables grown in this way, but I understand that organic produce is often twice the price. If you have read my previous book *The Undeniable TRUTH About FOOD*, you would know that I am a big advocate for growing your own. Ditch the flowerbed and establish a vegetable garden and put in some fruit trees.

If you must buy commercial produce, buy seasonally and don't assume that something is necessarily from this season. Stores can buy previous seasons stock cheaper and then put it on 'special' for you. If you're not sure ask. I would rather spend a couple of dollars more, knowing that the fruit I am buying has not sat in cold storage since last year.

Try to buy whole produce that has not been pre-cut. Fruit and vegetables continue to respire after they have been picked, once the flesh has been cut into, the life force is liberated and it is.....dead. There are miraculous phytochemicals and live enzymes in plant food that only survive for a maximum of twenty minutes once it has been cut. Research shows that these amazing compounds exhibit antioxidant and anti-cancer properties. However, they are very fragile and don't survive for long, especially when subjected to heat or freezing.

Meat

Approximately eighty percent of supermarket meat and forty percent of butcher meat come from intensive farming operations. The animals are confined, fed an unnatural diet and slaughtered factory-style. Even if you are not concerned with animal welfare, meat produced in 'feed lots' have lower nutrient compositions and inferior amino acid profiles. In order to build muscle effectively, animals must be able to move. Meat is then vacuum-sealed and is up to three months old when it is sold as 'fresh'. Vacuum sealing eliminates oxygen so that bacteria cannot thrive. However, amines are able to thrive, as they do not require oxygen. Amines are derivatives from ammonia and are compounds that are inevitable in the presence of cellular death - they are the result of decay or protein denature (oxygen causes the foul odour). Not all amines are bad; in fact many such as amino acids are vital for bodily function. However, others can accumulate in the body causing toxic effects. Everyone's tolerance for amines is different, but the end result is intoxication. Hay fever is an example of how people react differently to histamines. Everyone's tolerance for amines is different. The boiling point of amines is very high and therefore heat stable during normal cooking.

I recommend buying free-range meat from a butcher and don't be afraid to ask about the date of slaughter and the presence of food additives. They are perfectly reasonable questions and most butchers are happy to oblige.

Avoid buying marinated or crumbed meat as they are likely to contain food additives and they are usually made from the previous day's meat that didn't sell.

Milk

Despite what we are told, milk really doesn't promote health or contribute to bone density. Milk is high in phosphate, which causes the body to become acidic. In order to maintain the body's pH, it draws minerals, namely calcium from the bone and soft tissue. Bone in particular, acts as a buffer, delivering calcium ions, but over time this process leads to the dissolution of bone minerals and bone density. According to numerous studies calcium intake from dairy has no beneficial effect on bone density. In a double-blind study conducted by Cambridge University (2010), one group was given calcium rich water and the other was given bicarbonate rich (alkaline) water. Those drinking the calcium water experienced no impact on bone density, where as those drinking the alkaline-rich bicarbonate water showed significant results. In addition, researchers have found that the consumption of dairy products is associated with a higher risk of colorectal cancer, prostate cancer, ovarian cancer and breast cancer.

Another interesting fact is that approximately fifteen percent of the world's population (mostly Caucasian) possess the enzyme lactase, which is necessary to breakdown lactose in milk after the age of four. This means that at least eighty-five percent of the Western population is likely to be lactose intolerant. Asian people are notorious for their avoidance of dairy products due to lactose intolerance, favouring soy instead. Approximately ninety-eight percent of Indigenous Australians are lactose intolerant. In fact many cultures stop drinking milk after the age of five and we are the only creatures on the planet that drink milk as adults.

As the Western world doesn't tend to breast feed to the age of five, nor do we have wet nurses anymore; another animal's milk is all that is on offer. I do recommend children consuming milk until five and then water should be substituted. I don't really think there is a need for adults to be drinking milk.

If you do want to drink milk, opt for A2 milk that is packaged in glass or tetra pack. A2 milk is the original type of milk, mostly from Jersey cows, that contains proteins which are easier for humans to digest. Unfortunately, a couple of centuries ago farmers were seduced by the high yielding A1 cows. The A1 cows were mostly the Friesian breeds that produce higher quantities of milk that are of a lower quality. Today with cross-breeding, a cow must be biochemically tested in order to determine the type of proteins it produces. New Zealand has phased out its A1 cows and it is becoming trendy in Australia also.

The other benefit of drinking A2 milk is there is no additives or permeates added. Permeates are a biological substance produced from the whole milk, when making other dairy products such as cheese. The Permeates are then added back into the milk supply and in effect 'water it down'. This is standard practice. Unless the milk states that it is additive free, assume that it isn't. There are several small dairies producing organic permeate free milk and the likes of Pura Gold. The biggest brand that is easily obtained is the A2 milk company.

Alternatively, almond milk is an excellent substitute, which is naturally nutrient dense and tastes delicious.

Oil

There is a lot of hype about different types of oil, but it is important to understand that they all yield virtually the same amount of energy. The most important consideration when choosing oil is packaging. NEVER buy cooking oil packaged in plastic. Only choose from those that come in glass or metal. Most of the chemicals that a plastic bottle is made from can leach out, given enough time, heat or acidity. However, oil or a high fat substance needs little time or heat to affect a plastic bottle or packaging as many of the chemicals are fat soluble. These chemicals are carcinogenic.

In terms of health I recommend grapeseed oil, rice bran oil, sunflower oil, macadamia oil or olive oil. Each has their own unique benefit, but none are so special, that the others should be discounted.

Oil also is notorious for containing undeclared additives such as 320 or 319. Very rarely are the additives labelled. Please note that genetically modified canola is permitted in Australia and New Zealand and there is a lot of conflicting evidence about its safety.

Pasta

Commercial pasta is all pretty much the same, except for the use of eggs; most are made from flour and water. There are some interesting varieties like spelt, plus there are wholemeal and organic brands.

I recommend making your own........I know you've seen them making it on Master Chef......It only takes about half an hour!

If that concept is beyond you, choose organic. Most supermarkets have their own brand for approximately a dollar more than the regular.

Rice

I am a big fan of brown rice; it has more nutrients, fibre, flavour and makes you feel full for longer. However, some dishes really call for white rice and it isn't a huge issue. What is important to remember it that rice is very energy dense. Use the rule of thumb of about half a cup of rice per person (uncooked).

Sugar

Always buy organic, preferably raw sugar as it is the only sugar that is alkaline. The body's pH has a major impact on gut health, immune function and the onset of chronic disease. Sugar is a major contributor to acidity of the body. I'm a big fan of stevia as an alternative.

BABY FOODS

Generally baby foods are produced well. Food additives are strictly controlled and manufacturing procedures are very stringent. The advantage of mass produced baby food is that it is cooked and cooled quickly, which reduces the likelihood of food-borne illness. Research shows that home cooked baby food tends to be "left out on the bench", which provides the ideal conditions for pathogens to thrive. Food prepared at home also tends to be stored in plastic containers or ice-cube trays; where as commercial brands are usually stored in glass.

I am in no way encouraging or suggesting mothers opt for commercial baby foods, I am always going to recommend fresh food prepared daily. However, I have raised four children, three of which are very close in age and I do understand the need for convenience at times.

Brands I currently believe are the best choices are *Only Organic, Holle Organic, Organic Bubs* and *Green Monkeys*.

Baby Mum Mum

Product Name	Energy	Major Nutrients	Food Additives	Nutritious Rating
Rusks	1695kJ	✓	✓	Average

Bellamy's Organic

Product Name	Energy	Major Nutrients	Food Additives	Nutritious Rating

Product Name	Energy	Major Nutrients	Food Additives	Nutritious Rating
Cereal, apple & cinnamon	155kJ	✓	✓	Good
Cereal, rice	153kJ	✓	✓	Good
Porridge	153kJ	✓	✓	Good
Rice cakes	1480kJ	✓	✓	Average
Toothipegs	1480kJ	✓	✓	Average
Apple snacks	1540kJ	✓	✓	Average
Apple & pear snacks	1260kJ	✓	✓	Average
Apple & banana snacks	1427kJ	✓	✓	Average
Pinkie apple, banana & pea	1407kJ	↑ Sugar	160b	Average
Pinkie apple, strawberry & mango	1436kJ	↑ Sugar	160b	Average

Farex

Product Name	Energy	Major Nutrients	Food Additives	Nutritious Rating
Cereal, rice 4+	190kJ	✓	✓	Good
Cereal, pear & banana	200kJ	✓	✓	Good
Cereal, original 7+	185kJ	✓	✓	Good
Muesli, apple 9+	590kJ	✓	✓	Good
Porridge, fruit	580kJ	✓	✓	Good
RTE peach & apricot	295kJ	✓	✓	Good
RTE porridge 7+	300kJ	✓	✓	Good
Muesli, pear & banana	275kJ	✓	✓	Good

Food 4 Kids

Product Name	Energy	Major Nutrients	Food Additives	Nutritious Rating
Banana & custard	1480kJ	↑ Sugar	422	Average
Apple & custard	1350kJ	↑ Sugar	422	Average

Golden Circle

Product Name	Energy	Major Nutrients	Food Additives	Nutritious Rating
Juice, apple &	67kJ	✓	✓	Average

blackcurrant				
Juice, tropical	67kJ	✓	✓	Average
Juice, apple	67kJ	✓	✓	Average

Green Monkeys

Product Name	Energy	Major Nutrients	Food Additives	Nutritious Rating
Pumpkin, silverbeet & sweet potato	145kJ	✓	✓	Good
NZ beef, apple, beetroot & pumpkin	211kJ	✓	✓	Good
NZ lamb, carrot & sweet potato	189kJ	✓	✓	Good

Healtheries

Product Name	Energy	Major Nutrients	Food Additives	Nutritious Rating
Wiggles bikkies banana	1580kJ	↑ Fat ↑ Sugar	✓	Poor
Wiggles bikkies, honey	1560kJ	↑ Fat ↑ Sugar	✓	Poor
Wiggles bikkies, strawberry	1630kJ	↑ Fat ↑ Sugar	120	Poor
Wiggles fruit fills, apples	1380kJ	↑ Sugar	420	Average
Wiggles fruit fills, apricot	1380kJ	↑ Sugar	✓	Average
Wiggles ricey bites cheese	1840kJ	↑ Fat	YE, 223	Poor

Heinz

Product Name	Energy	Major Nutrients	Food Additives	Nutritious Rating
Apples 10-15 months	255kJ	✓	✓	Good
Apple & mango 4-6m	260kJ	✓	✓	Good
Chicken & noodles 4-6m	270kJ	✓	✓	Average
Fruity apple 4-6m	255kJ	✓	✓	Good
Fruity pear 4-6m	260kJ	✓	✓	Good

Pear & banana 4-6m	290kJ	✓	✓	Good
Pumpkin & corn 4-6m	220kJ	✓	✓	Good
Pumpkin, potato & beef 4-6months	240kJ	✓	✓	Good
Strawberry, rice & yoghurt dessert 7-9m	290kJ	✓	✓	Average
Apple, mango & kiwi gel All Ages	185kJ	✓	407	Average
Apple & blackcurrant gel All Ages	205kJ	✓	407	Average
Fruits of forest gel All Ages	230kJ	↑ Sugar	407	Average
Summer fruits gel All Ages	230kJ	↑ Sugar	407	Average
Custard, caramel All Ages	265kJ	✓	✓	Poor
Custard, apple All Ages	335kJ	✓	✓	Poor
Custard, egg All Ages	270kJ	✓	✓	Poor
Custard, banana AA	455kJ	↑ Sugar	✓	Poor
Custard, choc AA	250kJ	✓	✓	Poor
Custard, fruit	355kJ	✓	✓	Poor
Custard, vanilla	265kJ	✓	✓	Poor
Fruit yoghurt All Ages		✓	✓	Poor
Strawberry & banana custard All Ages	265kJ	✓	✓	Poor
Strawberry yoghurt All Ages	300kJ	✓	✓	Poor
Apple & banana cereal All Ages	350kJ	✓	✓	Good
Apple oatmeal All Ages	285kJ	✓	✓	Good
Creamy banana porridge	260kJ	✓	✓	Good
Apple & blueberry muesli All Ages	275kJ	✓	✓	Good
Teething rusks	1530kJ	✓	✓	Average
Apple & blackcurrant	60kJ	✓	✓	Average

juice				
Apple & raspberry pudding delights	285kJ	✓	✓	Average
Homemade Heros chicken meatballs	350kJ	✓	YE	Average
Homemade Heros ravioli	350kJ	✓	✓	Average
Homemade Heros beef	260kJ	✓	✓	Average
Little Kids Yoghurt muesli fruit fingers	1460kJ	↑ Sugar	220	Average
Little Kids Yoghurt muesli fingers, apple & blackcurrant	1340kJ	↑ Sugar	220	Average
Little Kids Yoghurt muesli fruit fingers, fruit salad	1480kJ	↑ Sugar	220	Average
Little Kids Bikkies honey/oat/banana	1960kJ	↑ Fat ↑ Sugar	✓	Poor
Little Kids Breadsticks cheddar cheese	1770kJ	↑ Fat	YE	Poor
Little Kids Breadsticks cheeseymite	1755kJ	↑ Fat	YE	Poor
Little Kids soft fruit bars apricot	1440kJ	↑ Sugar	160b, 220	Average
Little Kids soft fruit bars strawberry	1370kJ	↑ Sugar	220, 120	Average
Little Kids yoghurt muesli fingers sultana apple	1460kJ	✓	220	Average
Little Kids pumpkin risotto & chicken	265kJ	✓	✓	Good
Little Kids macaroni meatballs	330kJ	✓	✓	Average
Little Kids vegetable beef risotto	255kJ	✓	✓	Good
Little Kids spaghetti	275kJ	✓	✓	Good

bolognaise				
Little Kids cereal bar apple blueberry	1430kJ	↑ Sugar	160b, 422	Average
Little Kids cereal bar apple cinnamon	1380kJ	↑ Sugar	160b, 422	Average
Little Kids cereal bar apple strawberry	1280kJ	↑ Sugar	160b, 422	Average
Little Kids mini corn cakes apple banana	1660kJ	✓	✓	Average
Little Kids mini corn cakes tomato	1760kJ	↑ Fat	YE, 160b	Average
Mum's Recipe alphabet pasta tomato beef	230kJ	✓	✓	Good
Mum's Recipe beef vegetable casserole	280kJ	✓	✓	Good
Mum's Recipe creamy tuna pasta	205kJ	✓	✓	Good
Mum's Recipe pumpkin couscous	240kJ	✓	✓	Good
Mum's Recipe cheesy pasta bolognaise	230kJ	✓	✓	Average
Mum's Recipe chicken, sweet corn & sweet potato	265kJ	✓	✓	Good
Organic cheese pasta bake	205kJ	✓	✓	Average
Organic spinach & pumpkin ricotta	215kJ	✓	✓	Good
Organic spring lamb & baby vegetables	250kJ	✓	✓	Good
Organic apple cinnamon porridge	315kJ	✓	✓	Good
Organic banana mango	325kJ	✓	✓	Good
Organic pumpkin, sweet potato & beef	230kJ	✓	✓	Good
Organic golden vegetables	225kJ	✓	✓	Good

Organic sweet baby vegetables	175kJ	✓	✓	Good
Organic smooth fruity pear & apricot	250kJ	✓	✓	Good
Organic apple berry blush	235kJ	✓	✓	Good
Organic banana & blueberry custard	335kJ	✓	✓	Average
Organic pear, apple & muesli	330kJ	✓	✓	Good
Organic baby bircher apple & banana	325kJ	✓	✓	Good
Organic pear & currant	355kJ	✓	✓	Good
Organic beef & vegetables	310kJ	✓	✓	Good
Organic butternut pumpkin pilaf	235kJ	✓	✓	Good
Organic chicken & sweet potato	250kJ	✓	✓	Good
Organic lamb shepherds pie	240kJ	✓	✓	Good
Organic Provencale chicken pasta	260kJ	✓	✓	Good
Organic oats, fig & sultana	390kJ	✓	✓	Good
Organic custard vanilla cereal	505kJ	✓	✓	Average
Organic rice cakes apple	1570kJ	✓	✓	Average
Fruit juice pear	70kJ	✓	✓	Average
Fruit juice, apple & cranberry	75kJ	✓	✓	Average
Simply Apple oatmeal	230kJ	✓	✓	Good
Simply Apple, peach & mango	290kJ	✓	✓	Good
Simply banana custard	310kJ	✓	✓	Average
Simply pear, banana	295kJ	✓	✓	Good

	Energy	Major Nutrients	Food Additives	Nutritious Rating
& apple				
Simply pumpkin, potato & carrot	155kJ	✓	✓	Good
Simply pea, pumpkin & sweet potato	180kJ	✓	✓	Good

Holle Organic

Product Name	Energy	Major Nutrients	Food Additives	Nutritious Rating
Apple & blueberry	347kJ	✓	✓	Good
Apple & peach	278kJ	✓	✓	Good
Pear	277kJ	✓	✓	Good
Apple & pear	335kJ	✓	✓	Good
Mixed Vegetables	132kJ	✓	✓	Good
Broccoli & wholegrain rice	144kJ	✓	✓	Good
Pumpkin & chicken	237kJ	✓	✓	Good
Baby muesli	1457kJ	✓	✓	Good
3 grain porridge	1585kJ	✓	✓	Good
Rolled oats porridge	1619kJ	✓	✓	Good
Baby spelt rusks	1619kJ	✓	✓	Average
Baby spelt biscuits	1823kJ	✓	✓	Average

Little Bellies

Product Name	Energy	Major Nutrients	Food Additives	Nutritious Rating
Fruity choo chews organic apple, apricot & date	1480kJ	✓	✓	Good
Fruity choo chews organic apple & berry	1480kJ	✓	✓	Good

Nestle

Product Name	Energy	Major Nutrients	Food Additives	Nutritious Rating
Cerelac Stage 1 rice cereal	232kJ	✓	✓	Good
Cerelac Stage 2 wheat cereal	228kJ	✓	✓	Good

Only Organic

Product Name	Energy	Major Nutrients	Food Additives	Nutritious Rating
Chicken bolognaise	200kJ	✓	✓	Good
Apple & berry ripple	242kJ	✓	✓	Good
Apple custard	213kJ	✓	✓	Average
Chicken & vegetable risotto	210kJ	✓	✓	Good
Mango & yoghurt brekkie	319kJ	✓	✓	Good
Banana, berries & yoghurt	364kJ	✓	✓	Good
Orchard apple	156kJ	✓	✓	Good
Pumpkin & sweet corn	231kJ	✓	✓	Good
Pumpkin & wild rice	144kJ	✓	✓	Good
Fruit muesli	237kJ	✓	✓	Good
Mango & banana bliss	311kJ	✓	✓	Good
Pasta bolognaise	203kJ	✓	✓	Good
Pear & rice cereal	296kJ	✓	✓	Good
Pumpkin, potato & beef	244kJ	✓	✓	Good
Pear, banana & apple	290kJ	✓	✓	Good
Cottage pie		✓	✓	Good
Banana & apple smoothie	328kJ	✓	✓	Good
Banana, raspberry & vanilla smoothie		✓	✓	Good
Vanilla bean custard	288kJ	✓	✓	Average
Mango custard	265kJ	✓	✓	Average
Golden fruit porridge	310kJ	✓	✓	Good
Mango rice pudding	287kJ	✓	✓	Average
Kumera & sweet corn	299kJ	✓	✓	Good
Rusks	1528kJ	✓	✓	Average

Organic Bubs

Product Name	Energy	Major Nutrients	Food Additives	Nutritious Rating
Apple cinnamon	248kJ	✓	✓	Good
Mango, peach & banana	343kJ	✓	✓	Good
Pear & white grape	319kJ	✓	✓	Good
Pumpkin, apricot & fig		✓	✓	Good
Raspberry, apple & rosehip	370kJ	✓	✓	Good
Sweet potato, carrot & pumpkin	316kJ	✓	✓	Good
Blueberry, quinoa & banana	462kJ	✓	✓	Good
Apple & raspberry bircher muesli	357kJ	✓	✓	Good
Banana & apricot porridge	362kJ	✓	✓	Good
Pumpkin & kumera couscous	260kJ	✓	✓	Good
Sweet corn, pumpkin & chia	355kJ	✓	✓	Good
Vegetable & rice congee	167kJ	✓	✓	Good

Rafferty's Garden

Product Name	Energy	Major Nutrients	Food Additives	Nutritious Rating
Chicken, basil & tomato pasta	294kJ	✓	✓	Good
Rissoni pasta & garden vegetables	166kJ	✓	✓	Good
Macaroni bolognaise	197kJ	✓	✓	Good
Sweet potato & lamb casserole	290kJ	✓	✓	Good
Italian lasagne	257kJ	✓	✓	Good
Shepherds pie	251kJ	✓	✓	Good

Baked beans	345kJ	✓	✓	Average
Spaghetti hoops	549kJ	✓	✓	Average
Apple, pear & cinnamon	147kJ	✓	✓	Good
Banana, pear & mango	243kJ	✓	✓	Good
Blueberry, banana & apple	235kJ	✓	✓	Good
Sweet potato, carrot & apple	182kJ	✓	✓	Good
Pumpkin, apple & corn	207kJ	✓	✓	Good
Pear & apricot	246kJ	✓	✓	Good
RTE rice cereal banana	451kJ	✓	✓	Good
RTE rice cereal pear, mango & milk	389kJ	✓	✓	Good
Bangers, mash & vegetable	220kJ	✓	✓	Good
Smoothie Apple & raspberry	244kJ	✓	✓	Good
Smoothie banana & blueberry	314kJ	✓	✓	Good
Smoothie banana &mango	339kJ	✓	✓	Good
Cereal apricot & banana	301kJ	✓	✓	Good
Multigrain cereal	304kJ	✓	✓	Good
Chicken & apricot puree	414kJ	✓	✓	Good
Creamy chicken & vegetable puree	245kJ	✓	✓	Good
Hearty beef & vegetable puree	240kJ	✓	✓	Good
Old fashioned chocolate custard	437kJ	✓	✓	Poor
Old fashioned chocolate & banana custard	423kJ	↑ sugar	✓	✓
Tuna rice & vegetables	279kJ	✓	✓	Good
Spinach, apple, broccoli & peas	170kJ	✓	✓	Good
Porridge & banana flakes	301kJ	✓	✓	Good
Super hero apple & mango	155kJ	✓	✓	Good

Super hero carrot, apple & sweet corn	191kJ	✓	✓	**Good**
Super hero beetroot & vegetable puree	142kJ	✓	✓	**Good**
Super hero pear, banana & avocado	305kJ	✓	✓	**Good**
Super hero lamb & vegetable risotto	431kJ	✓	✓	**Good**
Super hero mango & chicken puree	337kJ	✓	✓	**Good**
Super hero carrot & cheddar puree	211kJ	✓	✓	**Good**
Snack bars banana	1490kJ	↑fat ↑ sugar	160b	Poor
Snack bars apple	1510kJ	↑fat ↑ sugar	160b	Poor
Milk rusks banana	1480kJ	✓	✓	Average
Organic baby rice cereal	339kJ	✓	✓	**Good**

Breakfast Cereals

There are a wide variety of cereals on the market, more than ever in history. Yet we are creatures of habit and studies show that people are often reluctant to try new breakfast cereals, even when another is "on special". It is important not to discount muesli and porridge as they are often high in kilojoules. These breakfast varieties contain diverse nutrients and are a challenge for the body to digest, making one feel fuller for longer. It is portion size that must be considered when eating muesli or porridge – half a cup when dry is plenty.

Other cereals to consider are the pressed flakes, like weet-bix and vita bits. The ones to avoid are those with 'clusters', which is a nice way of saying biscuits. I understand they are sweet and tasty, but I'm not sure when it became acceptable to eat biscuits for brekky. There are also compressed powder varieties, such as *cheerios* and *nutri-grain*. These are not a challenge for the body to digest and cause huge blood-sugar spikes and earlier hunger pangs.

Food additives are also of consideration. Dried fruit is almost always preserved with sulphites and humectants unless you select the organic or health food varieties. Annatto extracts and food colourings are of concern, particularly with kids going to school. In addition, there are the synthetic antioxidants in the vegetable oils used in many breakfast cereals.

Our biggest mistake with breakfast cereal packaging was swapping the wax paper bags for plastic inserts. My picks are *Be Natural, Carman's, Food for health, Monster and McKenzies.*

Abundant Earth

Product Name	Energy	Major Nutrients	Food Additives	Nutritious Rating
Puffed rice	1610kJ	✓	✓	Good
Puffed kumut	1310kJ	✓	✓	Good
Puffed corn cereal	1610kJ	✓	✓	Average
Puffed rice cereal	1500kJ	✓	✓	Good

Anchor

Product Name	Energy	Major Nutrients	Food Additives	Nutritious Rating
Classic Swiss muesli	1383kJ	↑ sugar	220	Good
Quick oats	1600kJ	↑fat	✓	Good
Rolled oats	1600kJ	↑fat	✓	Good
Semolina	1479kJ	✓	✓	Good

Arnold's Farm

Product Name	Energy	Major Nutrients	Food Additives	Nutritious Rating
Apricot & yoghurt muesli	1570kJ	↑ sugar	220	Good
Full o fruit muesli	1810kJ	↑fat ↑ sugar	220	Good
Strawberry & yoghurt muesli	1610kJ	↑ sugar	220	Good
Toasted farmhouse	1700kJ	↑ sugar	220	Good

Basco Gluten Free

Product Name	Energy	Major Nutrients	Food Additives	Nutritious Rating
Apricot & apple cereal	1510kJ	↑ sugar	220, 221	Good
Honey rings	1470kJ	↑ sugar	✓	Average

Be Natural

Product Name	Energy	Major Nutrients	Food Additives	Nutritious Rating
5 Wholegrain flake cereal	1530kJ	↑ sugar	✓	Good
Cashew hazelnut, coconut & almond cereal	1790kJ	↑ sugar ↑ fat	✓	Good
Pink lady & flame raisin cereal	1610kJ	↑ sugar	✓	Good
Multigrain porridge	1600kJ	↑ fat	✓	Good
Vanilla & almond porridge sachets	1680kJ	↑ sugar ↑ fat	✓	Good

Biogenic

Product Name	Energy	Major Nutrients	Food Additives	Nutritious Rating
Yeast & wheat free muesli	1857kJ	↑ fat	220	Good
Wheat & gluten free muesli	1579kJ	✓	220, 202	Good

Carman's

Product Name	Energy	Major Nutrients	Food Additives	Nutritious Rating
Classic fruit muesli	1865kJ	↑ sugar ↑ fat	✓	Good
Classic fruit muesli tub	1865kJ	↑ sugar ↑ fat	✓	Good
Deluxe fruit muesli	1829kJ	↑ sugar ↑ fat	✓	Good
Natural bircher muesli	1730kJ	↑ sugar ↑ fat	✓	Good
Fruit free muesli	1990kJ	↑fat	✓	Good
Traditional Australian oats	1620kJ	✓	✓	Good
Honey roasted nut porridge sachets	1690kJ	↑ sugar ↑ fat	✓	Good

Natural fruit & seed porridge sachets	1800kJ	↑ sugar ↑ fat	✓	Good

Back To Nature

Product Name	Energy	Major Nutrients	Food Additives	Nutritious Rating
Cookie bitez, choc chip	1480kJ	↑ sugar	220	Average
Cookie bitez, corn & maple	1566kJ	↑ salt	✓	Average

Bibo

Product Name	Energy	Major Nutrients	Food Additives	Nutritious Rating
Semolina	1380kJ	✓	✓	Good

Bobs Red Mill

Product Name	Energy	Major Nutrients	Food Additives	Nutritious Rating
Oats, rolled	795kJ	✓	✓	Good
Oats, steel cut	795kJ	✓	✓	Good

Coles

Product Name	Energy	Major Nutrients	Food Additives	Nutritious Rating
Bran start cereal	1130kJ	↑ sugar	160b	Good
Sultana bran flakes	1430kJ	↑ sugar	✓	Good
Cocoa puffs	1650kJ	↑ sugar	✓	Average
Corn flakes	1530kJ	↑ salt	✓	Average
Honey crunch flakes	1697kJ	↑ sugar	✓	Average
Frooty rings	1610kJ	↑ sugar	100, 110, 122, 133	Average
Mighty grain cereal	1610kJ	↑ sugar	160b	Good
Rice puffs	1580kJ	↑ salt	✓	Average
Right start cereal	1470kJ	↑ sugar	220, 422	Good
Special flakes	1556kJ	↑ sugar	✓	Average
Whole wheat biscuits	1590kJ	✓	✓	Good
Flavoured oats	1571-	↑ sugar	220	Good

Product Name	Energy	Major Nutrients	Food Additives	Nutritious Rating
sachets	1662kJ			
Apricot, almond & date muesli	1560kJ	↑ sugar ↑ fat	220	Good
Low fat muesli	1420kJ	↑ sugar	220	Good
Summer fruits muesli	1570kJ	↑ sugar ↑ fat	220	Good
Original toasted muesli	1770kJ	↑ sugar ↑ fat	220	Good
Quick oat sachets	1600kJ	✓	✓	Good
Organic instant oats	1671kJ	✓	✓	Good
Right start cereal fruit & fibre	1520kJ	↑ sugar	422	Good
Smart buy wheat biscuits	1525kJ	✓	✓	Good
Smart buy muesli	1538kJ	↑ sugar	220	Good
Smart buy Oat bran	1600kJ	✓	✓	Good
Smart buy quick oats	1600kJ	✓	✓	Good
Smart buy rolled oats	1600kJ	✓	✓	Good
Smart buy wheat bran	1360kJ	↑ sugar	✓	Good

Dick Smith

Product Name	Energy	Major Nutrients	Food Additives	Nutritious Rating
Bush foods breakfast cereal	866kJ	↑ sugar	422	Good

Farmer's Choice

Product Name	Energy	Major Nutrients	Food Additives	Nutritious Rating
Apricot & almond cereal	1425kJ	↑ sugar	✓	Good
Apple, cranberry & cinnamon cereal	1396kJ	↑ sugar	✓	Good

Food for Health

Product Name	Energy	Major	Food	Nutritious

		Nutrients	Additives	Rating
Fruit free cluster cereal	1801kJ	↑ sugar ↑ fat	✓	Good
Cleansing muesli fibre	1720kJ	↑ fat	✓	Good
Gluten free muesli	1245kJ	↑ sugar	✓	Good
Liver cleansing muesli	1820kJ	↑ fat	✓	Good

Freedom Foods

Product Name	Energy	Major Nutrients	Food Additives	Nutritious Rating
Gluten & wheat fee muesli breakfast bars	1610kJ	↑ sugar ↑ fat	220, 223	Good
Cocoa puffs	1530kJ	↑ sugar	✓	Average
Cornflakes with psyllium low salt	1630kJ	✓	✓	Average
Gluten free muesli	1730kJ	↑ sugar ↑ fat	✓	Good
Rice flakes	1590kJ	✓	✓	Average
Rice puffs	1540kJ	✓	✓	Average
Tropicos gluten free cereal	1560kJ	↑ sugar	✓	Good
Ultra rice maple crunch cereal	1580kJ	↑ sugar	✓	Average
Freelicious cornflakes	1610kJ	✓	✓	Average

Goodness Superfoods

Product Name	Energy	Major Nutrients	Food Additives	Nutritious Rating
Digestive 1st cereal	1500kJ	↑ sugar	420, 220	Good
Heart 1st cereal	1630kJ	↑ sugar ↑ fat	420, 220	Good
Protein 1st cereal	1500kJ	↑ sugar	420, 220	Good
Fibre boost	1370kJ	✓	✓	Good

Healtheries

Product Name	Energy	Major Nutrients	Food Additives	Nutritious Rating
Bircher muesli, apple & raisin	1650kJ	↑ sugar ↑ fat ↑ salt	220	**Good**
Bircher muesli, deluxe	1710kJ	↑ fat	422, 220	**Good**

Heritage Mill

Product Name	Energy	Major Nutrients	Food Additives	Nutritious Rating
Toasted country muesli	1700kJ	↑ sugar	220	Good
Toasted muesli with fruit	1810kJ	↑ sugar ↑ fat	220	Good
Strawberry & yoghurt muesli	1610kJ	↑ sugar	220	**Good**

IGA Signature & Purely Organic

Product Name	Energy	Major Nutrients	Food Additives	Nutritious Rating
Almond & honey nut clusters	1630kJ	↑ sugar ↑ fat	✓	Good
Cornflakes	1580kJ	↑ salt	✓	Average
Quick oats	1600kJ	↑ fat	✓	Good
Quick oats, sachets	1600kJ	✓	✓	Good
Nutty Clusters	1820kJ	↑ sugar ↑ fat	✓	Average
Purely organic, rolled oats	1600kJ	↑ fat	✓	Good
Strawberry & yoghurt clusters	2090kJ	↑ sugar ↑ fat	✓	Average
Wheat flakes	1520kJ	✓	✓	Average

IGA Black & Gold

Product Name	Energy	Major Nutrients	Food Additives	Nutritious Rating
Wheat Biscuits	1470kJ	✓	✓	Average

Corn flakes	1600kJ	✓	✓	Average
Fruity rings	1600kJ	↑ sugar	122, 110, 133	Average
Cocoa orbits	1680kJ	↑ sugar	✓	Average
Rolled oats	1580kJ	✓	✓	Good
Quick oats	1600kJ	✓	✓	Good
Tropical muesli	1600kJ	↑ sugar	220	Good
Toasted museli	1500kJ	✓	220	Good

Kellogg's

Product Name	Energy	Major Nutrients	Food Additives	Nutritious Rating
All bran	1370kJ	↑ sugar	✓	Good
All bran, honey & almond	1530kJ	↑ sugar	✓	Good
All bran wheat flakes	1430kJ	✓	✓	Good
All bran, apple crunch	1510kJ	↑ sugar	✓	Good
Cocoa pops	1610kJ	↑ sugar ↑ salt	✓	Average
Cocoa pops bowl	1610kJ	↑ sugar ↑ fat	✓	Average
Cocoa pop chex	1590kJ	↑ sugar ↑ fat	✓	Average
Corn flakes	1580kJ	↑ salt	✓	Average
Crispix, honey	1630kJ	↑ sugar ↑ salt	✓	Average
Crunch nut clusters	1720kJ	↑ sugar	✓	Average
Crunchy nut cornflakes	1660kJ	↑ sugar	✓	Average
Froot loops	1640kJ	↑ sugar	110, 129, 133	Average
Guardian cereal	1440kJ	↑ sugar	✓	Good
Just right, original	1490kJ	↑ sugar	220, 420	Good
Just right, grain & clusters	1570kJ	↑ sugar	✓	Good
Just right, barley berry	1490kJ	↑ sugar	420	Good
Mini wheats,	1490kJ	↑ sugar	422	Good

blackcurrant				
Mini wheats, 5 grains	1490kJ	↑ sugar	422	Good
Mini wheats, mixed berry	1450kJ	↑ sugar	422	Good
Nutri grain	1600kJ	↑ sugar ↑ salt	✓	Average
Nutri grain bowl	1600kJ	↑ sugar ↑ salt	✓	Average
Rice bubbles	1600kJ	↑ sugar	✓	Average
Special K	1570kJ	↑ salt ↑ sugar	✓	Average
Special K advantage	1480kJ	↑ sugar	✓	Good
Special K, forest berries	1570kJ	↑ sugar	✓	Good
Special K, honey & almond	1660kJ	↑ sugar ↑ salt	✓	Good
Special K, fruit n nut	1410kJ	↑ sugar	160b, 422	Good
Sultana bran	1410kJ	↑ sugar	420	Good
Sultana bran buds	1410kJ	↑ sugar	422	Average
Sultana bran crunch	1460kJ	↑ sugar	422	Average
Sustain, original	1570kJ	↑ sugar	220	Good

Little Bellies

Product Name	Energy	Major Nutrients	Food Additives	Nutritious Rating
Number cereal, peach	1380kJ	✓	✓	Good

Lowan

Product Name	Energy	Major Nutrients	Food Additives	Nutritious Rating
Cocoa bombs	1630kJ	↑ sugar	✓	Average
Apricot & almond muesli	1620kJ	↑ sugar ↑fat	220, 223	Good
Original muesli	1680kJ	↑fat	✓	Good

Swiss muesli	1570kJ	↑ sugar	221	Good
Tropical fruit muesli	1620kJ	↑ sugar	220. 223	Good
Orchard fruit porridge	1390kJ	↑ sugar	220	Good
Whole grain rolled oats	1610kJ	↑fat	✓	Good
Natural oat bran	1610kJ	↑fat	✓	Good
Quick oats	1610kJ	↑fat	✓	Good

McKenzies

Product Name	Energy	Major Nutrients	Food Additives	Nutritious Rating
Natural whole oats	1600kJ	↑fat	✓	Good
Natural minute oats	1600kJ	↑fat	✓	Good
Natural instant oats	1600kJ	↑fat	✓	Good
Natural creamy oatmeal	1600kJ	↑fat	✓	Good
Natural oat bran	1600kJ	✓	✓	Good
Natural unprocessed bran	1110kJ	✓	✓	Good

Monster

Product Name	Energy	Major Nutrients	Food Additives	Nutritious Rating
Free & lo muesli	942kJ	✓	✓	Good
Multi grain porridge	1330kJ	✓	✓	Good
Free & fruity muesli	975kJ	↑ sugar	✓	Good

Morning Sun

Product Name	Energy	Major Nutrients	Food Additives	Nutritious Rating
Natural apricot & almond muesli	1520kJ	↑ sugar	220, 422	Good
Natural peach & pecan muesli	1560kJ	↑ sugar ↑fat	220, 422	Good
97% FF Fruit muesli	1430kJ	↑ sugar	220, 422	Good

Nature First

Product Name	Energy	Major Nutrients	Food Additives	Nutritious Rating
Organic rolled oats creamy style	1600kJ	↑fat	✓	Good
Organic muesli	1592kJ	↑fat	✓	Good
Organic instant rolled oats	1592kJ	↑fat	✓	Good

Nestle

Product Name	Energy	Major Nutrients	Food Additives	Nutritious Rating
Milo cereal	1630kJ	↑ sugar	319	Good
Milo cereal, duo	1620kJ	↑ sugar	319	Good
Milo oats sachets	1610kJ	↑ sugar	✓	Good
Nesquik cereal	1610kJ	↑ sugar	319	Good

Norganic

Product Name	Energy	Major Nutrients	Food Additives	Nutritious Rating
Organic cornflakes	1570kJ	↑ salt	✓	Average
Crunchola, apple & blueberry	1660kJ	↑ sugar	✓	Good
Crunchola, apple & cinnamon	1670kJ	↑ sugar	✓	Good
Crunchola, berry & vanilla	1730kJ	↑ sugar ↑ fat	✓	Good
Breakfast bar, apple & blueberry	1370kJ	✓	220	Good
Breakfast bar, chewy apple & cinnamon	1380kJ	✓	220	Good
Breakfast bar, apricot	1340kJ	✓	220	Good

Nu Vit

Product Name	Energy	Major Nutrients	Food Additives	Nutritious Rating
Gluten free muesli, fruit & flakes	1371kJ	↑ sugar	220, 223, 129	Good

Low fat fruity muesli	1500kJ	↑ sugar	220	Good
Linseed	2234kJ	↑ fat	✓	Good
LSA mix	2380kJ	↑ fat	✓	Good
Mega high protein muesli	1580kJ	↑ fat ↑ sugar	220, 223	Good
Gluten free muesli	2264kJ	↑ fat	✓	Good
Phyto soy LSA mix	2188kJ	↑ fat	✓	Good
Wheat germ	1281kJ	✓	✓	Good
Semolina	1560kJ	✓	✓	Good
Rice bran	1690kJ	↑ fat	✓	Good
Fibre powder	1532kJ	↑ fat	✓	Good

Olympic Fine Foods

Product Name	Energy	Major Nutrients	Food Additives	Nutritious Rating
Muesli, apricot & almond natural	1607kJ	↑ sugar	220	Good
Muesli, fruity	1570kJ	↑ sugar ↑ fat	220	Good
Muesli, honey toasted	1716kJ	↑ sugar ↑ fat	220	Good
Muesli, tropical natural	1538kJ	↑ sugar	220	Good
Oats, quick	1480kJ	✓	✓	Good
Oats, rolled	1540kJ	✓	✓	Good

Orgran

Product Name	Energy	Major Nutrients	Food Additives	Nutritious Rating
O's Itsy bitsy cocoa	1370kJ	↑ sugar	✓	Average
O's, wildberry	1310kJ	↑ sugar	✓	Average
Supergrain O's, quinoa	1620kJ	✓	✓	Good
Puffed amaranth	1700kJ	✓	✓	Good

Planet

Product Name	Energy	Major Nutrients	Food Additives	Nutritious Rating
Organic gluten free porridge	1500kJ	✓	✓	Good

Purina

Product Name	Energy	Major Nutrients	Food Additives	Nutritious Rating
Toasted muesli	1835kJ	↑ fat ↑ sugar	319, 220	Good

Sanitarium

Product Name	Energy	Major Nutrients	Food Additives	Nutritious Rating
Honey weets	1550kJ	↑ sugar	220	Average
Light n tasty, berry	1500kJ	↑ sugar	✓	Good
Light n tasty, apricot & almond	1540kJ	↑ sugar	160b, 420, 220	Good
Light n tasty, macadamia & honey	1620kJ	↑ sugar	✓	Good
Puffed wheat	1520kJ	✓	✓	Average
Weet bix bites, crunchy honey	1580kJ	↑ sugar	✓	Average
Weet bix bites, wildberry	1390kJ	↑ sugar	422	Average
Weet bix	1490kJ	✓	✓	Average
Weet bix fruity bites, apricot	1390kJ	↑ sugar	422	Average
Weet bix bites, golden crumb	1630kJ	↑ sugar	319	Average
Weet bix bites, cocoa malt	1620kJ	↑ sugar	✓	Average
Weet bix organic	1490kJ	✓	✓	Average
Weet bix, multigrain	1590kJ	✓	✓	Average
Weet bix kids	1480kJ	✓	✓	Average
Weet bix, high bran	1490kJ	✓	✓	Good
Golden oats fruit	1830kJ	↑ sugar	160b, 420,	Good

Product Name	Energy	Major Nutrients	Food Additives	Nutritious Rating
muesli		↑ fat	220	
Granola clusters, berry delicious	1680kJ	↑ sugar	420, 220	Average
Granola clusters, vanilla & almond	1760kJ	↑ sugar ↑ fat	319, 221	Average
Berry coated flakes & muesli	1560kJ	↑ sugar	120, 220, 420	Good
Fruit & five grain muesli	1540kJ	↑ sugar	220, 420	Good
Up & go, vive banana	320kJ	✓	407	Good
Up & go, vive, wildberry	320kJ	✓	407	Good
Up & go, energise chocolate	320kJ	✓	407	Good
Up & go, energise vanilla	330kJ	✓	407	Good
Up & go, strawberry	330kJ	✓	407	Good
Up & go, banana	320kJ	✓	407	Good
Up & go, choc ice	320kJ	✓	407	Good

Sun Sol

Product Name	Energy	Major Nutrients	Food Additives	Nutritious Rating
Bircher muesli	1500kJ	↑ sugar ↑ fat	220, 223	Good
Breakfast lite	**1538kJ**	**↑ sugar**	**✓**	**Good**
Breakfast plus	1660kJ	↑ sugar ↑ fat	220, 223	Good
Deluxe linseed muesli	1600kJ	↑ sugar ↑ fat	129, 223, 220	Good
Fruity muesli	1550kJ	↑ sugar ↑ fat	129, 223, 220	Good
Gluten free muesli	1500kJ	↑ sugar	129, 223, 220	Good
Low fat apple & berry muesli	1410kJ	↑ sugar	129, 223, 220, 120, 122, 124	Good
Natural muesli	1352kJ	↑ sugar	129, 223, 220	Good
Original muesli	1660kJ	↑ sugar	129, 223, 220	Good

		↑ fat		

The Muesli Company

Product Name	Energy	Major Nutrients	Food Additives	Nutritious Rating
Natural muesli	150kJ	↑ sugar	220	Good

Uncle Toby's

Product Name	Energy	Major Nutrients	Food Additives	Nutritious Rating
Cheerios	1580kJ	↑ sugar	160b, 220, 319	Average
Cheerio's, honey & oat	1590kJ	↑ sugar	160b, 319	Average
Heathwise for heart & circulatory system	1600kJ	↑ sugar	220, 420	Good
High fibre bites, honey	**1455kJ**	**↑ sugar**	✓	**Average**
High fibre bites, brown sugar & cinnamon	1450kJ	↑ sugar	220	Average
Nut feast	1640kJ	↑ sugar	220	Average
Oat crisps, almond	1720kJ	↑ sugar ↑ fat	160b, 220	Average
Oat crisps, honey	1660kJ	↑ sugar	160b, 220	Average
Oat flakes	**1640kJ**	**↑ sugar**	✓	**Average**
Oatbrits	**1570kJ**	✓	✓	**Average**
Plus, antioxidant lift	1510kJ	↑ sugar	420, 220	Good
Plus, essential for woman	1520kJ	↑ sugar	120	Good
Plus, fibre	1430kJ	↑ sugar	220	Good
Plus, muesli flakes	1508kJ	↑ sugar	220	Good
Plus, omega 3 lift	1610kJ	↑ sugar	220	Good
Plus, protein lift	**1550kJ**	**↑ sugar**	✓	**Good**
Plus, sports lift	1470kJ	↑ sugar	220	Good
Shredded wheat	**1490kJ**	✓	✓	**Good**
Vita brits	**1510kJ**	✓	✓	**Average**
Vita brits wheeties	**1520kJ**	✓	✓	**Average**
Fruity bites,	1560kJ	↑ sugar	420, 220	Average

wildberry				
Gourmet selection oats, cranberry & raspberry	1570kJ	↑ sugar	220	Good
Gourmet selection oats, hazelnut & almond	**1670kJ**	**↑ sugar ↑ fat**	✓	**Good**
Gourmet selection oats, sultana, apple & honey	1580kJ	↑ sugar	220	Good
Natural style muesli	1530kJ	↑ sugar	220, 420	Good
Oats, brown sugar & cinnamon microwavable bowl	1600kJ	↑ sugar	✓	Good
Oats, creamy honey microwavable bowl	1630kJ	↑ sugar	✓	Good
Oats, multigrain	1550kJ	✓	✓	Good
Oats, original microwavable bowl	1590kJ	↑ fat	✓	Good
Oats, traditional porridge	1590kJ	↑ fat	✓	Good
Quick oats	1590kJ	↑ fat	✓	Good
Quick oats, brown sugar	1600kJ	↑ sugar	✓	Good
Quick oats, creamy honey	1640kJ	↑ sugar	✓	Good
Quick oats sachets	1590kJ	↑ sugar	✓	Good
Oats so tasty, honey buzz	1610kJ	↑ sugar	✓	Good
Oats so tasty, smooth	1610kJ	↑ sugar	✓	Good
Oats, weightwise	1540kJ	✓	✓	Good

Vogel

Product Name	Energy	Major Nutrients	Food Additives	Nutritious Rating
Grain cluster crunch	1820kJ	↑ sugar ↑ fat	160b, 220	Average
Bran, soy & linseed	1400kJ	↑ sugar	160b	Good

cereal				

Weight Watcher's

Product Name	Energy	Major Nutrients	Food Additives	Nutritious Rating
Fruit & fibre tropical muesli	1510kJ	↑ sugar	220	Good

Woolworths/Safeways

Product Name	Energy	Major Nutrients	Food Additives	Nutritious Rating
Select Berry bircher muesli	1480kJ	↑ sugar	220	Good
Select Swiss bircher	1390kJ	↑ sugar	220	Good
Select Berry blend muesli	1600kJ	↑ sugar	223	Good
Select Classic muesli	1790kJ	↑ sugar ↑ fat	223, 420, 160b, 220	Good
Select vanilla almond clusters	1730kJ	↑ sugar	223, 220	Good
Select great start bran & sultana	**1440kJ**	↑ sugar	✓	**Good**
Select great start berry	1560kJ	↑ sugar	422	Good
Select great start original	1580kJ	↑ sugar	422, 160b	Good
Select light choice	**1600kJ**	↑ sugar	✓	**Good**
Select special choice	**1600kJ**	↑ sugar	✓	**Good**
Homebrand wheat biscuits	1510kJ	✓	✓	Average
Homebrand cocoa puffs	1630kJ	↑ sugar	✓	Average
Homebrand Rice pops	1580kJ	✓	✓	Average
Homebrand corn flakes	1530kJ	✓	✓	Average
Homebrand fruit rings	1580kJ	↑ sugar	122, 110, 133	Average

Homebrand traditional muesli	1580kJ	✓	220	Good
Homebrand fruit & nut muesli	1660kJ	↑ fat ↑ sugar	220	Good
Homebrand oat bran	1560kJ	✓	✓	Good
Homebrand semolina	1500kJ	✓	✓	Good
Homebrand natural bran	1280kJ	✓	✓	Good
Homebrand processed bran	1170kJ	↑ sugar	✓	Good
Homebrand rolled oats	1620kJ	✓	✓	Good
Homebrand quick oats	1590kJ	✓	✓	Good

Pantry Items

Canned Fruit

Most brands are similar, so go with what is on special and preferably locally produced. Just be wary that steel cans leach BPA.

Admiral

Product Name	Energy	Major Nutrients	Food Additives	Nutritious Rating
Mangoes sliced in natural juice	266kJ	✓	✓	Good
Black cherries, stoneless	380kJ	↑ sugar	✓	Good
Lychees, syrup	366kJ	↑ sugar	✓	Good
Berry combo, syrup	399kJ	↑ sugar	✓	Good
Passionfruit, syrup	424kJ	↑ sugar	✓	Good
Mandarin segments	257kJ	✓	✓	Good

Ardmona

Product Name	Energy	Major Nutrients	Food Additives	Nutritious Rating
Bakers pie filling, apricot	188kJ	✓	✓	Good
Apples sliced	190kJ	✓	✓	Good

Coles

Product Name	Energy	Major Nutrients	Food Additives	Nutritious Rating
Apricot halves in fruit juice	187kJ	✓	✓	Good
Blueberries in syrup	353kJ	↑ sugar	✓	Good
Cherries, pitted in syrup	355kJ	↑ sugar	✓	Good
Peach slices in	206kJ	✓	✓	Good

natural juice				
Pear halves in fruit juice	228kJ	✓	✓	Good
Fruit salad in natural juice	209kJ	✓	127	Good
Pineapple pieces in juice	260kJ	↑ sugar	✓	Good
Pineapple sliced in juice	280kJ	↑ sugar	✓	Good
Plums in juice	271kJ	↑ sugar	✓	Good
Two fruits in juice	218kJ	✓	✓	Good
Strawberries	420kJ	↑ sugar	✓	Good
Raspberries	392kJ	↑ sugar	✓	Good
Lychees, pitted in syrup	230kJ	↑ sugar	✓	Good
Mandarin segments	272kJ	↑ sugar	✓	Good
Mango slices in syrup	368kJ	↑ sugar	✓	Good
Mixed berries	343kJ	↑ sugar	✓	Good
Passionfruit pulp	460kJ	↑ sugar	✓	Good
Snack pack, mandarin in syrup 4pk	267kJ	↑ sugar	✓	Good
Snack pack, pears in syrup 4pk	267kJ	↑ sugar	✓	Good
Pineapple in syrup 4pk	234kJ	↑ sugar	✓	Good
Fruit salad in syrup 4pk	267kJ	↑ sugar	✓	Good
Peaches in syrup 4pk	267kJ	↑ sugar	✓	Good
Jelly fruit, mandarin in orange jelly 4pk	341kJ	↑ sugar	120	Good
Jelly fruit, peaches in mango jelly 4pk	278kJ	↑ sugar	120, 160b	Good
Jelly fruit, two fruit in strawberry jelly 4pk	311kJ	↑ sugar	120, 160b	Good
Jelly fruit, two	311kJ	↑ sugar	✓	Good

fruit in tropical jelly 4pk				
Smart buy apricot halves in syrup	287kJ	↑ sugar	✓	Good
Smart buy fruit salad in syrup	262kJ	↑ sugar	127	Good
Smart buy peach slices in syrup	328kJ	↑ sugar	✓	Good
Smart buy Pear halves in syrup	264kJ	↑ sugar	✓	Good
Smart buy pineapple pieces in syrup	272kJ	↑ sugar	✓	Good
Smart buy pineapple sliced in syrup	272kJ	↑ sugar	✓	Good

Delish

Product Name	Energy	Major Nutrients	Food Additives	Nutritious Rating
Guava halves	367kJ	↑ sugar	✓	Good

Dole

Product Name	Energy	Major Nutrients	Food Additives	Nutritious Rating
Chunks of tropical fruit	318kJ	↑ sugar	✓	Good
Pineapple chunks	234kJ	↑ sugar	✓	Good
Pineapple slices	195kJ	↑ sugar	✓	Good

D'oro

Product Name	Energy	Major Nutrients	Food Additives	Nutritious Rating
Mango in light syrup	332kJ	↑ sugar	✓	Good
Fruit salad traditional in natural juice	235kJ	↑ sugar	✓	Good
Fruit salad traditional in syrup	345kJ	↑ sugar	✓	Good
Pineapple, crushed in natural juice	240kJ	↑ sugar	✓	Good

Pineapple, crushed in syrup	335kJ	↑ sugar	✓	Good
Pineapple, pieces in natural juice	240kJ	↑ sugar	✓	Good
Pineapple, pieces in syrup	335kJ	↑ sugar	✓	Good
Pineapple, slices in natural juice	240kJ	↑ sugar	✓	Good
Pineapple, slices in syrup	335kJ	↑ sugar	✓	Good
Pineapple, slices thin in natural juice	240kJ	↑ sugar	✓	Good
Pineapple, slices thin in syrup	335kJ	↑ sugar	✓	Good

Golburn Valley

Product Name	Energy	Major Nutrients	Food Additives	Nutritious Rating
Apple Puree snack pack	232kJ	✓	✓	Good
Apple & strawberry snack pack	224kJ	✓	120	Good
Fruit salad in natural juice snack pack	249kJ	↑ sugar	✓	Good
Peach & mango in natural juice snack pack	277kJ	↑ sugar	✓	Good
Peaches in natural juice snack pack	212kJ	↑ sugar	✓	Good
Apple & berry puree snack pack	264kJ	↑ sugar	✓	Good
Two fruits snack pack	246kJ	↑ sugar	✓	Good
Apricots snack pack	259kJ	↑ sugar	✓	Good
Pears in juice snack pack	242kJ	↑ sugar	✓	Good
Peach & pineapple snack pack	255kJ	↑ sugar	✓	Good

Two fruits in natural juice	207kJ	✓	✓	Good
Apricot halves in natural juice	280kJ	✓	✓	Good
Plums in natural juice	282kJ	↑ sugar	✓	Good
Fruit salad in natural juice	223kJ	✓	127	Good
Pear slices in natural juice	209kJ	✓	✓	Good
Peach slices in natural juice	251kJ	↑ sugar	✓	Good
Peach in mango puree	234kJ	✓	✓	Good

Great Lakes

Product Name	Energy	Major Nutrients	Food Additives	Nutritious Rating
Blueberries	390kJ	↑ sugar	✓	Good
Strawberries	346kJ	↑ sugar	124, 129	Good

Heinz

Product Name	Energy	Major Nutrients	Food Additives	Nutritious Rating
Splat, apple & mango	250kJ	↑ sugar	✓	Good
Splat, apple & strawberry	280kJ	↑ sugar	✓	Good

IGA/Franklins

Product Name	Energy	Major Nutrients	Food Additives	Nutritious Rating
Signature peaches, natural juice	206kJ	✓	✓	Good
Signature pear halves, natural juice	228kJ	✓	✓	Good
Signature fruit salad, natural juice	223kJ	✓	127	Good
Signature died two	218kJ	✓	✓	Good

fruits, natural juice				
Signature apricot halves	277kJ	↑ Sugar	✓	Good
Black & Gold pineapple slices	260kJ	✓	✓	Good
Black & Gold apricots, syrup	260kJ	↑ Sugar	✓	Good
Black & Gold pears, syrup	264kJ	↑ Sugar	✓	Good
Black & Gold fruit salad, syrup	262kJ	↑ Sugar	✓	Good
Black & Gold peaches, syrup	255kJ	↑ Sugar	✓	Good
Black & Gold two fruits, syrup	260kJ	↑ Sugar	✓	Good

SPC

Product Name	Energy	Major Nutrients	Food Additives	Nutritious Rating
Apricots halves in syrup	260kJ	↑ Sugar	✓	Good
Diced peaches, sliced lite	189kJ	✓	✓	Good
Peaches sliced in natural juice	252kJ	↑ Sugar	✓	Good
Fruit salad in juice	209kJ	✓	127	Good
Fruit salad in syrup	262kJ	↑ Sugar	127	Good
Peach slices in syrup	255kJ	↑ Sugar	✓	Good
Peaches in mango juice	285kJ	↑ Sugar	✓	Good
Pear halves in syrup	264kJ	↑ Sugar	✓	Good
Pears sliced, in juice	247kJ	✓	✓	Good
Apple puree 4pk	237kJ	✓	✓	Good
Fruit crush-ups, strawberry	280kJ	↑ Sugar	✓	Good
Fruit crush-ups, tropical	296kJ	↑ Sugar	✓	Good
Fruit snacks, grape in	313kJ	↑ Sugar	120	Good

apple jelly				
Fruit snacks, peaches in mango jelly	303kJ	↑ Sugar	160b	Good
Fruit snacks, pears in lime jelly	**315kJ**	**↑ Sugar**	✓	**Good**
Fruit snacks, pears in raspberry jelly	320kJ	↑ Sugar	120	Good
Fruit snacks, peaches in pineapple jelly	310kJ	↑ Sugar	120	Good
Fruit squeezies, apple & banana	**318kJ**	**↑ Sugar**	✓	**Good**
Fruit squeezies, banana, pear & passionfruit	**403kJ**	**↑ Sugar**	✓	**Good**
Fruit squeezies, apple & raspberry	**357kJ**	**↑ Sugar**	✓	**Good**
Power pulp, mixed berry	**282kJ**	**↑ Sugar**	✓	**Good**
Power pulp, tropical	**296kJ**	**↑ Sugar**	✓	**Good**
Jelly & fruit splits, mango & pineapple	**336kJ**	**↑ Sugar**	✓	**Good**

Tania

Product Name	Energy	Major Nutrients	Food Additives	Nutritious Rating
Sliced mango in syrup	**266kJ**	**↑ sugar**	✓	**Good**
Cherries	160kJ	↑ sugar	202, 211, 129	Good

Weight Watchers

Product Name	Energy	Major Nutrients	Food Additives	Nutritious Rating
Apricot halves	110kJ	✓	952, 954	Good
Fruit salad	145kJ	✓	952, 954	Good
Peaches	135kJ	✓	952, 954	Good
Peaches in mango syrup	140kJ	✓	952, 954	Good
Two fruits	140kJ	✓	952, 954	Good
Apricots snack pack	118kJ	✓	952, 954	Good

Peaches snack pack	109kJ	✓	952, 954	Good
Two fruits snack pack	116kJ	✓	952, 954	Good
Fruit salad snack pack	116kJ	✓	952, 954	Good
Two fruits in tropical jelly	62kJ	✓	120, 952, 954, 961	Good
Peaches in mango in orange jelly	66kJ	✓	952, 954, 961, 160b, 327	Good
Pears in fruits of the forest jelly	60kJ	✓	120, 952, 954, 961	Good

Woolworths

Product Name	Energy	Major Nutrients	Food Additives	Nutritious Rating
Select, sliced apple	177kJ	✓	✓	Good
Select, passionfruit pulp	489kJ	↑ Sugar	✓	Good
Select, blackberries	395kJ	↑ Sugar	✓	Good
Select, blueberries	409kJ	↑ Sugar	✓	Good
Select, pineapple slices	244kJ	↑ Sugar	✓	Good
Select, pineapple pieces	189kJ	✓	✓	Good
Select, apricot halves in juice	202kJ	✓	✓	Good
Select, pear slices in juice	252kJ	↑ Sugar	✓	Good
Select, chunky fruit salad	209kJ	↑ Sugar	127	Good
Select, peaches in juice	260kJ	↑ Sugar	✓	Good
Select snack tub, diced peaches in juice	210kJ	↑ Sugar	✓	Good
Select snack tub, diced two fruits in juices	210kJ	↑ Sugar	✓	Good

Select snack tub, diced fruit salad in juice	220kJ	↑ Sugar	✓	Good
Select snack tub, apple puree assortment	210-230kJ	↑ Sugar	120	Good
Select, pears in lime jelly	270kJ	↑ Sugar	✓	Good
Select, pears in raspberry jelly	270kJ	↑ Sugar	120	Good
Select, two fruits in tropical jelly	280kJ	↑ Sugar	✓	Good
Homebrand, pineapple slices in juice	189kJ	✓	✓	Good
Homebrand, peach slices in syrup	280kJ	↑ Sugar	✓	Good
Homebrand, pear halves in syrup	258kJ	↑ Sugar	✓	Good
Homebrand, fruit salad in syrup	309kJ	↑ Sugar	127	Good
Homebrand, apricot halves in syrup	298kJ	↑ Sugar	✓	Good
Homebrand, mango slices in syrup	320kJ	↑ Sugar	✓	Good

Canned Vegetables

Canned vegetables are very comparable. Be wary of the hidden sugar and salt content as well as the BPA in the steel can.

Always Fresh

Product Name	Energy	Major Nutrients	Food Additives	Nutritious Rating
Artichoke hearts, whole	147kJ	✓	✓	Good
Asparagus spears in spring water	111kJ	✓	✓	Good
Bamboo shoots, sliced	68kJ	✓	✓	Good
Champignons, whole	139kJ	✓	✓	Good
Sauerkraut, German	124kJ	✓	✓	Good
Water chestnuts, whole	143kJ	✓	✓	Good
Asparagus, balsamic	216kJ	✓	220	Good
Asparagus, marinated & crisp	134kJ	✓	✓	Good
Bean sprouts	76kJ	✓	✓	Good

Annalisa

Product Name	Energy	Major Nutrients	Food Additives	Nutritious Rating
Italian diced tomatoes	95kJ	✓	✓	Good
Italian whole tomatoes	95kJ	✓	✓	Good
4 bean mix	547kJ	✓	✓	Good
Chick peas	579kJ	✓	✓	Good
Red kidney beans	418kJ	✓	✓	Good
Butter beans	288kJ	✓	✓	Good
Lentils	483kJ	✓	✓	Good
Borlotti beans	547kJ	✓	✓	Good

Cannelini beans	515kJ	✓	✓	Good
White beans	547kJ	✓	✓	Good

Ardmona

Product Name	Energy	Major Nutrients	Food Additives	Nutritious Rating
Rich & thick bolognese chopped tomatoes	157kJ	✓	HVP	Good
Rich & thick chopped capsicum	140kJ	✓	✓	Good
Rich & thick tomatoes, garlic & basil	136kJ	✓	✓	Good
Rich & thick tomatoes, chopped herbs	110kJ	✓	✓	Good
Rich & thick tomatoes, chopped onion & garlic	116kJ	✓	✓	Good
Rich & thick tomatoes, ITA parmigana	120kJ	✓	✓	Good
Rich & thick tomatoes, chopped finely	110kJ	✓	✓	Good
Tomatoes chopped , no added salt	102kJ	✓	✓	Good
Tomatoes, whole peeled	102kJ	✓	✓	Good
Tomatoes, crushed	107kJ	✓	✓	Good
Tomato puree	177kJ	✓	✓	Good

Bachelors

Product Name	Energy	Major Nutrients	Food Additives	Nutritious Rating
Mushy peas, chip shop style	294kJ	✓	133	Good
Mushy peas, original	294kJ	✓	133	Good

Peas, small processed marrowfat	251kJ	✓	133	Good

Bask-a-Jon

Product Name	Energy	Major Nutrients	Food Additives	Nutritious Rating
Whole baby beets	161kJ	✓	✓	Good
Beetroot, grated	272kJ	↑Salt	✓	Good

Bibo

Product Name	Energy	Major Nutrients	Food Additives	Nutritious Rating
Tomatoes, Italian whole peeled	105kJ	✓	✓	Good
Mushrooms, whole	170kJ	✓	✓	Good
Mushrooms, pieces & stems	170kJ	✓	✓	Good

Bio Nature

Product Name	Energy	Major Nutrients	Food Additives	Nutritious Rating
Organic cannellini beans	397kJ	✓	✓	Good
Organic red kidney beans	419kJ	✓	✓	Good
Organic brown lentils	359kJ	✓	✓	Good
Organic chick peas	568kJ	✓	✓	Good
Organic chopped tomatoes	97kJ	✓	✓	Good

Capricio

Product Name	Energy	Major Nutrients	Food Additives	Nutritious Rating
Italian diced tomatoes	88kJ	✓	✓	Good
Italian whole tomatoes	91kJ	✓	✓	Good
Artichokes, brine	143kJ	✓	✓	Good

Product Name	Energy	Major Nutrients	Food Additives	Nutritious Rating
Chick peas	311kJ	✓	✓	Good
Fagioli rossi	413kJ	✓	✓	Good
Butter beans	288kJ	✓	✓	Good
Lentils	368kJ	✓	✓	Good
Borlotti beans	403kJ	✓	✓	Good
Cannelini beans	368kJ	✓	✓	Good

Cecilia

Product Name	Energy	Major Nutrients	Food Additives	Nutritious Rating
Lima beans	481kJ	✓	✓	Good
4 bean mix	451kJ	✓	✓	Good
Chick peas	502kJ	✓	✓	Good
Lentils	386kJ	✓	✓	Good
Borlotti beans	389kJ	✓	✓	Good
Cannelini beans	381kJ	✓	✓	Good

Classic Asian

Product Name	Energy	Major Nutrients	Food Additives	Nutritious Rating
Straw mushrooms	176kJ	✓	✓	Good
Shitake mushrooms	176kJ	✓	✓	Good

Coles

Product Name	Energy	Major Nutrients	Food Additives	Nutritious Rating
Asparagus, cuts & tips	87kJ	✓	✓	Good
Asparagus, spears	87kJ	✓	✓	Good
Baby beets	211kJ	✓	✓	Good
Beetroot, sliced	211kJ	✓	✓	Good
Baby corn, cuts & tips	113kJ	✓	✓	Good
Baby carrots	93kJ	✓	✓	Good
Butter beans	384kJ	✓	✓	Good
Lentils	290kJ	✓	✓	Good
Mexican chilli beans	304kJ	✓	✓	Good
Chick peas	384kJ	✓	✓	Good

Kidney beans	370kJ	✓	✓	Good
Cannelini beans	301kJ	✓	✓	Good
Four bean mix	299kJ	✓	✓	Good
Organic four bean mix	299kJ	✓	✓	Good
Organic butter beans	349kJ	✓	✓	Good
Organic chick peas	391kJ	✓	✓	Good
Organic red kidney beans	370kJ	✓	✓	Good
Champignons, pieces & stems	120kJ	✓	✓	Good
Champignons, whole	120kJ	✓	✓	Good
Mushrooms, sliced in butter sauce	146kJ	✓	✓	Good
Mushrooms, sliced in butter sauce no added salt	150kJ	✓	✓	Good
Asparagus, spears no salt	87kJ	✓	✓	Good
Corn kernels	275kJ	✓	✓	Good
Corn kernels, no added salt	275kJ	✓	✓	Good
Corn spears, young	113kJ	✓	✓	Good
Corn, creamed	286kJ	✓	✓	Good
Organic corn kernels	360kJ	✓	✓	Good
Organic tomatoes, diced	80kJ	✓	✓	Good
Organic tomatoes, whole peeled	80kJ	✓	✓	Good
Tomatoes, crushed with mixed herbs	122kJ	✓	✓	Good
Tomatoes, diced Italian	76kJ	✓	✓	Good
Tomatoes, whole peeled	84kJ	✓	✓	Good
Baby peas	320kJ	✓	✓	Good
Potatoes, whole	215kJ	✓	✓	Good
Potato salad	395kJ	✓	✓	Good

Water chestnuts	80kJ	✓	✓	Good
Smart buy beetroot, sliced	211kJ	✓	✓	Good
Smart buy corn kernels	276kJ	✓	✓	Good
Smart buy instant mashed potatoes	365kJ	✓	320, 223	Good
Smart buy mushy green peas	450kJ	✓	✓	Good
Smart buy dehydrated peas	275kJ	✓	✓	Good
Smart buy tomatoes, diced	92kJ	✓	✓	Good
Smart buy tomatoes, whole	100kJ	✓	✓	Good

Cucina

Product Name	Energy	Major Nutrients	Food Additives	Nutritious Rating
Chick peas	455kJ	✓	✓	Good
Lentils	234kJ	✓	✓	Good
Borlotti beans	432kJ	✓	✓	Good

Deb

Product Name	Energy	Major Nutrients	Food Additives	Nutritious Rating
Instant mashed potatoes, onion	331kJ	✓	220, 319, 160b	Good
Instant mashed potatoes, plain	333kJ	✓	220, 319, 160b	Good

D'oro

Product Name	Energy	Major Nutrients	Food Additives	Nutritious Rating
Asparagus spears, green	59kJ	✓	✓	Good
Asparagus tips & cuts	100kJ	✓	✓	Good
Corn kernels	277kJ	✓	✓	Good

Product Name	Energy	Major Nutrients	Food Additives	Nutritious Rating
Mushrooms, whole	130kJ	✓	✓	Good
Mushrooms, pieces & stems	170kJ	✓	✓	Good

Edgell

Product Name	Energy	Major Nutrients	Food Additives	Nutritious Rating
Asparagus spears, green	77kJ	✓	✓	Good
Asparagus tips & cuts	79kJ	✓	✓	Good
Baby peas	282kJ	✓	✓	Good
Baby peas & super sweet corn	350kJ	✓	✓	Good
Peas, corn & carrots	246kJ	✓	✓	Good
Peas & carrots	208kJ	✓	✓	Good
Green beans & carrots	115kJ	✓	✓	Good
Garden peas, minted	282kJ	✓	✓	Good
Green beans, sliced	94kJ	✓	✓	Good
Beetroot, sliced	224kJ	✓	✓	Good
Beetroot, whole	250kJ	✓	✓	Good
Beetroot, summer style	265kJ	✓	✓	Good
Capsicum, diced	135kJ	✓	✓	Good
Chick peas	532kJ	✓	✓	Good
Corn, creamed	356kJ	✓	✓	Good
Corn kernels	448kJ	✓	✓	Good
Corn kernels, no added salt	307kJ	✓	✓	Good
Corn kernels, super sweet	313kJ	✓	✓	Good
Four bean mix	497kJ	✓	✓	Good
Four bean mix, no added salt	524kJ	✓	✓	Good
Red kidney beans	499kJ	✓	✓	Good
Red kidney beans, no added salt	494kJ	✓	✓	Good
Three bean & corn	355kJ	✓	✓	Good

mix with balsamic vinegar				
Three bean & corn mix, honey wholegrain mustard	421kJ	✓	320	Good
Three bean & corn mix, Thai sweet chilli	378kJ	✓	407	Good
Instant mashed potato	315kJ	✓	222	Good
Tiny taters	287kJ	✓	✓	Good
Tiny taters, minted	287kJ	✓	✓	Good
Mushrooms, sliced in butter sauce	146kJ	✓	✓	Good
Sauerkraut	55kJ	✓	220	Good
Mixed vegetables	222kJ	✓	✓	Good
Tomato supreme	195kJ	✓	✓	Good

Farrows

Product Name	Energy	Major Nutrients	Food Additives	Nutritious Rating
Marrow fat peas	377kJ	✓	✓	Good

Global Organics

Product Name	Energy	Major Nutrients	Food Additives	Nutritious Rating
Red kidney beans	569kJ	✓	✓	Good
Lentils, brown	327kJ	✓	✓	Good
Borlotti beans	426kJ	✓	✓	Good
Cannelini beans	327kJ	✓	✓	Good

Golden Circle

Product Name	Energy	Major Nutrients	Food Additives	Nutritious Rating
Baby beets, whole	250kJ	✓	✓	Good
Australian baby beetroot in juice	190kJ	✓	✓	Good
Baby beetroot, whole	250kJ	✓	✓	Good
Beetroot, sliced	250kJ	✓	✓	Good

Beetroot, diced	250kJ	✓	✓	Good
Beetroot, wedges	250kJ	✓	✓	Good
Corn & peas	360kJ	✓	✓	Good
Corn kernels	360kJ	✓	✓	Good
Corn, creamed	305kJ	✓	✓	Good
Peas, green	375kJ	✓	✓	Good
Garden corn, peas & carrots	370kJ	✓	✓	Good
Garden sweet corn	430kJ	✓	✓	Good
Garden green peas	360kJ	✓	✓	Good

Greenland

Product Name	Energy	Major Nutrients	Food Additives	Nutritious Rating
Mexican chilli beans	400kJ	✓	✓	Good
Corn cuts	76kJ	✓	✓	Good
Corn kernels	320kJ	✓	✓	Good
Asparagus spears	90kJ	✓	✓	Good
Carrots	80kJ	✓	✓	Good
Champignons	170kJ	✓	✓	Good
Bean sprouts	70kJ	✓	✓	Good
Bamboo shoots	70kJ	✓	✓	Good
Spinach	110kJ	✓	✓	Good
Stir fry mix	85kJ	✓	✓	Good
Baby asparagus	90kJ	✓	✓	Good
Water chestnuts	150kJ	✓	✓	Good
Cucumber slices	600kJ	↑Salt	✓	Good

Heinz

Product Name	Energy	Major Nutrients	Food Additives	Nutritious Rating
Beetroot jar	172kJ	✓	202	Good
Minted peas	350kJ	↑Salt	102, 133	Good

IGA/Franklins

Product Name	Energy	Major Nutrients	Food Additives	Nutritious Rating
Country Ridge,	110kJ	✓	✓	Good

asparagus				
Country Ridge, sliced beetroot	211kJ	✓	✓	Good
Country Ridge, corn cuts	80kJ	✓	✓	Good
Country Ridge, 4 bean mix	530kJ	✓	✓	Good
Signature, asparagus	110kJ	✓	✓	Good
Signature, sliced beetroot	211kJ	✓	✓	Good
Signature, corn kernels	180kJ	✓	✓	Good
Signature, sliced mushrooms in gravy	130kJ	✓	✓	Good
Signature, roma tomatoes	100kJ	✓	✓	Good
Signature, tomato puree	130kJ	✓	✓	Good
Signature, whole tomatoes	102kJ	✓	✓	Good
Black & Gold, sliced beetroot	211kJ	✓	✓	Good
Black & Gold, asparagus spears	110kJ	✓	✓	Good
Black & Gold, asparagus cuts	110kJ	✓	✓	Good
Black & Gold, corn kernels	347kJ	✓	✓	Good
Black & Gold, creamed corn	230kJ	✓	✓	Good
Black & Gold, baby carrots	88kJ	✓	✓	Good
Black & Gold, whole baby potatoes	271kJ	✓	✓	Average
Black & Gold, potato salad	503kJ	✓	320	Average
Black & Gold, champignons whole	170kJ	✓	✓	Good

	Energy	Major Nutrients	Food Additives	Nutritious Rating
Black & Gold, champignons stems & pieces	170kJ	✓	✓	Good
Black & Gold, garden peas	370kJ	✓	✓	Good
Black & Gold, quick cook peas	275kJ	✓	✓	Good
Purely Organic, chick peas	395kJ	✓	✓	Good
Purely Organic, whole tomatoes	73kJ	✓	✓	Good
Purely Organic, diced tomatoes	73kJ	✓	✓	Good

Jean Nicolas

Product Name	Energy	Major Nutrients	Food Additives	Nutritious Rating
Chopped spinach	106kJ	✓	✓	Good
Chick peas	519kJ	✓	✓	Good

La Gina

Product Name	Energy	Major Nutrients	Food Additives	Nutritious Rating
Tomatoes, whole	100kJ	✓	✓	Good
Tomatoes, diced	93kJ	✓	✓	Good
Tomatoes, crushed	93kJ	✓	✓	Good

La Nova

Product Name	Energy	Major Nutrients	Food Additives	Nutritious Rating
4 bean mix	552kJ	✓	✓	Good
Red kidney beans	366kJ	✓	✓	Good
Chick peas	595kJ	✓	✓	Good
Cannelini beans	283kJ	✓	✓	Good
Borlotti beans	570kJ	✓	✓	Good
Soya beans	364kJ	✓	✓	Good
Butter beans	536kJ	✓	✓	Good
Lentils	426kJ	✓	✓	Good
Artichoke hearts	108kJ	✓	✓	Good

La Verde

Product Name	Energy	Major Nutrients	Food Additives	Nutritious Rating
Tomatoes, whole	83kJ	✓	✓	Good
Tomatoes, diced	83kJ	✓	✓	Good
Tomatoes, diced, oregano & basil	86kJ	✓	✓	Good
Tomatoes, diced, olives	192kJ	✓	✓	Good
Tomatoes, diced, capsicum & onion	117kJ	✓	✓	Good
Tomatoes, diced, gourmet	95kJ	✓	✓	Good
Artichoke, whole	105kJ	✓	✓	Good

Rainbow

Product Name	Energy	Major Nutrients	Food Additives	Nutritious Rating
Corn, kernels	326kJ	✓	✓	Good
Corn, creamed	204kJ	✓	✓	Good
Corn, baby	127kJ	✓	✓	Good

Romanella

Product Name	Energy	Major Nutrients	Food Additives	Nutritious Rating
4 bean mix	431kJ	✓	✓	Good
Red kidney beans	372kJ	✓	✓	Good
Cannelini beans	455kJ	✓	✓	Good
Borlotti beans	393kJ	✓	✓	Good
Butter beans	393kJ	✓	✓	Good
Lentils	234kJ	✓	✓	Good

Russo

Product Name	Energy	Major Nutrients	Food Additives	Nutritious Rating
Borlotti beans	306kJ	✓	✓	Good
Butter beans	290kJ	✓	✓	Good
Cannellini beans	305kJ	✓	✓	Good

Red kidney beans	309kJ	✓	✓	Good
Chick peas	343kJ	✓	✓	Good
Lentils	284kJ	✓	✓	Good

SPC

Product Name	Energy	Major Nutrients	Food Additives	Nutritious Rating
Tomatoes, whole	102kJ	✓	✓	Good
Tomatoes, diced onion, basil & garlic	127kJ	✓	✓	Good
Tomatoes, crushed	107kJ	✓	✓	Good
Tomatoes, crushed, basil & oregano	110kJ	✓	✓	Good

Sunsol

Product Name	Energy	Major Nutrients	Food Additives	Nutritious Rating
Green split peas	1247kJ	✓	✓	Good
Supreme soup mix	1290kJ	✓	✓	Good
red lentils	1148kJ	✓	✓	Good
Yellow split peas	1194kJ	✓	✓	Good
Pearl barley	1327kJ	✓	✓	Good
Lentils	1097kJ	✓	✓	Good

Surprise

Product Name	Energy	Major Nutrients	Food Additives	Nutritious Rating
Dehydrated peas	375kJ	✓	✓	Good
Dehydrated peas, minted	375kJ	✓	✓	Good

Tania

Product Name	Energy	Major Nutrients	Food Additives	Nutritious Rating
Asparagus, whole white	96kJ	✓	✓	Good
Asparagus, whole spears green	94kJ	✓	✓	Good
Beetroot, whole	182kJ	✓	✓	Good

pickled				

Trident

Product Name	Energy	Major Nutrients	Food Additives	Nutritious Rating
Asparagus spears	118kJ	✓	✓	Good
Asparagus cuts	82kJ	✓	✓	Good
Chinese mixed vegetables	88kJ	✓	✓	Good
Baby corn	105kJ	✓	✓	Good
Baby corn spears	108kJ	✓	✓	Good

Windsor Farm

Product Name	Energy	Major Nutrients	Food Additives	Nutritious Rating
Petite potatoes	271kJ	✓	✓	Average
Mushy peas	368kJ	✓	142, 102	Good
Sliced mushrooms in butter sauce	134kJ	✓	320	Good
Sliced mushrooms in pepper sauce	134kJ	✓	✓	Good

Woolworths/Safeways

Product Name	Energy	Major Nutrients	Food Additives	Nutritious Rating
Select, tomatoes whole	95kJ	✓	✓	Good
Select, tomatoes diced	95kJ	✓	✓	Good
Select, tomatoes diced no salt	95kJ	✓	✓	Good
Select, tomatoes diced herbs & basil	90kJ	✓	✓	Good
Select, corn kernels	336kJ	✓	✓	Good
Select, corn kernels no added salt	348kJ	✓	✓	Good
Select, super sweet corn	314kJ	✓	✓	Good
Select, creamed	235kJ	✓	✓	Average

corn				
Select, baby corn spears	192kJ	✓	✓	Good
Select, baby corn cuts	192kJ	✓	✓	Good
Select, beetroot sliced	257kJ	✓	✓	Good
Select, asparagus spears	87kJ	✓	✓	Good
Select, asparagus cuts & tips	93kJ	✓	✓	Good
Select, garden peas	306kJ	✓	✓	Good
Select, peas & corn	293kJ	✓	✓	Good
Select, peas & carrots	241kJ	✓	✓	Good
Select, baby carrots	115kJ	✓	✓	Good
Select, beans sliced	129kJ	✓	✓	Good
Select, mushrooms sliced in butter	146kJ	✓	320	Good
Select, five bean mix	548kJ	✓	✓	Good
Select, five bean mix no added salt	418kJ	✓	✓	Good
Select, chick peas	568kJ	✓	✓	Good
Select, chick peas no added salt	568kJ	✓	✓	Good
Select, red kidney beans	418kJ	✓	✓	Good
Select, red kidney beans no added salt	418kJ	✓	✓	Good
Select, butter beans	401kJ	✓	✓	Good
Homebrand, 3 bean mix	377kJ	✓	✓	Good
Homebrand, red kidney beans	465kJ	✓	✓	Good
Homebrand, chick peas	522kJ	✓	✓	Good

Homebrand, corn kernels	336kJ	✓	✓	Good
Homebrand, creamed corn	225kJ	✓	✓	Good
Homebrand, corn spears	192kJ	✓	✓	Good
Homebrand, baby corn cuts	192kJ	✓	✓	Good
Homebrand, beetroot sliced	222kJ	✓	✓	Good
Homebrand, Italian roma tomatoes	74kJ	✓	✓	Good
Homebrand, tomatoes diced	74kJ	✓	✓	Good
Homebrand, asparagus spears	88kJ	✓	✓	Good
Homebrand, asparagus cuts	88kJ	✓	✓	Good
Homebrand, water chestnuts	120kJ	✓	✓	Good
Homebrand, peas	334kJ	✓	✓	Good
Homebrand, peas minted	299kJ	✓	102, 133	Good
Homebrand, sliced beans	97kJ	✓	✓	Good
Homebrand, champignons whole	115kJ	✓	✓	Good
Homebrand, champignons pieces & stems	140kJ	✓	✓	Good
Homebrand, sliced mushrooms	146kJ	✓	✓	Good
Homebrand, sliced mushrooms no salt	143kJ	✓	✓	Good

Coconut Milk/Cream

Coconut milk can be made very easily at home at a fraction of the price with desiccated coconut and water blended for a few minutes.

Ayam

Product Name	Energy	Major Nutrients	Food Additives	Nutritious Rating
Premium coconut cream	1261kJ	↑Fat	✓	Good
Premium coconut cream, light	1287kJ	↑Fat	✓	Good
Premium coconut milk	1024kJ	↑Fat	✓	Good
Premium coconut milk, organic	1024kJ	↑Fat	✓	Good
Premium coconut water	96kJ	✓	223	Good
Premium coconut powder	2930kJ	↑Fat	✓	Average

Ceres Organic

Product Name	Energy	Major Nutrients	Food Additives	Nutritious Rating
Coconut milk	731kJ	↑Fat	✓	Good
Coconut cream	877kJ	↑Fat	✓	Good

Classis Asian

Product Name	Energy	Major Nutrients	Food Additives	Nutritious Rating
Coconut milk	664kJ	↑Fat	✓	Good
Coconut milk, lite	613kJ	↑Fat	✓	Good
Coconut cream	821kJ	↑Fat	✓	Good
Coconut cream, lite	756kJ	↑Fat	✓	Good

Pandaroo

Product Name	Energy	Major Nutrients	Food Additives	Nutritious Rating
Coconut milk	472kJ	↑Fat	✓	Good
Coconut milk, lite	210kJ	✓	✓	Good
Coconut cream	658kJ	↑Fat	✓	Good

Spiral Organic

Product Name	Energy	Major Nutrients	Food Additives	Nutritious Rating
Coconut milk	252kJ	↑Fat	✓	Good
Coconut cream	752kJ	↑Fat	✓	Good

Trident

Product Name	Energy	Major Nutrients	Food Additives	Nutritious Rating
Coconut milk	750kJ	↑Fat	✓	Good
Coconut milk, lite	358kJ	✓	✓	Good
Coconut cream	1080kJ	↑Fat	✓	Good
Coconut cream, lite	363kJ	✓	✓	Good

Canned Meat

My picks are *Seakist, Tassal, Brunswick, Ally, Sirena, Coles and Woolworths select.*

When selecting tuna, try to opt for the pole & line varieties, as they cause the least environmental impact.

Ally

Product Name	Energy	Major Nutrients	Food Additives	Nutritious Rating
Pink salmon	634kJ	✓	✓	Good

Always Fresh

Product Name	Energy	Major Nutrients	Food Additives	Nutritious Rating
Anchovies, flat fillets	773kJ	↑Fat ↑Salt	✓	Good
Mussels, smoked	947kJ	↑Fat	✓	Good
Oysters, smoked in oil	989kJ	↑Fat	✓	Good
Prawns	422kJ	↑Salt	223	Good
Crab meat	252kJ	↑Salt	223	Good

Brunswick

Product Name	Energy	Major Nutrients	Food Additives	Nutritious Rating
Sardines in olive oil	871kJ	↑Fat	✓	Good
Sardines in spring water	643kJ	✓	✓	Good
Sardines in spring water, no added salt	643kJ	✓	✓	Good
Sardines in tomato sauce	558kJ	✓	✓	Good
Seafood snack, kippers	654kJ	↑Fat ↑Salt	✓	Good

Chop Chop

Product Name	Energy	Major Nutrients	Food Additives	Nutritious Rating
Chicken chunks in sea salt & water	456kJ	✓	✓	Average
Chicken shredded with chilli & lite mayo	646kJ	✓	✓	Average
Chicken shredded with lite mayo	655kJ	✓	✓	Average
Chicken shredded with mustard & lite mayo	682kJ	↑Fat	✓	Average
Chicken shredded with pepper & lite mayo	670kJ	↑Fat	✓	Average
Chicken shredded with sundried tomato & lite mayo	666kJ	↑Fat	✓	Average

Coles

Product Name	Energy	Major Nutrients	Food Additives	Nutritious Rating
Corned beef	933kJ	↑Fat ↑Salt	250	Average
Deli style chicken	568kJ	↑Salt	✓	Average
Ham	596kJ	↑Salt	250, 407	Average
Crab meat	305kJ	↑Salt	223	Good
Prawn in brine	368kJ	↑Salt	223	Good
Pink salmon	670kJ	✓	✓	Good
Pink salmon, no added salt	670kJ	✓	✓	Good
Pink salmon, skinless & boneless	568kJ	✓	✓	Good
Red salmon	769kJ	↑Fat	✓	Good
Red salmon, no added salt	795kJ	↑Fat	✓	Good
Red salmon, skinless & boneless	711kJ	↑Fat	✓	Good

Sandwich tuna in olive oil blend	623kJ	✓	✓	Average
Tuna chunks in brine	576kJ	✓	✓	Average
Tuna chunks in spring water	481kJ	✓	✓	Average
Pole & line tuna chunks in spring water	481kJ	✓	✓	Average
Pole & line tuna chunks in brine	443kJ	✓	✓	Average
Pole & line tuna chunks in olive oil	623kJ	✓	✓	Average
Tuna chunks in oil	741kJ	↑Fat	✓	Average
Tuna, Italian style	259kJ	✓	✓	Average
Tuna, Thai red curry	665kJ	↑Fat	✓	Average
Tuna, lemon pepper	531kJ	✓	✓	Average
Tuna, lemon & cracked pepper	330kJ	✓	✓	Average
Tuna, lime & cracked pepper	367kJ	✓	✓	Average
Tuna, zesty vinaigrette	556kJ	✓	✓	Average
Tuna, rosemary & sundried tomato	514kJ	✓	220	Average
Tuna, tomato & basil	560kJ	✓	✓	Average
Tuna, tomato & chilli	381kJ	✓	✓	Average
Tuna, spicy chilli style	681kJ	↑Fat	✓	Average
Tuna, sweet seeded mustard	589kJ	✓	223	Average
Tuna, Spanish style	295kJ	✓	✓	Average
Tuna, Japanese style	392kJ	↑Salt	✓	Average
Tuna, onion & savoury sauce	581kJ	✓	✓	Average
Tuna, sweet corn &	510kJ	✓	✓	Average

mayo				
Tuna, smoked flavour	493kJ	✓	✓	Average
Tuna, Mexican style	303kJ	✓	✓	Average
Tuna, Moroccan style	307kJ	✓	✓	Average
Tuna, mild Indian curry	518kJ	✓	✓	Average
Smart Buy, tuna in brine	443kJ	✓	✓	Average
Smart Buy, tuna in vegetable oil	653kJ	✓	✓	Average
Smart Buy, pink salmon	670kJ	✓	✓	Good
Smart Buy, sardines in tomato sauce	647kJ	↑Fat	✓	Good
Smart Buy, sardines in olive oil	807kJ	↑Fat	✓	Good

Delicius

Product Name	Energy	Major Nutrients	Food Additives	Nutritious Rating
Anchovy fillets, capers	728kJ	↑Salt	✓	Good
Anchovy fillets, hot chilli	996kJ	↑Salt ↑Fat	✓	Good
Mackerel fillets, olive oil	783kJ	↑Fat	✓	Good

Deli Menu

Product Name	Energy	Major Nutrients	Food Additives	Nutritious Rating
Malaysian laksa chicken	728kJ	↑Salt	✓	Average
Satay tuna & rice	996kJ	↑Fat	✓	Average
Teriyaki rice & chicken	783kJ	✓	✓	Average
Italian pasta & tuna	445kJ	✓	✓	Average

Hamper

Product Name	Energy	Major Nutrients	Food Additives	Nutritious Rating
Corned beef	975kJ	↑Salt ↑Fat	250, 407	Average
Corned beef, easy slice	975kJ	↑Salt ↑Fat	250, 407	Average
Corned beef, lite	835kJ	↑Salt ↑Fat	250, 407	Average
Lamb tongues	860kJ	↑Salt ↑Fat	250	Average
Camp pie	685kJ	↑Salt ↑Fat	250, HVP	Poor

Heinz

Product Name	Energy	Major Nutrients	Food Additives	Nutritious Rating
Chicken, shredded with lite mayo	665kJ	✓	✓	Average
Chicken with sweet chilli	710kJ	↑Fat	✓	Average
Chicken with sweet corn & mayo	670kJ	↑Salt ↑Fat	✓	Average
Chicken, natural smoked	360kJ	✓	✓	Average
Chicken in sea salt & water	395kJ	✓	✓	Average
Chicken with tomato & onion	600kJ	✓	✓	Average
Chicken with mustard & mayo	745kJ	↑Salt ↑Fat	224	Average
Chicken tandoori	480kJ	✓	✓	Average
Breast slices, natural smoke	470kJ	✓	✓	Average
Breast slices, spring water	480kJ	✓	✓	Average

Hormel

Product Name	Energy	Major Nutrients	Food Additives	Nutritious Rating
Luncheon meat	1045kJ	↑Salt ↑Fat	250, 160b, 1520	Poor

IGA

Product Name	Energy	Major Nutrients	Food Additives	Nutritious Rating
Signature, tuna in canola	750kJ	✓	✓	Average
Signature, tuna in spring water	490kJ	✓	✓	Average
Signature, tuna in brine	502kJ	↑Salt	✓	Average
Signature, tuna & tomato & basil	998kJ	↑Fat	✓	Average
Signature, tuna & chilli	948kJ	↑Salt ↑Fat	✓	Average
Signature, tuna & tomato & onion	647kJ	↑Fat	✓	Average
Signature, tuna & lemon pepper	1062kJ	↑Fat	✓	Average
Black & Gold, tuna in brine	502kJ	✓	✓	Average
Black & Gold, pink salmon	630kJ	✓	✓	Good
Black & Gold, mussels	1540kJ	↑Fat	✓	Good
Black & Gold, oysters	1260kJ	↑Fat	✓	Good
Black & Gold, sardines in tomato	342kJ	✓	✓	Good
Black & Gold, corned beef	1000kJ	↑Salt ↑Fat	250, 407	Average
Black & Gold, spiced ham	1390kJ	↑Salt ↑Fat	250	Average

John West

Product Name	Energy	Major Nutrients	Food Additives	Nutritious Rating
Tuna & beans, 3 beans	671kJ	↑Fat	✓	Good
Tuna & beans, capsicum, sweet corn, red kidney beans & chilli	645kJ	↑Fat	✓	Good
Tuna & beans, roast capsicum & 3 beans	478kJ	↑Fat	✓	Good
Tuna to go, tuna	963kJ	↑Fat ↑Salt	✓	Average
Tuna to go, tomato & basil	978kJ	↑Fat ↑Salt	✓	Average
Tuna to go, sweet chilli	976kJ	↑Fat ↑Salt	✓	Average
Tuna slices, spring water	484kJ	✓	✓	Average
Tuna slices, olive oil	804kJ	↑Fat	✓	Average
Tuna slices, smoked	804kJ	↑Fat	✓	Average
Tuna slices, sweet chilli	603kJ	✓	✓	Average
Tuna no drain, spring water	551kJ	✓	✓	Average
Tuna no drain, brine	551kJ	✓	✓	Average
Tuna no drain, olive oil	723kJ	✓	✓	Average
Chunk style tuna, spring water	443kJ	✓	✓	Average
Chunk style tuna, olive oil	918kJ	↑Fat	✓	Average
Chunk style tuna, brine	482kJ	✓	✓	Average
Tuna tempters, mild Indian curry	519kJ	✓	✓	Average
Tuna tempters, lemon & cracked pepper	632kJ	↑Fat	223	Average
Tuna tempters, zesty	610kJ	↑Fat	220	Average

vinaigrette				
Tuna tempters, chilli	787kJ	↑Fat	✓	Average
Tuna tempters, sweet chilli	787kJ	↑Fat	✓	Average
Tuna tempters, tomato salsa	619kJ	↑Fat	✓	Average
Tuna tempters, sweet seed mustard	814kJ	↑Fat	223, 160b	Average
Tuna tempters, mango chilli	543kJ	✓	✓	Average
Tuna tempters, sweet corn	523kJ	✓	✓	Average
Tuna tempters, oven dried tomato & basil	596kJ	✓	✓	Average
Tuna tempters, naturally smoked	588kJ	✓	✓	Average
Tuna tempters, onion & tomato	494kJ	✓	✓	Average
Tuna tempters, garlic & soy	691kJ	↑Fat	✓	Average
Tuna tempters, sea salt & pepper	649kJ	✓	✓	Average
Tuna tempters, chilli & lime	692kJ	✓	223	Average
Tuna tempters light, onion & tomato	345kJ	✓	220	Average
Salmon tempters, spring water	394kJ	✓	✓	Good
Salmon tempters, natural smoked	574kJ	✓	✓	Good
Salmon tempters, lemon & cracked pepper	677kJ	↑Fat ↑Salt	223	Good
Salmon tempters, chilli & lime	452kJ	↑Salt	223	Good
Salmon tempters, mayonnaise	572kJ	✓	✓	Good
Alaskan salmon	485kJ	✓	✓	Good

tempter, spring water				
Alaskan salmon tempter, lemon & sea salt	705kJ	↑Fat	223	Good
Alaskan salmon tempter, salt & cracked pepper	**700kJ**	**↑Fat**	✓	**Good**
Alaskan salmon tempter, onion& tomato	602kJ	✓	220	Good
Alaskan salmon tempter, sundried tomato& basil	740kJ	↑Fat	220	Good
Salmon slices, spring water	**485kJ**	✓	✓	**Good**
Salmon slices, smoked	**446kJ**	✓	✓	**Good**
Salmon slices, olive oil	**762kJ**	↑Fat	✓	**Good**
Alaskan salmon, pink	**634kJ**	✓	✓	**Good**
Alaskan salmon, red	**692kJ**	✓	✓	**Good**
Canadian salmon, pink	**634kJ**	✓	✓	**Good**
Sardines, spring water	**946kJ**	↑Fat	✓	**Good**
Sardines, oil	**1100kJ**	↑Fat	✓	**Good**
Sardines, tomato sauce	576kJ	↑Fat ↑Salt	220	Good
Smoked kippers, brine	**691kJ**	↑Fat ↑Salt	✓	**Good**
Mackerel fillets, brine	**1110kJ**	↑Fat ↑Salt	✓	**Good**
Anchovies, olive oil	**770kJ**	↑Fat ↑Salt	✓	**Good**
Oysters, BBQ sauce	**673kJ**	↑Salt	✓	**Good**
Oysters, vegetable oil	**1050kJ**	↑Fat	✓	**Good**
Herring fillets,	797kJ	↑Fat	220	Good

tomato sauce				

King Oscar

Product Name	Energy	Major Nutrients	Food Additives	Nutritious Rating
Sardines, olive oil	1100kJ	↑Fat	✓	Good
Sardines, oil	721kJ	↑Fat	✓	Good
Sardines, tomato sauce	730kJ	↑Fat	✓	Good

Paramount

Product Name	Energy	Major Nutrients	Food Additives	Nutritious Rating
Red salmon	631kJ	✓	✓	Good
Pink salmon	704kJ	↑Fat	✓	Good

Plumrose

Product Name	Energy	Major Nutrients	Food Additives	Nutritious Rating
Cocktail frankfurts	792kJ	↑Fat ↑Salt	250, 155	Poor
Deli ham	605kJ	↑Fat ↑Salt	250, 407	Poor
Leg ham	575kJ	↑Salt	250, 407	Poor
Skinless hotdogs	792kJ	↑Fat ↑Salt	250, 155	Poor
Luncheon meat	990kJ	↑Fat ↑Salt	250, 155	Poor
Shoulder ham	605kJ	↑Fat ↑Salt	250, 407	Poor

Safcol

Product Name	Energy	Major Nutrients	Food Additives	Nutritious Rating
Salmon, premium skinless & boneless	535kJ	✓	✓	Good
Salmon, spring water	745kJ	↑Fat	✓	Good
Salmon, lemon &	577kJ	✓	211, 223	Good

pepper				
Salmon, natural wood smoke	744kJ	↑Fat	✓	Good
Salmon, red chilli	508kJ	↑Salt	✓	Good
Tuna, Thai green curry	527kJ	✓	✓	Average
Tuna, Thai Penang curry	602kJ	✓	✓	Average
Tuna, sweet chilli sauce	405kJ	✓	✓	Average
Tuna, spicy chilli	444kJ	✓	✓	Average
Tuna, spring water	403kJ	✓	✓	Average
Gourmet on the go, tuna spring water & lemon	528kJ	↑Salt	211, 223	Average
Gourmet on the go, tuna premium yellowfin	616kJ	✓	✓	Average
Gourmet on the go, salmon Mediterranean style	770kJ	↑Fat	223	Good
Gourmet on the go, salmon lemon & dill	660kJ	✓	221, 223	Good
Gourmet on the go salmon, mild red chilli	830kJ	↑Fat ↑Salt	✓	Good

Seakist

Product Name	Energy	Major Nutrients	Food Additives	Nutritious Rating
Tuna, spring water	406kJ	✓	✓	Average
Tuna, brine	406kJ	✓	✓	Average
Lunch kit, sweet chilli	923kJ	↑Fat	✓	Average
Lunch kit, sweet corn	1060kJ	↑Fat	✓	Average
Lunch kit, thousand island	753kJ	↑Fat	✓	Average

Sirena

Product Name	Energy	Major Nutrients	Food Additives	Nutritious Rating
Tuna slices, Italian style	675kJ	✓	✓	Average
Tuna slices, chilli & oil with beans	675kJ	↑Salt	✓	Average
Tuna, oil Italian style	675kJ	↑Salt	✓	Average
Tuna, spring water	458kJ	✓	✓	Average
Tuna, chilli & oil	675kJ	✓	✓	Average
Tuna, lemon pepper	932kJ	✓	✓	Average
Tuna, puttanesca	941kJ	↑Fat	✓	Average
Tuna, tomato & onion	525kJ	✓	✓	Average
Tuna, basil infused	668kJ	✓	✓	Average
Tuna, rosemary infused	668kJ	✓	✓	Average
Tuna, sweet chilli sauce	502kJ	✓	✓	Average
Tuna, lemon & spring water	458kJ	✓	223	Average
Tuna, lite chilli	546kJ	✓	✓	Average
Tuna, light oil	529kJ	↑Salt	✓	Average
Tuna & rice, spicy tomato	548kJ	✓	✓	Average

Spam

Product Name	Energy	Major Nutrients	Food Additives	Nutritious Rating
Ham with real bacon	1344kJ	↑Fat ↑Salt	250	Poor
Ham, classic	1286kJ	↑Fat ↑Salt	250,	Poor
Spiced ham, less salt	1286kJ	↑Fat ↑Salt	250	Poor
Spiced ham, lite	845kJ	↑Fat ↑Salt	250	Poor
Turkey oven roasted	597kJ	↑Fat	250, 160b,	Poor

		↑Salt	1520	

Tassal

Product Name	Energy	Major Nutrients	Food Additives	Nutritious Rating
Tasmanian salmon, canola	975kJ	↑Fat	✓	Good
Tasmanian salmon, spring water	675kJ	↑Fat	✓	Good
Tasmanian salmon, Asian style sweet chilli	904kJ	↑Fat	✓	Good
Tasmanian salmon, lemon & cracked pepper	870kJ	↑Fat	223	Good

Tatteys

Product Name	Energy	Major Nutrients	Food Additives	Nutritious Rating
Tuna, spring water	606kJ	✓	✓	Average
Tuna, olive oil	567kJ	✓	✓	Average

Woolworths/Safeways

Product Name	Energy	Major Nutrients	Food Additives	Nutritious Rating
Select, chicken & mayo	563kJ	✓	✓	Average
Select, chicken in spring water	358kJ	↑Salt	✓	Average
Select, chicken smoked flavour	346kJ	↑Salt	✓	Average
Select, chicken & mustard mayo	602kJ	↑Salt	✓	Average
Select, chicken & tomato & onion	655kJ	↑Fat ↑Salt	✓	Average
Select, chicken & sweet chilli	776kJ	↑Fat ↑Salt	✓	Average
Select, tuna chunks in spring water	460kJ	✓	✓	Average

Select, tuna chunks in olive oil	800kJ	↑Fat	✓	Average
Select, tuna chunks in brine	460kJ	✓	✓	Average
Select, sandwich tuna in olive oil	800kJ	↑Fat	✓	Average
Select, flaked tuna smoked	667kJ	↑Fat	✓	Average
Select, flaked tuna chilli	538kJ	✓	✓	Average
Select, flaked tuna sweet chilli	538kJ	✓	✓	Average
Select, flaked tuna lime & cracked pepper	334kJ	✓	✓	Average
Select, flaked tuna tomato & basil	523kJ	✓	✓	Average
Select, flaked tuna savoury onion	576kJ	✓	✓	Average
Select, flaked tuna sweet mustard	613kJ	✓	223	Average
Select, flaked tuna tomato salsa	612kJ	↑Salt	✓	Average
Select, yellow fin slices sweet chilli	635kJ	✓	✓	Average
Select, yellow fin slices lemon pepper	642kJ	✓	✓	Good
Select, pink salmon	505kJ	✓	✓	Good
Select, red salmon	683kJ	✓	✓	Good
Homebrand, corned beef	880kJ	↑Fat ↑Salt	250	Good
Homebrand, mackerel in tomato sauce	572kJ	✓	✓	Good
Homebrand, smoked oysters	1330kJ	↑Fat	✓	Good
Homebrand, smoked mussels	1090kJ	↑Fat	✓	Good
Homebrand,	409kJ	✓	✓	Good

sardines in spring water				
Homebrand, sardines & tomato	457kJ	✓	✓	Good
Homebrand, tuna chunks in spring water	444kJ	✓	✓	Average
Homebrand, tuna chunks in brine	398kJ	✓	✓	Average
Homebrand, tuna chunks in oil	788kJ	↑Fat	✓	Average
Homebrand, yellow fin tuna in spring water	500kJ	✓	✓	Average
Homebrand, light tuna in olive oil	444kJ	✓	✓	Average
Homebrand, tuna & sweet chilli	471kJ	↑Salt	✓	Average
Homebrand, tuna tomato & onion	663kJ	↑Fat	✓	Average
Homebrand, tuna & lemon pepper	701kJ	↑Fat	211, 223	Average
Homebrand, pink salmon	569kJ	✓	✓	Good
Homebrand, red salmon	682kJ	✓	✓	Good

Ready Meals

Ready meals are either produced reasonably well or horrendously bad! Top picks

are: *Ceres organics, Tasty bite, Minute chef, SPC and Stag.*

Ceres Organics

Product Name	Energy	Major Nutrients	Food Additives	Nutritious Rating
Baked beans	347kJ	✓	✓	Good

Coles

Product Name	Energy	Major Nutrients	Food Additives	Nutritious Rating
Beef curry	503kJ	✓	✓	Average
Beef stroganoff	435kJ	✓	635, 202, HVP, YE	Average
Chicken curry	346kJ	✓	635	Average
Chilli, beef & beans	518kJ	✓	✓	Average
Steak & vegetables	311kJ	✓	635, 202, HVP, YE	Average
Baked beans, tomato	363kJ	✓	✓	Good
Baked beans, BBQ	483kJ	✓	✓	Good
Bean beans, ham	389kJ	✓	250	Good
Baked bean, organic	363kJ	✓	✓	Good
Spaghetti, organic	232kJ	✓	✓	Average
Spaghetti	322kJ	✓	✓	Average
Smart Buy, baked bean	420kJ	✓	✓	Good
Smart buy, spaghetti	260kJ	✓	✓	Average
Burrito seasoning	1350kJ	↑Salt	VP	Poor
Burrito tortillas	1240kJ	↑Salt ↑Fat	320, 282, 200	Poor
Taco shells	1940kJ	↑Fat	319	Poor
Mexican sauce	175kJ	↑Salt	220	Average

Enjoyo

Product Name	Energy	Major Nutrients	Food Additives	Nutritious Rating
Beef stroganoff	497kJ	✓	621, 627, 635, YE	Average
Malaysian curry chicken	490kJ	✓	621, 627, 635, YE	Average
Apricot chicken	406kJ	✓	220, 621, YE 160b	Average
Indian butter chicken	456kJ	✓	621, 627, 635, YE	Average

Fray Bentos

Product Name	Energy	Major Nutrients	Food Additives	Nutritious Rating
Steak & kidney pie with pastry	748kJ	↑Fat	HVP	Average

Global Organics

Product Name	Energy	Major Nutrients	Food Additives	Nutritious Rating
Baked beans	347kJ	✓	HVP	Average

Harvest

Product Name	Energy	Major Nutrients	Food Additives	Nutritious Rating
Beef & red wine	256kJ	✓	635	Average
Braised steak & onions	300kJ	↑Salt	HVP, 621	Average
Hearty Irish stew	281kJ	✓	YE, 621	Average
Lamb hot pot	259kJ	✓	621	Average
Mild curry beef & vegetables	**297kJ**	✓	✓	**Average**
Ravioli beef	354kJ	✓	YE, 635	Average
Tortellini bolognaise	337kJ	✓	635, YE	Average
Vegetables & sausages	324kJ	✓	250, HVP	Average
Vegetables & steak	300kJ	↑Salt	HVP	Average

Heinz

Product Name	Energy	Major Nutrients	Food Additives	Nutritious Rating
Big eat big n beefy casserole	225kJ	✓	YE	Average
Big eat breakfast all day	460kJ	↑Salt	250	Average
Big eat peppered steak & onions	255kJ	✓	HVP, YE	Average
Big eat ravioli bolognaise	380kJ	✓	YE	Average
Big eat spaghetti bolognaise	365kJ	✓	YE	Average
Tortellini 3 cheese, Italian style	335kJ	✓	627, 631	Average
Tortellini 3 cheese, creamy pumpkin & garlic	340kJ	✓	627, 631, YE	Average
Tortellini 3 cheese, mushroom & bacon	365kJ	✓	YE, 620, 250, 319	Average
Spaghetti	245kJ	✓	160b	Average
Spaghetti, reduced salt	250kJ	✓	160b	Average
Spaghetti, extra cheese	240kJ	✓	160b	Average
Spaghetti, Bolognese sauce	270kJ	✓	HVP	Average
Thomas pasta shapes	290kJ	✓	✓	Average
Wiggles pasta shapes	270kJ	✓	✓	Average
Ben 10 pasta shapes	290kJ	✓	✓	Average
Dora pasta shapes	290kJ	✓	✓	Average
Alpha spaghetti	255kJ	✓	✓	Average
Oops	260kJ	↑Salt	✓	Average
Baked beans	380kJ	✓	160b	Good
Baked beans, ham sauce	395kJ	✓	250, 160b, YE	Good

Baked beans, reduced salt	365kJ	✓	✓	Good
Baked beans, no salt	355kJ	✓	✓	Good
Baked beans, sweet chilli	405kJ	✓	✓	Good
Baked beans, BBQ sauce	430kJ	✓	YE	Good
Baked beans, cheesy tomato	385kJ	✓	YE	Good
Baked beans, English recipe	385kJ	✓	✓	Good

Hormel

Product Name	Energy	Major Nutrients	Food Additives	Nutritious Rating
Compleats, chicken breast & gravy	295kJ	✓	627, 631, HVP, YE, 621, 222, 160b	Average
Compleats, roast beef & gravy	325kJ	✓	627, 631, HVP, 621, 222	Average
Compleats, beef stew	369kJ	✓	✓	Average
Compleats, meat loaf	428kJ	✓	YE	Average
Compleats, sesame chicken	384kJ	✓	627, 631	Average
Kidz Kitchen, mini beef ravioli	488kJ	✓	631, 627	Average
Kidz Kitchen, spaghetti mini meat balls	465kJ	✓	✓	Average
Kidz Kitchen, cheesy mac n beef	441kJ	✓	✓	Poor

IGA/ Franklins

Product Name	Energy	Major Nutrients	Food Additives	Nutritious Rating
Taco shells	1940kJ	↑Fat	319	Poor
Purely Organic, spaghetti	243kJ	✓	✓	Average
Purely Organic, baked beans	369kJ	✓	160b	Good
Signature, spaghetti	350kJ	✓	✓	Average
Signature, baked beans	322kJ	✓	✓	Good
Black & Gold, spaghetti with cheese	280kJ	✓	✓	Average
Black & Gold, vegetables & sausages	305kJ	✓	223	Average
Black & Gold, Irish stew	240kJ	✓	120, 621, 223	Average
Black & Gold, braised steak & onions	425kJ	✓	HVP, 621, 627	Average
Black & Gold, vegetables & steak	360kJ	✓	HVP, 223	Average

Maharajah's Choice

Product Name	Energy	Major Nutrients	Food Additives	Nutritious Rating
Chappatti, plain	1320kJ	↑Salt ↑Fat	✓	Average

Minute Chef

Product Name	Energy	Major Nutrients	Food Additives	Nutritious Rating
Chicken korma	663kJ	✓	✓	Average
Black Pepper beef	568kJ	✓	✓	Average
Spaghetti bolognaise	628kJ	✓	✓	Average

Mission

Product Name	Energy	Major Nutrients	Food Additives	Nutritious Rating
Burrito tortillas	1243kJ	↑Salt ↑Fat	282, 200, 320	Poor
Corn chips, extreme cheese	2023kJ	↑Fat	319, 621, 635, 202, YE, VP	Poor
Corn chips, white corn	2030kJ	↑Fat	319	Poor
Corn chips, chilli & lime	2130kJ	↑Fat	202, YE, HVP, 621, 627, 631	Poor
Indian chapallis, garlic	1250kJ	↑Salt ↑Fat	200, 282, 320	Poor
Indian chapallis, plain	1227kJ	↑Salt ↑Fat	200, 282, 320	Poor
Naan bread, plain	1330kJ	↑Salt	282, 320	Poor
Naan bread, garlic & herb	1330kJ	↑Salt	282, 320	Poor
Naan bread, yoghurt & mint	1330kJ	↑Salt	282, 320	Poor
Tortillas, hi fibre	1190kJ	↑Salt	200, 282, 320	Poor
Tortillas, low fat 96%	1110kJ	↑Salt	200, 282, 320	Poor
Tortillas, multigrain	1240kJ	↑Salt ↑Fat	200, 282, 320	Poor
Tortillas, salsa	1410kJ	↑Salt ↑Fat	200, 282, 320	Poor
Tortillas, white corn	902kJ	✓	200, 282	Poor
Tortillas, wholegrain	1280kJ	↑Salt	200, 282, 320, 223, 422	Poor

Old El Paso

Product Name	Energy	Major Nutrients	Food Additives	Nutritious Rating
Beans, mexi	299kJ	✓	223	Good
Beans, refried	318kJ	✓	223	Good

Beans, refried with chilli	306kJ	✓	223	Good
Burrito seasoning mix	**1207kJ**	**↑Salt**	✓	**Poor**
Burrito tortillas	1420kJ	↑Salt ↑Fat	422, 282, 202, 223	Poor
Burrito tortillas, jumbo	1420kJ	↑Salt ↑Fat	422, 282, 202, 223	Poor
Tortillas, mini	1420kJ	↑Salt ↑Fat	422, 282, 202, 223	Poor
Tortillas, healthy fiesta extra light	1257kJ	✓	422, 282, 202, 223	Poor
Tortillas, light	1190kJ	↑Salt	422, 282, 202	Poor
Nacho sauce	251kJ	✓	220	Poor
Taco shells	**1903kJ**	**↑Fat**	✓	**Poor**
Taco shells, jumbo	**1903kJ**	**↑Fat**	✓	**Poor**
Taco shells, stand n stuff	**1903kJ**	**↑Fat**	✓	**Poor**
Taco shells, soft	1420kJ	↑Fat	422, 282, 202, 223	Poor
Taco seasoning mix	**1222kJ**	**↑Salt**	✓	**Poor**
Taco seasoning mix, salt reduced	**1324kJ**	**↑Salt**	✓	**Poor**
Taco sauce mild	**128kJ**	**↑Salt**	✓	**Poor**
Taco sauce, medium	**141kJ**	**↑Salt**	✓	**Poor**
Taco sauce, hot	**130kJ**	**↑Salt**	✓	**Poor**
Chilli jalapenos	62kJ	↑Salt	220	Good
Chunky tomato salsa, mild	133kJ	✓	220	Good
Chunky tomato salsa, medium	137kJ	✓	220	Good
Enchilada sauce	**160kJ**	**↑Salt**	✓	**Good**
Enchilada tortillas	1290kJ	✓	422, 282, 202, 223	Poor
Fajita tortillas	1420kJ	↑Salt ↑Fat	422, 282, 202, 223	Poor
Fajita seasoning	1331kJ	↑Salt	202	Poor
Crispy chicken	1461kJ	↑Salt	160b, YE	Poor

seasoning				
Gaucamole seasoning	1460kJ	↑Salt	202	Poor

Podravka

Product Name	Energy	Major Nutrients	Food Additives	Nutritious Rating
Beef goulash	496kJ	↑Salt	621	Average

Southern Cross

Product Name	Energy	Major Nutrients	Food Additives	Nutritious Rating
Baked beans	394kJ	✓	✓	Good
Spaghetti	280kJ	✓	✓	Average

SPC

Product Name	Energy	Major Nutrients	Food Additives	Nutritious Rating
Baked beans	369kJ	✓	✓	Good
Baked beans, salt reduced	343kJ	✓	✓	Good
Baked beans, cheesy cheese	342kJ	✓	✓	Good
Baked beans, hot chilli	294kJ	✓	✓	Good
Baked beans, ham	436kJ	✓	635, 621	Good
Baked beans, steakhouse	372kJ	✓	✓	Good
Spaghetti	318kJ	✓	✓	Average
Spaghetti, tomato & cheese	322kJ	✓	✓	Average
Spaghetti, salt reduced	318kJ	✓	✓	Average
Spaghetti, cheesy cheddar	332kJ	✓	✓	Average
Spagasaurus	326kJ	✓	✓	Average
Spaghetti, number	297kJ	✓	✓	Average

St Dalfour

Product Name	Energy	Major Nutrients	Food Additives	Nutritious Rating
Ready to eat gourmet to go, wild salmon & veg	381kJ	✓	✓	Good
Ready to eat gourmet to go, tuna & pasta	424kJ	✓	✓	Average

Stag

Product Name	Energy	Major Nutrients	Food Additives	Nutritious Rating
Classic chilli	555kJ	✓	✓	Average
Chilli, dynamite hot	571kJ	✓	✓	Average
Chilli, lean beef	428kJ	✓	✓	Average
Chilli, chunky beef	545kJ	✓	HVP	Average

Tasty Bite

Product Name	Energy	Major Nutrients	Food Additives	Nutritious Rating
Agra peas & greens	412kJ	✓	✓	Good
Bengal chickpeas	465kJ	✓	✓	Good
Bombay potatoes	294kJ	✓	✓	Good
Jaipur vegetables	501kJ	✓	✓	Good
Jodhpar yellow dahl	312kJ	✓	✓	Good
Kashmir spinach	383kJ	✓	✓	Good
Madras lentil	353kJ	✓	✓	Good
Mumbai mushrooms	316kJ	✓	✓	Good

Tom Piper

Product Name	Energy	Major Nutrients	Food Additives	Nutritious Rating
Sausages & vegetables	310kJ	✓	HVP, 223	Average
Braised steak & onions	335kJ	✓	627, 631, HVP	Average
Braised steak & vegetables	310kJ	✓	627, 223, HVP	Average

Homestyle Irish stew	270kJ	✓	621, 627, 631	Average
Savoury mince & vegetables	315kJ	✓	223, 631, HVP	Average

Watties

Product Name	Energy	Major Nutrients	Food Additives	Nutritious Rating
Baked beans	420kJ	✓	✓	Good
Baked beans & sausages	530kJ	✓	✓	Good
Spaghetti	260kJ	✓	✓	Average
Spaghetti, extra cheese	285kJ	✓	✓	Average
Spaghetti, cheesy meatballs	320kJ	✓	621, 635, 200	Average
Spaghetti, meatballs	405kJ	✓	✓	Average
Spaghetti, sausages	395kJ	✓	✓	Average

Woolworths

Product Name	Energy	Major Nutrients	Food Additives	Nutritious Rating
Select, nacho kit	2050kJ	↑Salt ↑Fat	319	Poor
Select, chunky salsa mild	144kJ	✓	220	Average
Select, chunky salsa medium	147kJ	✓	220	Average
Select, taco shells	1940kJ	↑Fat	319	Poor
Select, tortillas	1200kJ	↑Salt ↑Fat	282, 200	Poor
Select, tortillas jumbo	1200kJ	↑Salt ↑Fat	282, 200	Poor
Select, tortillas corn	1050kJ	✓	282, 200, 280	Poor
Homebrand, taco shells	1940kJ	↑Fat	319	Poor
Homebrand, tortillas	1290kJ	↑Salt ↑Fat	282, 200	Poor

Weight Watchers

Product Name	Energy	Major Nutrients	Food Additives	Nutritious Rating
Baked beans	376kJ	✓	✓	Good

Soup & Legumes

Generally the tomato soup varieties are the most reliable as additive free. I recommend *Orgran cup soups, La Zuppa and Rosella.*

Baxters

Product Name	Energy	Major Nutrients	Food Additives	Nutritious Rating
French Onion	284kJ	✓	VE, YE	Average
Cream of chicken	498kJ	↑Salt	YE	Average
Cream of mushroom	481kJ	↑Salt	YE, VE, 202, 220	Average
Cream of tomato	**547kJ**	✓	✓	**Average**
Lentil & bacon	391kJ	↑Salt	250	Average
Minestrone	298kJ	✓	YE	Average
Potato & leek	525kJ	✓	YE	Average
Pea & ham	539kJ	✓	250	Average

Campbell's

Product Name	Energy	Major Nutrients	Food Additives	Nutritious Rating
Chunky fully loaded, hearty chicken	261kJ	✓	220, 635, YE, VPE	Average
Chunky fully loaded, chilli beef	321kJ	✓	635, VPE, YE	Average
Chunky fully loaded, outback steak & bacon	267kJ	✓	250, 220, VPE, 635, YE,	Average
Chunky fully loaded, lamb hotpot	270kJ	✓	VPE, 635, YE, 160b?	Average
Chunky fully loaded, peppered steak & gravy	244kJ	✓	VPE, 635, YE	Average
Chunky fully loaded, rigatoni meatballs	**340kJ**	✓	✓	**Average**
Chunky fully loaded, roast lamb &	260kJ	✓	VPE, YE	Average

rosemary				
Chunky fully loaded, stockman lamb casserole	312kJ	✓	VPE, YE	Average
Chunky fully loaded microwavable, chilli beef	321kJ	✓	VPE, YE, 635	Average
Chunky fully loaded, outback steak & bacon	268kJ	✓	VPE, YE, 635, 250, 220	Average
Chunky fully loaded, stockman lamb casserole	312kJ	✓	VPE, YE	Average
Chunky microwavable, beef	222kJ	✓	VPE, YE	Average
Chunky microwavable, hearty Irish stew	242kJ	✓	VPE, YE, 635	Average
Chunky microwavable, pea & ham	255kJ	✓	250, YE	Average
Chunky microwavable, roast chicken & vegetables	209kJ	✓	VPE, YE, 635	Average
Chunky microwavable, stockpot	221kJ	✓	VPE, YE	Average
Chunky, beef	218kJ	✓	VPE, YE	Average
Chunky, beef & potato curry	296kJ	✓	VPE, YE, 635, 223	Average
Chunky, roast chicken & vegetables	211kJ	✓	VPE, 635	Average
Chunky, hearty Irish stew	242kJ	✓	VPE, 635	Average
Chunky, pea & ham	293kJ	✓	VPE, 250	Average
Chunky, potato & bacon	342kJ	✓	VPE, 250, 635	Average
Chunky, stockpot	208kJ	✓	VPE, YE	Average
Chunky, hearty chicken & corn	241kJ	✓	VPE, YE, 635	Average
Condensed, beef & vegetable	112kJ	✓	VPE, YE, 635	Average

Condensed, chicken noodle	114kJ	✓	VPE, 635, YE	Average
Condensed, cream of asparagus	205kJ	✓	VPE	Average
Condensed, cream of celery	**225kJ**	✓	✓	**Average**
Condensed, cream of chicken	220kJ	✓	VPE, 635	Average
Condensed, cream of chicken & mushroom	185kJ	✓	VPE, 635	Average
Condensed, cream of chicken & corn	237kJ	✓	VPE, 635, YE	Average
Condensed, cream of mushroom	185kJ	✓	YE	Average
Condensed, rich tomato	**134kJ**	✓	✓	**Average**
Condensed, split pea & ham	232kJ	✓	250	Average
Condensed, tomato	**133kJ**	✓	✓	**Average**
Country ladle microwavable, creamy pumpkin & chives	**195kJ**	✓	✓	**Average**
Country ladle microwavable spring vegetable & chicken	**136kJ**	✓	✓	**Average**
Country ladle microwavable, winter vegetable medley	225kJ	✓	YE	Average
Country ladle microwavable, vine ripened tomato with parmesan & herbs	**221kJ**	✓	✓	**Average**
Country ladle microwavable, butternut pumpkin	159kJ	✓	635	Average
Country ladle microwavable, chicken & sweet corn	190kJ	✓	VPE, 635	Average

Country ladle microwavable, minestrone	160kJ	✓	VPE, 635	Average
Country ladle, beef & vegetable	165kJ	✓	VPE, 620, 635, YE	Average
Country ladle, butternut pumpkin	159kJ	✓	635	Average
Country ladle, chicken & sweet corn	191kJ	✓	VPE, YE	Average
Country ladle, chicken & vegetable with wholegrain	137kJ	✓	VPE, 635, YE	Average
Country ladle, chicken pasta	169kJ	✓	407, YE, 220, VPE, 635	Average
Country ladle, minestrone with wholegrain pasta	160kJ	✓	VPE, 635	Average
Country ladle, pea & ham	260kJ	✓	250, 220	Average
Country ladle, potato & leek	289kJ	✓	YE	Average
Country ladle, potato & sweet corn chowder	276kJ	✓	YE	Average
Country ladle, pumpkin rich & creamy	200kJ	✓	YE, 223	Average
Country ladle, roast chicken & winter vegetables	241kJ	✓	VPE, VPE, 635	Average
Country ladle, traditional minestrone	160kJ	✓	635, YE	Average
Country ladle, spring lamb & vegetable	143kJ	✓	VPE, 635, YE	Average
Country ladle, chicken & mushroom with wholegrain pasta	222kJ	✓	VPE, 635, 220	Average
Country ladle,	143kJ	✓	YE	Average

farmhouse vegetable				
Country ladle, chicken noodle	205kJ	✓	VPE, 635, YE	Average
Country ladle, creamy chicken	210kJ	✓	VPE, 635, 220, YE	Average
Country ladle, creamy mushroom & pepper	255kJ	✓	220, VPE	Average
Country ladle, pumpkin with sour cream	233kJ	✓	VPE, YE	Average
Country ladle, rustic vegetable & herb	212kJ	✓	160b, YE	Average
Country ladle, spiced autumn vegetables	171kJ	✓	YE	Average
Country ladle, vine ripened tomato	228kJ	✓	✓	Average
Country ladle, smashed butternut pumpkin	180kJ	✓	VE	Average

Coles

Product Name	Energy	Major Nutrients	Food Additives	Nutritious Rating
Condensed, cream of chicken	207kJ	✓	✓	Average
Condensed, cream of mushroom	193kJ	✓	YE	Average
Condensed, cream of pumpkin	214kJ	✓	✓	Average
Condensed, tomato	136kJ	✓	✓	Average
Microwavable, beef & vegetables	241kJ	✓	✓	Average
Microwavable, creamy butternut pumpkin	224kJ	✓	✓	Average
Microwavable, creamy chicken & sweet corn	244kJ	✓	✓	Average
Microwavable,	240kJ	✓	YE	Average

Product Name	Energy	Major Nutrients	Food Additives	Nutritious Rating
creamy mushroom				
Microwavable, minestrone	160kJ	✓	✓	Average
Microwavable, creamy tomato	**349kJ**	✓	✓	**Average**
Cup a soup, chicken noodle	56kJ	✓	YE, 202	Average
Cup a soup, cream of chicken with croutons	150kJ	✓	202, 220,YE, HVP	Average
Cup a soup, cream of mushroom with croutons	173kJ	✓	202, 220, YE, VP	Average
Cup a soup, cream of pumpkin with croutons	179kJ	✓	202, 220 YE, HVP, 222	Average
Cup a soup, cream of tomato with croutons	199kJ	✓	202, 220, YE	Average
Instant chicken noodle	62kJ	✓	627, 631, 635, YE, HVP, VP	Average
Instant French onion	47kJ	✓	160b, HVP, 627, 631, 635, VP	Average

Continental

Product Name	Energy	Major Nutrients	Food Additives	Nutritious Rating
Cup A Soup Asian laksa	240kJ	✓	220, HVP, 621, 635, 120	Average
Cup A Soup Asian chicken & sweet corn	213kJ	✓	220, HVP, 621, 635	Average
Cup A Soup Asian red Thai curry	220kJ	✓	220, HVP, 621, 627	Average
Cup A Soup chicken & corn with croutons	228kJ	✓	220, HVP, 621, 635, 220	Average
Cup A Soup chicken noodle	75kJ	✓	621, 627	Average
Cup A Soup hearty	259kJ	✓	220, HVP,	Average

vegetable			621, 635	
Cup A Soup cream of chicken	144kJ	✓	220, HVP, 621, 635, YE	Average
Cup A Soup cream of mushroom with croutons	195kJ	✓	220, HVP, 621	Average
Cup A Soup creamy chicken with croutons	243kJ	✓	HVP, 621, 635	Average
Cup A Soup cream of mushroom	137kJ	✓	220, HVP, 621	Average
Cup A Soup creamy potato & bacon with croutons	192kJ	✓	220, HVP, 621, 635, 220, 222	Average
Cup A Soup creamy pumpkin with croutons	192kJ	✓	220, HVP, 621, 635, 220, 222	Average
Cup A Soup hearty beef	85kJ	✓	220, HVP, 621, 635	Average
Cup A Soup hearty Italian minestrone	243kJ	✓	621, 635, 120	Average
Cup A Soup hearty roast chicken	277kJ	✓	220 HVP, 621, 635	Average
Cup A Soup lots of noodles beef	194kJ	✓	HVP, 621	Average
Cup A Soup lot of noodles chicken	190kJ	✓	HVP, 621	Average
Cup A Soup lots of noodle Chinese chicken & corn	239kJ	✓	621, 635, HVP, 220	Average
Cup A Soup lots of noodle chicken curry	209kJ	✓	202, 220, HVP, 621, 627	Average
Cup A Soup lots of noodle cream of chicken	221kJ	✓	202, 220, HVP, 621, 627	Average
Cup A Soup pea & ham	131kJ	✓	202, 220, HVP, 621, 627, YE	Average

Cup A Soup hearty Dutch curry	205kJ	✓	220, 202, HVP, 621, 627	Average
Cup A Soup hearty winter vegetables	217kJ	✓	220, 222, YE, 120, 220	Average
Cup A Soup pumpkin	130kJ	✓	627, 222, 120, YE	Average
Cup A Soup spring vegetable	94kJ	✓	621, 635, HVP	Average
Cup A Soup tomato	133kJ	✓	635, YE	Average
Cup A Soup Spanish tomato	230kJ	✓	YE, 621,635, HVP	Average
Cup A Soup, Vegiful 8 vegetables	169kJ	✓	627, 222, YE, 220	Average
Cup A Soup rich tomato	172kJ	✓	HVP, 621	Average
Cup A Soup potato & leek	157kJ	✓	220, 222, 621, 627	Average
Cup A Soup winter vegetables	167kJ	✓	635, 220, YE	Average
Instant soup, chicken noodle	75kJ	✓	635, 621, YE	Average
Instant soup, chicken noodle salt reduced	72kJ	✓	635, 621, YE	Average
Instant soup cream of chicken	1490kJ	↑Salt	YE	Average
Instant soup cream of mushrooms	1400kJ	↑Salt	621, 635	Average
Instant soup Dutch curry & rice	116kJ	✓	621, YE	Average
Instant soup French onion	54kJ	✓	635	Average
Instant soup French onion salt reduced	54kJ	✓	635, YE	Average
Instant soup spring vegetables	46kJ	✓	621, 635, YE, 627	Average
Instant soup thick vegetables	92kJ	✓	621, 627, YE	Average

Country Cup

Product Name	Energy	Major Nutrients	Food Additives	Nutritious Rating
Butternut pumpkin & ham with croutons	230kJ	✓	220, 160b, 621, 635	Average
Cream of chicken with croutons	211kJ	✓	220, 160b, 621, 635, YE	Average
Chicken & corn with croutons	207kJ	✓	220, 160b, 621, 635, YE	Average
Chicken & mushroom with croutons	188kJ	✓	220, 621, 635, YE	Average
Cream of pumpkin with croutons	218kJ	✓	220, 160b, 621, 635	Average
Cream of tomato with croutons	216kJ	✓	220, 160b, 621, 635	Average
Cream of vegetable	218kJ	✓	220, 160b, 621, 635	Average
Cream of mushroom & chives	183kJ	✓	220, 160b, 621, 635	Average
Pea & ham with croutons	211kJ	✓	160b, 621, 635	Average
Potato & bacon with croutons	216kJ	✓	220, 160b, 621, 635	Average
Roasted pumpkin & garlic with crouton	439kJ	✓	220, 160b, 621, 635, YE	Average
Asian, Tom yum in crouton	163kJ	✓	160b, 621, 635	Average
Beef with noodles	214kJ	✓	220, 621, 635	Average
Chicken with noodles	233kJ	✓	220, 160b, 621, 635, YE	Average
Chicken & corn with noodles	226kJ	✓	220, 160b, 621, 635, YE	Average
Asian chicken & corn	264kJ	✓	220, 160b, 621, 635	Average
Pepper steak & mushrooms with croutons	216kJ	✓	220, YE, 621, 635	Average
Chicken with	228kJ	✓	220, 160b,	Average

wholegrain noodles			621, 635, YE	
Beef & barley	205kJ	✓	✓	**Average**
Beef bolognese	320kJ	✓	YE	Average
Chilli & meatballs	195kJ	✓	✓	**Average**

Heinz

Product Name	Energy	Major Nutrients	Food Additives	Nutritious Rating
Big 'N' Chunky steak, bacon & potato	230kJ	✓	250, YE	Average
Big 'N' Chunky beef & vegetable	225kJ	✓	YE, HVP	Average
Big 'N' Chunky beef stockpot	220kJ	✓	YE	Average
Big 'N' Chunky butter chicken curry	375kJ	✓	✓	**Average**
Big 'N' Chunky chicken & corn	245kJ	✓	✓	**Average**
Big 'N' Chunky chicken & vegetable pasta	215kJ	✓	YE	Average
Big 'N' Chunky flamin chicken	215kJ	✓	✓	**Average**
Big 'N' Chunky ravioli with beef & tomato	335kJ	✓	✓	**Average**
Big 'N' Chunky steak & pepper	260kJ	✓	YE	Average
Big 'N' Chunky tex mex beef	350kJ	✓	✓	**Average**
Big red tomato condensed	125kJ	✓	✓	**Average**
Big red tomato condensed salt reduced	120kJ	✓	✓	**Average**
Condensed, cream of pumpkin	195kJ	✓	✓	**Average**
Condensed, cream of chicken	240kJ	✓	635	Average

Condensed, vegetable & beef	140kJ	✓	635, HVP	Average
Condensed, minestrone	**170kJ**	✓	✓	**Average**
Condensed, pea & ham	225kJ	✓	250, YE	Average
Condensed, vegetable	100kJ	✓	YE	Average
Classic chicken & sweet corn	245kJ	✓	YE	Average
Classic country chicken	220kJ	✓	621, 627, 631	Average
Classic creamy chicken	**235kJ**	✓	✓	**Average**
Classic chicken & mushroom	210kJ	✓	202, 220 YE	Average
Classic creamy pumpkin	225kJ	✓	635, 220	Average
Classic Italian minestrone	170kJ	✓	YE, 220	Average
Classic pea & ham	225kJ	✓	621, 631, 627, 250	Average
Classic winter vegetables	150kJ	✓	YE	Average
Soup for one big red tomato	**125kJ**	✓	✓	**Average**
Soup for one creamy tomato	**270kJ**	✓	✓	**Average**
Very Special 8 vegetables	105kJ	✓	YE	Average
Very Special beef, vegetables & pasta	150kJ	✓	YE	Average
Very Special potato & spinach	185kJ	✓	YE	Average
Very Special pumpkin minestrone	260kJ	✓	YE	Average
Very Special ripe tomato & basil	180kJ	✓	YE	Average
Very Special spicy lentil	275kJ	✓	YE, VE	Average

Very Special sweet potato & pumpkin	215kJ	✓	YE	Average
Very Special vegetable & barley	210kJ	✓	VE, YE	Average
Very Special, Irish lamb stew	180kJ	✓	HVP, YE, VE	Average
Very Special, pumpkin & bacon	245kJ	✓	250, 635, 220	Average
Heinz Organic, creamy tomato	210kJ	✓	✓	Average
Heinz Organic, creamy pumpkin	210kJ	✓	✓	Average
Heinz Organic, vegetable	155kJ	✓	YE	Average
Microwave, Tomato & basil	**160kJ**	✓	✓	**Average**
Microwave, creamy pumpkin	205kJ	✓	635	Average

IGA/Franklins

Product Name	Energy	Major Nutrients	Food Additives	Nutritious Rating
Black & Gold instant, French onion	22kJ	✓	220, 621, 635	Average
Black & Gold instant, chicken noodle	43kJ	✓	HVP, 621, 635	Average
Black & Gold soup mix	**1390kJ**	✓	✓	**Average**
Black & Gold cup, tomato	141kJ	✓	HVP, 621, 627, 631, 320	Average
Black & Gold cup, chicken & sweet corn	190kJ	✓	321, 320, 1520, 631, 627, 220	Average
Black & Gold cup, chicken noodle	57kJ	✓	1520, 320, YE	Average
Black & Gold cup, cream of chicken	159kJ	✓	621, 627, 631, 220	Average
Black & Gold cup, hearty beef	96kJ	✓	321, 320, 1520, 621,	Average

			HVP, 220, VPE	
Black & Gold condensed, vegetable	108kJ	✓	✓	Average
Black & Gold condensed, cream of chicken	152kJ	✓	HVP	Average
Black & Gold condensed, minestrone	91kJ	✓	HVP	Average
Signature RTE, pumpkin	221kJ	✓	✓	Average
Signature RTE, minestrone	204kJ	✓	✓	Average
Signature RTE, beef & vegetable	234kJ	✓	✓	Average
Signature RTE, chicken & corn	220kJ	✓	✓	Average

La Zuppa

Product Name	Energy	Major Nutrients	Food Additives	Nutritious Rating
Chicken & vegetable	146kJ	✓	✓	Average
Chicken & corn chowder	181kJ	✓	✓	Average
Hearty chicken & vegetable with rice	164kJ	✓	✓	Average
Lentil	176kJ	✓	✓	Average
Minestrone	167kJ	✓	✓	Average
Moroccan pumpkin & chickpea	206kJ	✓	✓	Average
Spinach & chickpea	188kJ	✓	✓	Average
Ribbolita	117kJ	✓	YE	Average
Sweet corn soup	176kJ	✓	✓	Average
Pumpkin	130kJ	✓	✓	Average

McKenzies

Product Name	Energy	Major Nutrients	Food Additives	Nutritious Rating
Lentils, whole green	1480kJ	✓	✓	Good
Lentils, red	1200kJ	✓	✓	Good
Lentils, French style	1260kJ	✓	✓	Good
Peas, dried	1300kJ	✓	✓	Good
Peas, green split	1320kJ	✓	✓	Good
Peas, yellow split	1320kJ	✓	✓	Good
Peas, chick	1530kJ	✓	✓	Good
Pearl barley	1360kJ	✓	✓	Good
Soup mix	1390kJ	✓	✓	Good
Four bean mix	1282kJ	✓	✓	Good
Italian style mix	1300kJ	✓	✓	Good

Orgran

Product Name	Energy	Major Nutrients	Food Additives	Nutritious Rating
Garden vegetable cup soup	48kJ	✓	✓	Average
Tomato cup soup	126kJ	✓	✓	Average

Podravka

Product Name	Energy	Major Nutrients	Food Additives	Nutritious Rating
Instant soup, spring vegetable	86kJ	✓	621, 627, YE	Average
Instant soup, Vienesse	97kJ	✓	621, 627, YE	Average
Instant soup, Swiss	111kJ	✓	621, 627, YE	Average
Instant soup, homemade meat	96kJ	✓	621, 627, YE	Average
Instant soup, cream of mushroom	134kJ	✓	621, 627, YE	Average
Instant soup, chicken noddle & meat	90kJ	✓	621, 627, YE	Average
Instant soup, beef noodle	90kJ	✓	621, 627, YE, HVP	Average
Instant soup, fish	1266kJ	↑ Salt	621, 627, YE	Average

Instant soup, cream of tomato	113kJ	✓	621, 627, YE	Average
Instant soup, chicken noodle	98kJ	✓	621, 627	Average

Rosella

Product Name	Energy	Major Nutrients	Food Additives	Nutritious Rating
Tomato condensed	136kJ	✓	✓	Average

Trident

Product Name	Energy	Major Nutrients	Food Additives	Nutritious Rating
Chicken Thai noodle instant soup	213kJ	✓	635, 621	Average
Tom yum Thai instant noodle soup	210kJ	✓	635, 621	Average

Whiles

Product Name	Energy	Major Nutrients	Food Additives	Nutritious Rating
Shots, pumpkin	168kJ	✓	160b, 627, 631, VPE, 220	Average
Shots, chicken	184kJ	✓	160b, 627, 631, VPE, 220	Average
Shots, tomato	169kJ	✓	160b, 627, 631, VPE, 220	Average

Woolworths

Product Name	Energy	Major Nutrients	Food Additives	Nutritious Rating
Select, winter vegetables	103kJ	✓	YE	Average
Select, creamy pumpkin	104kJ	✓	✓	Average
Select, beef & vegetables	193kJ	✓	YE	Average
Select, minestrone	152kJ	✓	YE	Average
Select, chicken &	224kJ	✓	YE	Average

sweet corn				
Select, pepper steak	178kJ	✓	YE	Average
Homebrand, condensed tomato	**162kJ**	✓	✓	**Average**
Homebrand, soup cup chicken & sweet corn	170kJ	✓	220, HVP, YE	Average
Homebrand, soup cup cream of chicken	138kJ	✓	220, YE	Average
Homebrand, soup cup chicken noodle	57kJ	✓	1520, YE	Average
Homebrand, instant chicken noodle	65kJ	✓	635, YE, HVP, 631, 627	Average

Instant Pasta/Noodle/Rice/Cous Cous & Sauce

This is a style of food that is usually low in nutrients, and high in food additives.

There are a few exceptions; the most notable is *Sunrice, Kantong, Ayum, and Pandaroo.*

Ainsley Harriot

Product Name	Energy	Major Nutrients	Food Additives	Nutritious Rating
Cous Cous, lemon, mint & parsley	812kJ	✓	YE, 202, 220, 223	Average
Cous Cous, spice sensation	698kJ	✓	YE	Average
Cous Cous, Moroccan medley	754kJ	✓	YE	Average
Cous Cous, roasted vegetables	798kJ	✓	YE, 202, 220	Average
Cous Cous, sundried tomato & garlic	828kJ	✓	YE, 202, 220	Average
Cous cous, wild mushroom	790kJ	✓	YE, 202, 220, 223	Average
Risotto, wild mushroom	690kJ	✓	YE, VPE	Average
Risotto, asparagus & leek	667kJ	✓	YE	Average

Ayam

Product Name	Energy	Major Nutrients	Food Additives	Nutritious Rating
Instant noodles, original	928kJ	↑Fat	✓	Poor
Instant noodles, 99% fat free	556kJ	✓	✓	Poor

Benjamins

Product Name	Energy	Major Nutrients	Food Additives	Nutritious Rating
Instant noodles, original	1916kJ	↑Fat	102	Poor
Bakmi goreng noodles	2922kJ	✓	✓	Poor
Chow mein noodles	3010kJ	✓	✓	Poor
Broad noodles	2968kJ	✓	✓	Poor
Thin noodles	1629kJ	↑Salt	✓	Poor

Changs

Product Name	Energy	Major Nutrients	Food Additives	Nutritious Rating
Long life noodles, original	1467kJ	✓	✓	Poor
Rice noodles, vermicelli	1505kJ	✓	✓	Poor
Egg noodles	1179kJ	✓	160b	Poor
Crunchy noodles	2298kJ	↑Salt ↑Fat	160b	Poor
Fried noodles, original	2092kJ	↑Salt ↑Fat	160b	Poor
Hokkien noodles, Mongolian style	466kJ	↑Salt	220, 102	Poor

Coles

Product Name	Energy	Major Nutrients	Food Additives	Nutritious Rating
2 minute noodles, beef	274kJ	✓	627, 631	Poor
2 minute noodles, chicken	284kJ	✓	627, 631	Poor
Smart buy 2 minute noodles, beef	470kJ	✓	621, 627, 631, 320, 321	Poor
Smart buy 2 minute noodles, chicken	450kJ	✓	621, 627, 631, 320, 321	Poor
Smart buy 2 minute	470kJ	✓	621, 627,	Poor

noodles, oriental			631, 320, 321	

Continental

Product Name	Energy	Major Nutrients	Food Additives	Nutritious Rating
Pasta & sauce, chicken curry	1529kJ	↑Salt	627, YE, 202, 220	Average
Pasta & sauce, cheese & black pepper	1539kJ	↑Salt	635, 223, 202	Average
Pasta & sauce, bacon carbonara	1566kJ	↑Salt	635, YE, 250, 202, 120	Average
Pasta & sauce, alfredo	1558kJ	↑Salt	627, YE, 202	Average
Pasta & sauce, chicken mushroom	1530kJ	↑Salt	635, 202	Average
Pasta & sauce, four cheeses	1582kJ	↑Salt	627, 120, YE, 202	Average
Pasta & sauce, macaroni cheese	1569kJ	↑Salt	120, 202, YE	Average
Pasta & sauce, mushroom & bacon	1550kJ	↑Salt	202, 220, YE, 635, 120, 250	Average
Pasta & sauce, savoury tomato & onion	1513kJ	↑Salt	YE	Average
Pasta & sauce, lite alfredo	1550kJ	✓	YE, 627, 202	Average
Pasta & sauce, lite carbonara	1614kJ	↑Salt	635, 120, YE, 250, 202, 220	Average
Pasta & sauce, lite chicken curry	381kJ	✓	202, 220, YE, 627	Average
Pasta & sauce, sour cream & chives	1591kJ	↑Salt	YE, 202	Average
Pasta & sauce, sour cream & mushroom	1580kJ	↑Salt	220, 202	Average
Rice, rich beef & mushroom	1580kJ	↑Salt	635, YE, 202, 220, 223	Average
Rice, chicken &	1560kJ	↑Salt	627, 202,	Average

			220, 223, YE	
Rice, cheesey	1610kJ	↑Salt	635, 202, 250, YE	Average
Rice, satay	1650kJ	↑Salt	202, 220, 223	Average
Rice, oriental	1550kJ	↑Salt	635, YE, 250, 223	Average
Rice, chicken	1550kJ	↑Salt	635, 202, 220	Average
Cous cous Mediterranean	1490kJ	↑Salt	627, YE	Average
Potato mash	1590kJ	↑Salt	222, 160b	Average

Fantastic

Product Name	Energy	Major Nutrients	Food Additives	Nutritious Rating
Noodles bowl, beef	305kJ	✓	621, 627, 631, 319	Poor
Noodles bowl, chicken	309kJ	✓	621, 627, 631, 319, YE	Poor
Noodles bowl, oriental	307kJ	✓	621, 627, 631, 319, 220, 202	Poor
Noodles cup, chicken chow mein	416kJ	✓	621, 627, 631, HVP, 320, YE	Poor
Noodles cup, crispy bacon	361kJ	✓	621, 627, 631, 320, 202, HVP	Poor
Noodles cup, beef	359kJ	✓	621, 627, 631, 319, HVP, 202	Poor
Noodles cup, chicken	364kJ	✓	621, 627, 631, 319, YE, 202	Poor
Noodles cup, chicken & corn	359kJ	✓	621, 627, 631, 319, 160b, 202	Poor
Noodles cup, oriental	363kJ	✓	621, 627,	Poor

			631, HVP, 320	
Noodles cup, pepperoni	356kJ	✓	621, 320, 635, 627, 631, YE, 223	Poor
Noodles cup, lamb kebab	345kJ	✓	621, 320, 635, 627, 631, YE, 223	Poor
Noodles cup, Portuguese peri peri	387kJ	✓	621, 320, 635, 627, 631, YE, 223	Poor
Noodles cup, bacon & cheese	421kJ	✓	250, 223, HVP, YE	Poor
Noodles cup, Indian vindaloo	377kJ	↑Salt	320, HVP, 635, 627, 631, 223	Poor
Noodles cup, macaroni & cheese	423kJ	✓	220, 202, YE	Poor
Noodles mighty bowl, heart beef	278kJ	✓	621, 627, 631, 319, YE, 202	Poor
Noodles mighty bowl, hearty chicken	285kJ	✓	621, 627, 631, 319, YE	Poor
Stir thru noodle bowl, mi goreng	1050kJ	↑Salt ↑Fat	621, 627, 631, 319	Poor
Xtra saucy noodles, mi goreng	411kJ	✓	320, 211, YE, 621, 627	Poor
Xtra saucy noodles, chow mein	390kJ	✓	621, 627, 631, 320, YE, 202, HVP	Poor
Xtra saucy noodles, hot & spicy	391kJ	✓	621, 627, 631, 320, YE, 202, HVP, 223	Poor
Xtra saucy noodles, roast chicken	388kJ	✓	320, 621, 202, HVP, 627, 631, YE, 223	Poor
2 minute noodles,	319kJ	✓	621, 627,	Poor

			631, 202, 319, 220	
2 minute noodles, chicken	316kJ	✓	621, 627, 631, 319	Poor

Fortune Noodles

Product Name	Energy	Major Nutrients	Food Additives	Nutritious Rating
Beef	372kJ	✓	621, 627, 631, 635 320, 321, HVP	Poor
Chicken	371kJ	✓	621, 627, 631, 320, 202, HVP, YE	Poor

Gong Noodles

Product Name	Energy	Major Nutrients	Food Additives	Nutritious Rating
Mi goreng BBQ chicken	890kJ	↑Fat	621, 627, 631, VP	Poor
Mi Goreng special fried	842kJ	↑Fat	621, 627, 631, VP	Poor
Mi Goreng oriental beef	912kJ	↑Fat	621, 627, 631, VP	Poor
Mi Goreng spicy chicken & coconut	849kJ	↑Fat	621, 627, 631, VP	Poor

IGA

Product Name	Energy	Major Nutrients	Food Additives	Nutritious Rating
Black & Gold noodle cup, beef	489kJ	✓	320, 321, 621, 627, 631, 223	Poor
Black & Gold noodle cup, beef	440kJ	✓	320, 321, 621, 627, 631, 223	Poor
Black & Gold instant noodles, beef	651kJ	✓	320, 321, 621, 627, 631, 223	Poor

Black & Gold instant noodles, chicken	410kJ	✓	320, 321, 621, 627, 631, 223	Poor
Black & Gold macaroni & cheese	554kJ	✓	621, 220, 202	Poor
IGA Wok Wizz, chicken	640kJ	✓	220 621, 223	Poor
IGA Wok Wizz, beef	640kJ	✓	220, 621, 223	Poor
IGA alfredo pasta	557kJ	✓	220, 202, 635	Poor

Indomie

Product Name	Energy	Major Nutrients	Food Additives	Nutritious Rating
Mi goreng instant noodles	1000kJ	↑Fat	319, 101, 621, 631, 627, YE, 211, 223	Poor
Mi goreng instant noodles, satay	940kJ	↑Fat	319, 101, 621, 631, 627, YE, 211, 223	Poor

Kantong

Product Name	Energy	Major Nutrients	Food Additives	Nutritious Rating
Shelf fresh, flat Thai noodles	687kJ	✓	✓	Poor
Shelf fresh, hokkein noodles	672kJ	✓	✓	Poor
Shelf fresh, udon noodles	712kJ	✓	✓	Poor
Shelf fresh, Singapore noodles	665kJ	✓	✓	Poor
Shelf fresh, rice noodles	585kJ	✓	✓	Poor

Kraft

Product Name	Energy	Major Nutrients	Food Additives	Nutritious Rating
Easy Mac bowl, carbonara	627kJ	✓	220, 202, 627, 631	Poor
Easy Mac bowl, chicken	601kJ	✓	220, 160b, 202	Poor
Easy Mac bowl, cheese	645kJ	✓	220, 202,160b, YE, HVP	Poor
Easy Mac, cheese	603kJ	✓	202, 220,160b, YE, HVP	Poor
Easy Mac, chilli cheese	594kJ	✓	220, 202, YE, HVP	Poor
Easy Mac, nacho cheese	604kJ	✓	220, 202, YE, HVP, 635	Poor
Easy Mac, chicken	595kJ	✓	220, 202	Poor
Easy Mac, bacon carbonara	599kJ	✓	220, 202, 627, 631	Poor
Easy Mac microwavable. cheese	603kJ	✓	220, 202,160b YE	Poor
Easy Mac microwavable, bacon carbonara	595kJ	✓	220, 202, 627, 631	Poor
Easy Mac microwavable. chicken	599kJ	✓	220, 202	Poor
Macaroni & cheese	762kJ	✓	202	Poor
Macaroni & cheese, deluxe dinner	661kJ	✓	202, 160b, 234	Poor

Maggi

Product Name	Energy	Major Nutrients	Food Additives	Nutritious Rating
2 minute noodles, chicken	360kJ	✓	319, 621, 635, 320, 220	Poor
2 minute noodles,	360kJ	✓	319, 621,	Poor

curry			635, 320, 326, 220	
2 minute noodles, beef	365kJ	✓	319, 621, 635, 320, YE	Poor
2 minute noodles, oriental	360kJ	✓	319, 621, 635, 320, 220	Poor
2 minute noodles, chicken & corn	360kJ	✓	319, 621, 635, 320	Poor
Fusion, satay	1100kJ	↑ Salt ↑ Fat	319, 621, 220	Poor
Fusion, soy mild & spice	1080kJ	↑ Salt ↑ Fat	319, 621, 635, 320, 220, 202	Poor
Noodle cup, fusion hot & spicy	935kJ	↑ Salt ↑ Fat	319, 621, 635, 320, 220, 202	Poor
Noodle cup, fusian soy & mild spice	925kJ	↑ Salt ↑ Fat	319, 621, 635, 320, 220, 202	Poor
Noodle cup, fusian satay	950kJ	↑ Salt ↑ Fat	319, 621, 635, 320, 220, 202	Poor
Noodle cup, Asian beef	310kJ	✓	319, 621, 635, 320, 220	Poor
Noodle cup, beef	310kJ	✓	319, 621, 635, 320, 220, YE	Poor
Noodle cup, chicken	310kJ	✓	319, 621, 635, 320, 220	Poor
Noodle cup, Indian curry	310kJ	✓	319, 621, 635, 320, 220	Poor
Noodle cup, laksa	315kJ	✓	319, 621, 635, 627, 631, 320, 220, 202	Poor

Noodle cup, oriental	315kJ	✓	319, 621, 635, 320, 220	Poor
Noodle cup, super chicken 98% fat free	300kJ	✓	319, 621, 631, 627, 320, 220, YE	Poor
Noodle cup, super beef 98% fat free	300kJ	✓	319, 621, 631, 627, 320, 220, YE	Poor

Pandaroo

Product Name	Energy	Major Nutrients	Food Additives	Nutritious Rating
Chow mein dried noodles	2063kJ	↑ Fat	102	Poor
Thai rice noodles	1482kJ	✓	✓	Poor
Rice sticks	1505kJ	✓	✓	Poor
Rice vermicelli	750kJ	✓	✓	Poor
Thin egg noodles	750kJ	✓	✓	Poor

Rice A Riso

Product Name	Energy	Major Nutrients	Food Additives	Nutritious Rating
Chicken	496kJ	✓	YE	Poor

San Remo

Product Name	Energy	Major Nutrients	Food Additives	Nutritious Rating
La Pasta, alfredo	1540kJ	↑ Salt	202, 220 YE, HVP, 627, 631	Poor
La Pasta, carbonara	1540kJ	↑ Salt	202, 220 YE, HVP, 627, 631	Poor
La Pasta, creamy bacon	1540kJ	↑ Salt	202, 220 YE, HVP, 627, 631	Poor
La Pasta, macaroni & cheese	1550kJ	↑ Salt	202, 220 YE, HVP, 627,	Poor

			631	
La Pasta, chicken curry	1450kJ	↑ Salt	202, 220, YE, HVP	Poor
La Pasta, creamy mushroom onion	1440kJ	↑ Salt	202, 220, YE, HVP, 223	Poor
La Pasta, sour cream & chives	1490kJ	↑ Salt	202, 220, YE, HVP, 223	Poor
La Pasta, four cheeses	1510kJ	↑ Salt	220, 202, YE, HVP	Poor
La Pasta, mushroom & herb	1500kJ	↑ Salt	627, 631, 160b, HVP, YE, 223, 202, 220	Poor
La Pasta, beef & black bean	1490kJ	↑ Salt	HVP, 223, VP, 627, 631	Poor
La Pasta, chicken chow mein	1490kJ	↑ Salt	HVP, VP, 627, 631	Poor

Suimin

Product Name	Energy	Major Nutrients	Food Additives	Nutritious Rating
Meal in a cup, hot & spicy	366kJ	✓	320, 627, 631, YE, 223	Poor
Meal in a cup, mi goreng	1100kJ	↑ Salt ↑ Fat	319, 627, 631, VP	Poor
Meal in a cup, braised beef	368kJ	✓	320, 627, 631, HVP, VP	Poor
Meal in a cup, chicken	368kJ	✓	320, 627, 631, VP,	Poor
Meal in a cup, chicken & sweet corn	374kJ	✓	320, 627, 631, HVP	Poor
Meal in a cup, curried prawn	378kJ	✓	320, 627, 631, HVP, VP	Poor
Meal in a cup, oriental chicken	373kJ	✓	320, 627, 631, HVP, VP	Poor
Meal in a cup, prawn & chicken	376kJ	✓	320, 627, 631, HVP, VP, 160b	Poor

Sunrice

Product Name	Energy	Major Nutrients	Food Additives	Nutritious Rating
Chinese beef & black bean	483kJ	✓	220	Average
Chinese Mongolian beef	490kJ	✓	220	Average
Chinese sweet & sour	550kJ	✓	✓	Average
Indian butter chicken	628kJ	✓	✓	Average
Indian korma curry	614kJ	✓	✓	Average
Indian tiki masala	628kJ	✓	✓	Average
Napolitana penne	749kJ	✓	✓	Average
Thai chicken curry satay	720kJ	✓	✓	Average
Thai green curry	533kJ	✓	✓	Average
Thai mussaman curry	667kJ	✓	✓	Average
Thai red curry	596kJ	✓	✓	Average
Thai vegetable curry	618kJ	✓	✓	Average
Tuscan tomato fusilli	816kJ	↑ Salt	223	Average

Tandaco

Product Name	Energy	Major Nutrients	Food Additives	Nutritious Rating
One pan dinner, savoury noodle	1400kJ	↑ Salt	223	Poor
Tomato lasagne	1470kJ	↑ Salt	202, YE, 223	Poor

Trident

Product Name	Energy	Major Nutrients	Food Additives	Nutritious Rating
2 minute noodles, hot & spicy	387kJ	✓	621, 635	Poor
Hokkein noodles	559kJ	✓	✓	Poor
Rice stick noodles	750kJ	✓	✓	Poor
Pad Thai noodles	561kJ	↑Salt	223 621, 202	Poor

Rice vermicelli	1500kJ	✓	✓	Poor
Noodle man bowl, beef	403kJ	✓	621, 631, 202, 223	Poor
Noodle man bowl, chicken	394kJ	↑Salt	621, 631, 202, 223	Poor
Mega cup noodles, satay	542kJ	✓	621, 631, 627, 202, 210, YE, 202, 1520	Poor
Mega cup noodles, tom yum	427kJ	✓	621, 635	Poor
Mega cup noodles, honey soy	427kJ	✓	621, 631, 627, 202, 210, YE, 202, 220, 223	Poor
Mega cup noodles, BBQ spare ribs	427kJ	✓	621, 631, 627, 202, 210, YE, 202, 220, 223	Poor

Uncle Bens

Product Name	Energy	Major Nutrients	Food Additives	Nutritious Rating
Express rice, Chinese style	660kJ	✓	YE	Average
Express rice, egg fried rice style	735kJ	✓	YE, 223	Average
Express rice, special fried rice style	709kJ	✓	YE, 223	Average
Express rice, mushroom style	**650kJ**	**↑Salt**	✓	**Average**
Express rice, tomato & basil style	732kJ	✓	220, YE	Average
Express rice, Mediterranean wholegrain style	730kJ	✓	160b	Average
Express rice, savoury chicken style	629kJ	✓	YE	Average
Express rice,	**672kJ**	✓	✓	**Average**

Mexican style				
Express rice, basmati style	**774kJ**	✓	✓	**Average**
Express rice, tomato & Italian risotto style	765kJ	✓	220, YE	Average
Express rice, chicken & mushroom risotto style	629kJ	✓	YE	Average

Wokka

Product Name	Energy	Major Nutrients	Food Additives	Nutritious Rating
Thai peanut satay noodles	681kJ	✓	220	Poor
Mi goreng noodles	**639kJ**	↑Salt	✓	**Poor**
Roasted peanut & honey noodles	756kJ	↑Salt	202, YE, 220	Poor
Pad Thai noodles	**726kJ**	✓	✓	**Poor**
Thin egg style noodles	546kJ	✓	102, 110	Poor
Golden hokkein noodles	495kJ	✓	1221, 102, 110	Poor
Singapore noodles	534kJ	✓	102, 110	Poor

Woolworths/Safeways

Product Name	Energy	Major Nutrients	Food Additives	Nutritious Rating
Select, baked beans	**376kJ**	✓	✓	**Good**
Select, spaghetti	**270kJ**	✓	✓	Average
Select, chicken flavoured rice	1600kJ	↑Salt	221, 320, 202	Average
Select, oriental fried rice	1560kJ	↑Salt	250, 221, YE, 202	Average
Select, rich beef & mushroom rice	1580kJ	↑Salt	HVP, 202, 220	Average
Select, chicken & vegetable rice	1580kJ	↑Salt	221, 202, 320, YE, HVP	Average
Select, satay	1670kJ	↑Salt	221, 220	Average

Select, cheesy rice	1700kJ	↑Salt	HVP, YE, 202	Average
Select, Moroccan cous cous	1570kJ	↑Salt	YE	Average
Select, Mediterranean cous cous	1560kJ	✓	160b, YE, 202	Average
Select, chicken & curry pasta & sauce	1630kJ	↑Salt	YE, 202, 221, 220	Average
Select, four cheeses pasta & sauce	1610kJ	↑Salt	HVP, YE, 220, 202	Average
Select, alfredo pasta & sauce	1570kJ	↑Salt	202, HVP, YE, 220	Average
Select, creamy carbonara pasta & sauce	1590kJ	↑Salt	YE, 250, HVP, 202	Average
Select, cheese & cracked pepper pasta & sauce	1590kJ	↑Salt	202, HVP, YE, 220	Average
Select, sour cream & chives pasta & sauce	1660kJ	↑Salt	220, 202	Average
Select, macaroni & cheese pasta & sauce	1600kJ	↑Salt	202, HVP, YE, 220	Average
Homebrand, 2 minute noodles beef	374kJ	✓	635, 620, HVP, YE	Poor
Homebrand, 2 minute noodles chicken	389kJ	✓	635, 620, HVP, YE	Poor
Homebrand, 2 minute noodles oriental	378kJ	✓	635, HVP, YE	Poor
Homebrand, noodle cup beef	362kJ	✓	635, 620, HVP	Poor
Homebrand, noodle cup oriental	383kJ	✓	635, HVP, YE	Poor
Homebrand, noodle cup chicken & corn	357kJ	✓	635, 620, HVP, YE	Poor
Homebrand, noodle cup chicken	366kJ	✓	635, 620, HVP, YE	Poor
Homebrand, carbonara pasta & sauce	1620kJ	↑Salt	202, 220, YE, HVP, 250, 621, 631	Poor

Homebrand, alfredo pasta & sauce	1590kJ	↑Salt	627, 631, HVP, YE, 220, 202	Poor

Yoodles

Product Name	Energy	Major Nutrients	Food Additives	Nutritious Rating
Prawn & chicken	352kJ	✓	621, 635, 223	Poor
Hearty beef	253kJ	✓	621, 635, 223	Poor
Country chicken	356kJ	✓	621, 635, 223	Poor
Spicy tom yum	356kJ	✓	621, 635, 223	Poor

Cooking Sauces, Pastes & Concentrates

Let's face it, cooking sauces can be a lifesaver on a busy day, but some are better than others. Topping the list is *Val verde, Russo di pomodoro, Passage to Italy, Maharajah's choice, Five brothers IGA purely organic and Paul Newmans.*

Barilla

Product Name	Energy	Major Nutrients	Food Additives	Nutritious Rating
Pasta sauce, arrabbiata chilli	247kJ	✓	✓	**Good**
Pasta sauce, napolitana	295kJ	↑Salt	✓	Good
Pasta sauce, pesto rosso	1398kJ	↑Salt	✓	Good
Pasta sauce, olives	347kJ	↑Salt	220	Good
Pasta sauce, ricotta	**383kJ**	**↑Salt**	✓	**Good**
Pasta sauce, puttanesca	**221kJ**	✓	✓	**Good**
Pasta sauce, basilico	244kJ	↑Salt	✓	Good
Pasta sauce, mozzarella & ricotta	383kJ	✓	223	Good
Pesto, red onion	1182kJ	↑Salt ↑Fat	220	Good
Pesto, sundried tomato	1390kJ	↑Salt ↑Fat	220	Good
Pesto Genovese	2144kJ	↑Salt ↑Fat	✓	Good

Bertolli

Product Name	Energy	Major Nutrients	Food Additives	Nutritious Rating
Pasta sauce, pecorino	237kJ	↑Salt	223	Good
Pasta sauce, parmigana	**320kJ**	✓	✓	**Good**
Pasta sauce, basilico	296kJ	✓	220	Good

Pasta sauce, prouvista sugo classica	158kJ	✓	✓	Good
Arrabiata	346kJ	✓	✓	Good

Campbell's

Product Name	Energy	Major Nutrients	Food Additives	Nutritious Rating
Pasta sauce, spaghetti beef	463kJ	✓	VPE, 635	Average

Coles

Product Name	Energy	Major Nutrients	Food Additives	Nutritious Rating
Pasta sauce, arrabbiata	241kJ	✓	✓	Good
Pasta sauce, basil	151kJ	✓	✓	Good
Pasta sauce, basilico	246kJ	✓	✓	Good
Pasta sauce, bolognese	250kJ	✓	YE	Good
Pasta sauce, napoletana	363kJ	✓	✓	Good
Pasta sauce, romana	442kJ	↑Salt	YE	Good
Pasta sauce, oregano	151kJ	✓	✓	Good
Organic, traditional pasta sauce	210kJ	✓	✓	Good
Stir thru, cherry tomato & chilli	326kJ	✓	✓	Good
Stir thru, sundried tomato & basil	508kJ	↑Fat	220	Good
Stir thru, tomato & char-grilled vegetables	382kJ	✓	✓	Good
Pesto, tomato	1216kJ	↑Salt ↑Fat	220	Good
Pesto, basil	1899kJ	↑Salt ↑Fat	220	Good
Smart buy, pasta	190kJ	✓	220	Good

	Energy		Food Additives	Nutritious Rating
sauce				
Smart buy, chunky tomato pasta sauce	190kJ	✓	220	Good
Smart buy, tomato & vegetable pasta sauce	203kJ	✓	220	Good
Smart buy stir fry sauce, sweet & sour	537kJ	↑Sugar	220	Good

Continental

Product Name	Energy	Major Nutrients	Food Additives	Nutritious Rating
Asian tonight, Thai sweet chilli	522kJ	↑Salt ↑Sugar	220	Average
Asian Chinese honey teriyaki	405kJ	↑Salt ↑Sugar	220	Average
Asian Chinese sweet & sour	410kJ	↑Sugar	120, 220	Average
Chicken tonight, apricot chicken	247kJ	✓	YE, 160b, 627	Average
Chicken tonight, chicken cacciatore	**236kJ**	**✓**	**✓**	**Good**
Chicken tonight, country French chicken	482kJ	↑Fat	220, 627	Average
Chicken tonight, creamy cheese & bacon	431kJ	✓	YE, 635, 627	Average
Chicken tonight, creamy lemon chicken	468kJ	✓	220, 223, YE	Average
Chicken tonight, curried chicken with vegetables	203kJ	✓	220, 627	Average
Chicken tonight, golden honey & mustard	603kJ	↑Fat	220, 223, YE, 627	Average
Chicken tonight, golden honey &	300kJ	✓	223, 160b	Average

mustard lite				
Chicken tonight, stroganoff	462kJ	✓	627, YE	Average
Chicken tonight, creamy chicken & mushroom lite	192kJ	✓	YE	Average
Chicken tonight, stroganoff lite	205kJ	✓	220, YE	Average
Chicken tonight, Indian butter chicken	472kJ	✓	223, 160b, 120	Good
Chicken tonight, Indian butter chicken 97% Fat Free	307kJ	✓	220, 120, 223	Good
Chicken tonight, Indian, creamy tandoori	380kJ	✓	220, 223	Good
Chicken tonight Indian tandoori lite	307kJ	✓	220, 223, 120	Good
Sausages tonight	242kJ	✓	220, 627	Average

Dolmio

Product Name	Energy	Major Nutrients	Food Additives	Nutritious Rating
Pasta sauce, extra garden vegetable	225kJ	✓	✓	Good
Pasta sauce, extra bolognese	254kJ	✓	✓	Good
Pasta sauce, extra Italian herbs	276kJ	✓	✓	Good
Pasta sauce, extra mushroom	202kJ	✓	YE	Good
Pasta sauce, extra red wine & Italian herbs	247kJ	✓	220	Good
Pasta sauce, extra garden vegetables	220kJ	✓	✓	Good
Pasta sauce, extra	249kJ	✓	✓	Good

four cheeses				
Pasta sauce, extra tomato onion & garlic	233kJ	✓	✓	**Good**
Pasta sauce, extra tomato onion & garlic salt reduced	236kJ	✓	YE	Good
Pasta sauce, bolognese	254kJ	✓	✓	**Good**
Pasta sauce, carbonara	442kJ	↑Salt	✓	Good
Pasta sauce, extra garlic	259kJ	✓	✓	**Good**
Pasta sauce, tomato & basil	272kJ	✓	✓	**Good**
Pasta sauce, lasagne extra cheese	493kJ	↑Fat	160b	Good
Pasta sauce, traditional classic tomato	288kJ	✓	✓	**Good**
Pasta sauce, traditional classic tomato salt reduced	280kJ	✓	✓	**Good**
Pasta bake, creamy mushroom	451kJ	↑Salt	220, YE	Average
Pasta bake, creamy tomato & mozzarella	419kJ	↑Salt	220	Good
Pasta bake, three cheeses	493kJ	↑Fat	✓	Average
Pasta bake, tomato extra cheese	372kJ	↑Salt	YE	Good
Pasta bake, tuna	506kJ	✓	YE	Good
Pasta bake, sundried tomato & garlic	359kJ	↑Salt	220	Good
Pasta bake, tomato & extra cheese	372kJ	↑Salt	YE	Good
Lasagne, thick tomato	323kJ	✓	✓	**Good**

Five Brothers (Bertolli)

Product Name	Energy	Major Nutrients	Food Additives	Nutritious Rating
Pasta sauce, grilled summer vegetables	259kJ	✓	✓	Good
Pasta sauce, five cheeses	246kJ	✓	✓	Average
Pasta sauce, summer tomato & basil	212kJ	✓	✓	Good
Pasta sauce, oven roasted garlic & wine	225kJ	✓	220	Good
Pasta sauce, oven roasted garlic & onion	216kJ	✓	✓	Good
Pasta sauce, portebello mushroom & garlic	214kJ	✓	✓	Good

Jensens

Product Name	Energy	Major Nutrients	Food Additives	Nutritious Rating
Pasta sauce, organic basil & garlic	312kJ	↑Salt	✓	Good
Pasta sauce, organic bolognese	329kJ	↑Salt	223	Good

Kan Tong

Product Name	Energy	Major Nutrients	Food Additives	Nutritious Rating
Butter chicken sauce	530kJ	↑Fat	160b, YE	Good
Black bean sauce	364kJ	↑Salt	YE	Average
Satay peanut sauce	512kJ	✓	YE	Average
Chinese BBQ sauce	418kJ	↑Salt ↑Sugar	YE, 120	Average
Honey, sesame & garlic sauce	535kJ	✓	YE, 220	Average
Lemon chicken sauce	421kJ	✓	YE, 220	Average
Sweet & sour	410kJ	↑Sugar	220	Average

pineapple sauce				
Sweet & sour plum sauce	367kJ	↑Sugar	220	Average
Sweet & sour vegetable sauce	359kJ	↑Sugar	220	Average
Sweet soy & garlic sauce	318kJ	↑Sugar ↑Salt	220 YE	Average
Inspirations honey chicken	**477kJ**	✓	✓	Average
Inspirations massaman curry	380kJ	↑Salt	✓	Good
Inspirations lemon chicken	477kJ	↑Sugar	220, YE	Average
Inspirations, chicken & cashew nut	766kJ	↑Sugar ↑Salt	YE, VPE	Average
Inspirations, honey soy & garlic	594kJ	↑Sugar ↑Salt	VPE, 220	Average
Inspirations, fragrant Thai green curry	347kJ	↑Sugar ↑Salt	223	Average
Inspirations, Malaysian satay	615kJ	↑Fat	YE	Average
Inspirations, sizzling Mongolian	482kJ	↑Sugar ↑Salt	YE	Average
Inspirations, teriyaki sesame	544kJ	↑Salt	✓	Average
Inspirations, sweet chilli noodles	573kJ	↑Sugar ↑Salt	✓	Average
Inspirations, black bean	336kJ	↑Salt	220	Average
Inspirations, sizzling Mongolian	437kJ	↑Sugar ↑Salt	YE	Average
Simply stir fry, chilli & lime	543kJ	↑Sugar	223	Average
Simply stir fry, chilli, garlic & soy	232kJ	✓	220	Average
Simply stir fry, lemongrass, lime & coriander	220kJ	✓	220	Average

Simply stir fry, sweet & sour	550kJ	↑Sugar	✓	Average
Simply stir fry, sweet & sour lite	301kJ	↑Sugar	220	Average
Simply stir fry teriyaki honey	661kJ	↑Sugar	220, VPE	Average

Kohinoor Cook in Sauce

Product Name	Energy	Major Nutrients	Food Additives	Nutritious Rating
Butter chicken	573kJ	↑Salt	✓	Good
Chicken Tikki	786kJ	↑Fat	✓	Good
Jalfrezi	589kJ	✓	220	Good
Korma	556kJ	↑Fat ↑Salt	✓	Good
Madras curry	577kJ	↑Fat	220, 223	Good
Rogan josh	808kJ	↑Fat ↑Salt	✓	Good
Vindaloo	623kJ	↑Fat	✓	Good

Leggos

Product Name	Energy	Major Nutrients	Food Additives	Nutritious Rating
Pasta sauce, alfredo	517kJ	↑Fat ↑Salt	YE	Average
Pasta sauce, bolognese chunky garlic & herb	318kJ	↑Salt	YE	Good
Pasta sauce, bolognese chunky with red wine	309kJ	↑Salt	220, YE,	Good
Pasta sauce, bolognese chunky with bacon	269kJ	✓	250, YE	Good
Pasta sauce, creamy tomato	364kJ	✓	YE	Good
Pasta sauce, hidden vegetable bolognese	206kJ	✓	YE	Good
Pasta sauce, hidden	214kJ	✓	YE	Good

vegetable cheesy tomato				
Pasta sauce, hidden vegetable classic tomato	201kJ	✓	YE	Good
Pasta sauce, carbonara	397kJ	↑Salt	250, YE	Average
Pasta sauce, chunky Napolitano	279kJ	✓	YE	Good
Pasta sauce, parmagana chunky	**219kJ**	✓	✓	**Good**
Pasta bake, béchamel	**561kJ**	**↑Fat**	✓	**Average**
Pasta bake, creamy sundried tomato & garlic	303kJ	↑Salt	YE, 160b, 220, 223	Average
Pasta bake, creamy tomato & mozzarella	294kJ	↑Salt	✓	Average
Pasta bake, tomato, ricotta & spinach	355kJ	✓	YE	Average
Pasta bake, tuna, spinach & garlic	409kJ	↑Salt	YE, 223	Good
Pasta bake, Tuscan	283kJ	↑Salt	YE	Good
Spaghetti sauce with beef	299kJ	↑Salt	HVP, 627, 631	Good
Pesto, traditional basil	1030kJ	↑Salt ↑Fat	✓	Good
Pesto, sundried tomato	898kJ	↑Salt ↑Fat	223	Good
Stir through pasta sauce, char grilled vegetables	495kJ	↑Salt ↑Fat	YE, 223	Good
Stir through pasta sauce, semi dried tomato, basil & parmesan	533kJ	✓	220	Good
Stir through pasta sauce, ricotta & spinach with pecorino	653kJ	↑Salt ↑Fat	YE, 220	Good

cheese				
Stir through pasta sauce, sundried tomato & roasted garlic	517kJ	↑Salt ↑Fat	220, 223, YE	Good
Stir through pasta sauce, tomato & bacon	454kJ	↑Salt	250, YE, 621	Good
Stir through pasta sauce, tomato, olive & chilli	590kJ	↑Salt ↑Fat	223	Good
Stir through pasta sauce, tomato & garlic with red wine	426kJ	✓	220	Good
Simmer sauce, chicken scaloppini	428kJ	↑Salt	220, 250, 627, 631	Good
Simmer sauce, chicken parmagana	263kJ	✓	YE	Good

IGA/Franklins

Product Name	Energy	Major Nutrients	Food Additives	Nutritious Rating
Black & Gold, sweet & sour sauce	532kJ	↑Sugar	220	Average
Black & Gold, pasta sauce	250kJ	✓	✓	Good
Black & Gold, pasta sauce with mushrooms	246kJ	↑Salt	✓	Average
Purely Organic, Tomato & herb pasta sauce	116kJ	✓	✓	Good
Purely Organic, Tomato & garlic pasta sauce	110kJ	✓	✓	Good

Maharajah's Choice

Product Name	Energy	Major Nutrients	Food Additives	Nutritious Rating

Butter chicken	594kJ	↑Fat	✓	Good
Dhal tadka	**567kJ**	✓	✓	**Good**
Tikki marsala	566kJ	↑Fat	✓	Good

Macro Organic

Product Name	Energy	Major Nutrients	Food Additives	Nutritious Rating
Pasta sauce, tomato & basil	255kJ	↑Salt	✓	Good
Pasta sauce, Mediterranean	224kJ	↑Salt	✓	Good
Pasta sauce, arrabbiata	205kJ	↑Salt	✓	Good

Nandos

Product Name	Energy	Major Nutrients	Food Additives	Nutritious Rating
Simmer sauce, curry coconut	258kJ	✓	220, 223	Good
Simmer sauce, peri peri mild	246kJ	✓	220	Good
Simmer sauce, peri peri tomato	211kJ	✓	220	Good

Outback Spirit

Product Name	Energy	Major Nutrients	Food Additives	Nutritious Rating
Simmer sauce, coconut, chilli & lemon myrtle	498kJ	↑Salt ↑Sugar	220	Good
Simmer sauce, creamy coconut lemon aspen	440kJ	↑Sugar	223, 220	Good

Passage to India

Product Name	Energy	Major Nutrients	Food Additives	Nutritious Rating
Simmer sauce, Korma curry	627kJ	↑Salt ↑Fat	220	Good

Simmer sauce, rogan josh	579kJ	↑Salt ↑Fat	✓	Good
Simmer sauce, balti	600kJ	↑Salt ↑Fat	220, 202	Good
Simmer sauce, vindaloo	544kJ	↑Salt ↑Fat	220	Good

Passage to Italy

Product Name	Energy	Major Nutrients	Food Additives	Nutritious Rating
Pasta sauce, bolognese	384kJ	✓	✓	Good
Pasta sauce, marinara	389kJ	✓	✓	Good
Pasta sauce, Napolitano	449kJ	↑Fat	✓	Good

Passage to Morocco

Product Name	Energy	Major Nutrients	Food Additives	Nutritious Rating
Simmer sauce, spiced honey & lamb	257kJ	↑Sugar	220	Good
Simmer sauce, spiced lemon chicken	459kJ	↑Salt	220	Good
Pasta sauce, honey lamb	548kJ	↑Salt ↑Sugar	220	Good
Pasta sauce, apricot chicken	683kJ	↑Sugar ↑Salt	YE, VP	Good

Patkas

Product Name	Energy	Major Nutrients	Food Additives	Nutritious Rating
Simmer sauce, butter chicken	501kJ	✓	223	Good
Simmer sauce, cashew masala	613kJ	↑Fat	220, 223	Good
Simmer sauce, korma mild	656kJ	↑Fat	220. 223	Good
Simmer sauce, oven	336kJ	✓	223	Good

bake biryani hot & spicy				
Simmer sauce, oven bake biryani mild & fruity	434kJ	✓	220, 223	Good
Simmer sauce, oven bake biryani medium aromatic	**321kJ**	✓	✓	**Good**
Simmer sauce, tiki marsala	493kJ	↑Fat	223	Good
Simmer sauce, rogan josh	260kJ	✓	223	Good
Mango chicken	**415kJ**	✓	✓	**Good**
Spicy butter chicken	482kJ	✓	223	Good

Paul Newman's Own

Product Name	Energy	Major Nutrients	Food Additives	Nutritious Rating
Pasta sauce, bolognese	**190kJ**	✓	✓	**Good**
Pasta sauce, classic tomato	210kJ	✓	YE	Good
Pasta sauce, roast garlic & basil	**210kJ**	✓	✓	**Good**

Raguletto

Product Name	Energy	Major Nutrients	Food Additives	Nutritious Rating
Pasta sauce, Napolitana	210kJ	✓	220	Good
Pasta sauce, red wine & basil	214kJ	✓	220	Good
Pasta sauce, bolognese	**162kJ**	✓	✓	**Good**
Pasta sauce, romano style	184kJ	✓	220	Good
Pasta sauce, venetian style	**219kJ**	✓	✓	**Good**
Pasta sauce, red	223kJ	✓	220	Good

wine & garlic				

Russo Di Pomodoro

Product Name	Energy	Major Nutrients	Food Additives	Nutritious Rating
Pasta sauce, passata	103kJ	✓	✓	Good
Pasta sauce, polpa	138kJ	✓	✓	Good

Sacla

Product Name	Energy	Major Nutrients	Food Additives	Nutritious Rating
Pasta sauce, cherry tomato & basil	567kJ	✓	✓	Good
Pasta sauce, cherry tomato arrabbiata	563kJ	↑Fat ↑Salt	✓	Good
Pesto, classic	1936kJ	↑Fat ↑Salt	✓	Good
Pesto, fiery chilli	1299kJ	↑Fat ↑Salt	220	Good
Stir through pasta sauce, capsicum & eggplant	1022kJ	↑Fat ↑Salt	220	Good
Stir thru, olive & tomato	747kJ	↑Fat ↑Salt	✓	Good
Stir thru, tomato & garlic	701kJ	↑Fat ↑Salt	220	Good
Stir thru, arrabbiata	1153kJ	↑Fat ↑Salt	220, 223	Good

San Remo

Product Name	Energy	Major Nutrients	Food Additives	Nutritious Rating
Pasta sauce, tomato, onion & pepper	306kJ	↑Salt	220	Good
Pasta sauce, tomato & basil	226kJ	↑Salt	✓	Good
Pasta sauce, tomato, onion &	226kJ	↑Salt	✓	Good

garlic				
Pasta sauce, mushroom & tomato	372kJ	↑Salt	✓	Good

Sharwood

Product Name	Energy	Major Nutrients	Food Additives	Nutritious Rating
Simmer sauce, butter chicken	479kJ	↑Salt	✓	Good
Simmer sauce, korma	649kJ	↑Fat	220	Good
Simmer sauce, Madras	408kJ	↑Fat	220	Good
Simmer sauce, biryani coconut & curry	229kJ	✓	220, 223	Good
Simmer sauce, biryani coriander & mint	192kJ	✓	220, 223	Good
Simmer sauce, tiki marsala	532kJ	↑Fat ↑Salt	220, 223	Good
Simmer sauce, rogan josh	438kJ	↑Salt	✓	Good

Taylors

Product Name	Energy	Major Nutrients	Food Additives	Nutritious Rating
Simmer sauce, butter chicken	243kJ	↑Salt	✓	Good
Simmer sauce, green curry	338kJ	↑Salt ↑Sugar	YE	Good
Simmer sauce, massaman curry	520kJ	↑Salt	223, HVP	Good
Simmer sauce, peanut satay	660kJ	↑Fat ↑Salt	160b	Average

Val Verde

Product Name	Energy	Major Nutrients	Food Additives	Nutritious Rating
Pasta sauce,	125kJ	✓	✓	Good

passata				

Woolworths

Product Name	Energy	Major Nutrients	Food Additives	Nutritious Rating
Select, Bolognese	247kJ	↑Salt	✓	Good
Select, tomato & basil	247kJ	↑Salt	✓	Good
Select, tomato & mushroom	174kJ	↑Salt	✓	Good
Select, arrabbiata	234kJ	✓	✓	Good
Homebrand, traditional pasta	256kJ	✓	✓	Good
Homebrand, chunky pasta	215kJ	✓	✓	Good
Homebrand, sweet & sour	389kJ	↑Sugar	220, 223	Average
Homebrand, honey mustard	715kJ	↑Salt ↑Fat	223	Average
Homebrand, satay	1020kJ	↑Salt ↑Fat ↑Sugar	✓	Average

Stocks, Marinades, Powders & Pastes

This is an area that is done quite poorly; there are a few scattered varieties, such as *Masterfoods, Coles, Kikoman, Leggos, Dolmios, Spencers and Patkas.*

Always Fresh

Product Name	Energy	Major Nutrients	Food Additives	Nutritious Rating
Pizza partner, grilled vegetables & oregano	399kJ	✓	220, 224	Average
Pizza partner, classic olive, tomato & basil	363kJ	✓	220, 224, 223	Average

Benjamins

Product Name	Energy	Major Nutrients	Food Additives	Nutritious Rating
Noodle sauce, black bean	412kJ	↑Salt ↑Sugar	211, 627, 631, YE, VPE	Poor
Noodle sauce, hokkien mee	661kJ	↑Salt ↑Sugar	627, 631, YE, VP	Poor
Noodle sauce, mi goreng	**543kJ**	**↑Salt**	**✓**	**Poor**
Noodle sauce, teriyaki	246kJ	↑Salt ↑Sugar	220	Poor

Borvil

Product Name	Energy	Major Nutrients	Food Additives	Nutritious Rating
Vegetable extract	689kJ	↑Salt	YE, 635, 202	Poor

Campbell's

Product Name	Energy	Major Nutrients	Food Additives	Nutritious Rating
Consomme, beef	150kJ	✓	YE	Poor
Consomme, chicken	82kJ	↑Salt	220, YE	Poor
Real stock, beef	37kJ	✓	220, YE	Poor
Real stock, chicken	43kJ	✓	220, YE	Poor

Real stock, fish	20kJ	✓	223, 220	Poor
Real stock, vegetable	**34kJ**	**↑Salt**	**✓**	**Poor**
Real stock, beef salt reduced	37kJ	✓	220, YE	Poor
Real stock, chicken salt reduced	43kJ	✓	220, YE	Poor
Real stock, vegetable salt reduced	**34kJ**	✓	✓	**Poor**
Real stock, beef paste	504kJ	↑Salt	YE	Poor
Real stock, chicken paste sachets	631kJ	↑Salt ↑Fat	YE	Poor
Real stock, vegetable paste sachets	502kJ	↑Salt	YE	Poor

Coles

Product Name	Energy	Major Nutrients	Food Additives	Nutritious Rating
Marinade, Aussie smokey BBQ	349kJ	↑Salt ↑Sugar	220, VP, 223, YE	Poor
Marinade, honey soy	**749kJ**	**↑Salt ↑Sugar**	✓	**Poor**
Marinade, Moroccan	480kJ	↑Salt ↑Sugar	202	Poor
Marinade, teriyaki	**715kJ**	**↑Salt ↑Sugar**	✓	**Poor**
Marinade, Thai sweet chilli	737kJ	↑Salt ↑Sugar	220, 223	Poor
Gravy mix, brown onion	175kJ	↑Salt	202, 220, HVP	Poor
Gravy mix, chicken	178kJ	↑Salt	202, 220, HVP	Poor
Gravy mix, roast meat	153kJ	✓	220, 223	Poor
Gravy mix, traditional	142kJ	✓	220, 223	Poor
Smart buy, white	559kJ	✓	202	Poor

sauce mix				
Smart buy, cheese sauce mix	**604kJ**	✓	✓	**Poor**
Tomato paste	428kJ	↑Sugar	✓	Average
Smart buy tomato paste	290kJ	✓	✓	Average
Liquid stock, beef	32kJ	✓	YE	Poor
Liquid stock, chicken	32kJ	✓	VPE, YE, VP	Poor
Liquid stock, vegetable	26kJ	↑Salt	YE, VP	Poor
Recipe base, beef strogonoff	410kJ	↑Salt	VP, 202, YE	Poor
Recipe base, curried sausages	**180kJ**	**↑Salt**	✓	**Poor**
Recipe base, Chinese beef stir-fry	321 kJ	↑Salt	YE, 202	Poor
Recipe base, honey mustard chicken	430kJ	↑Salt ↑Sugar	220, 224	Poor
Recipe base, Italian chicken casserole	308kJ	↑Salt	223	Average
Recipe base, teriyaki	544kJ	↑Salt ↑Sugar	YE, 202, 220	Poor
Recipe base, Tuscan meatballs	285kJ	↑Salt	220, VP	Average

Continental

Product Name	Energy	Major Nutrients	Food Additives	Nutritious Rating
Cook in the bag, honey BBQ chicken	1520kJ	↑Salt ↑Sugar	220, 950, 952	Poor
Cook in the bag, honey mustard chicken	**1470kJ**	**↑Salt ↑Sugar**	✓	**Poor**
Cook in the bag, lemon & herb chicken	1500kJ	↑Salt	220, 635	Poor
Cook in the bag, Portuguese chicken	1460kJ	↑Salt	220	Poor
Cook in the bag, smokey BBQ	1450kJ	↑Salt ↑Sugar	220	Poor

Cook in the bag, traditional roast chicken	1414kJ	↑Salt ↑Sugar	627, 202	Poor
Cook in the bag, teriyaki fish	1428kJ	↑Salt ↑Sugar	220, YE,	Poor
Cook in the bag, fish dill & lemon	1463kJ	↑Salt	220, 635	Poor
Cook in the bag, Mediterranean fish	1420kJ	↑Salt ↑Sugar	220	Poor
Cook in the bag, lamb roast	1420kJ	↑Salt ↑Sugar	220	Poor
Cook in the bag, lamb shanks	1430kJ	↑Salt ↑Sugar	220	Poor
Hot Pot, casserole curry	1513kJ	↑Salt ↑Sugar	202, 223, YE	Poor
Hot Pot, French onion	1450kJ	↑Salt ↑Sugar	202, YE	Poor
Hot Pot, savoury casserole	1480kJ	↑Salt ↑Sugar	202, 635, YE	Poor
Hot Pot, sweet & sour	1586kJ	↑Salt ↑Sugar	202, YE	Poor
Recipe Base, lite beef stroganoff	1655kJ	↑Salt ↑Sugar	220, 202, YE, 635, 120	Poor
Recipe Base, rissoles	1440kJ	↑Salt ↑Sugar	223, YE, 627	Poor
Recipe Base, red wine beef casserole	1430kJ	↑Salt ↑Sugar	220, YE, 202, 635	Poor
Recipe Base, stroganoff	1590kJ	↑Salt ↑Fat ↑Sugar	220, YE, 202, 635	Poor
Recipe Base, chilli con carne	1290kJ	↑Salt ↑Sugar	YE	Average
Recipe Base, chow mein mince	1430kJ	↑Salt ↑Sugar	635, YE	Poor
Recipe Base, creamy chicken curry	1640kJ	↑Salt ↑Fat	YE, 202, 220	Poor
Recipe Base, creamy chicken mushroom	1620kJ	↑Salt ↑Fat ↑Sugar	220, YE, 202, 635	Poor

Recipe Base, creamy tuna mornay	1630kJ	↑Salt ↑Fat	627, YE	Poor
Recipe Base, curried sausages	**1500kJ**	**↑Salt**	✓	**Average**
Recipe Base, devilled sausages	1400kJ	↑Salt ↑Sugar	YE	Poor
Recipe Base, mild mince curry	1680kJ	↑Salt ↑Fat ↑Sugar	220, YE, 202	Average
Recipe Base, beefy mince	1435kJ	↑Salt	YE, 202, 627	Average
Recipe Base, shepherds pie	1430kJ	↑Salt	YE, 202, 627	Average
Recipe Base, spaghetti bolognaise	1480kJ	↑Salt ↑Sugar	YE	Average
Recipe Base, rich beef casserole	1440kJ	↑Salt	YE, 202, 627	Average
Recipe Base, creamy Malaysian satay	1560kJ	↑Salt ↑Fat ↑Sugar	220, 202, YE, 627	Poor
Recipe Base, apricot chicken	1430kJ	↑Salt ↑Sugar	202	Poor
Instant stock powder, beef	21kJ	✓	635, 627, 202, YE, 220	Poor
Instant stock powder, chicken	22kJ	✓	202, YE, 635	Poor
Instant stock powder, vegetable	23kJ	✓	202, YE, 635	Poor
Instant stock powder, chicken salt reduced	24kJ	✓	202, YE, 635	Poor
Instant stock powder, beef salt reduced	24kJ	✓	202, YE, 635	Poor
Stock cubes, beef	15kJ	✓	202, YE, 635	Poor
Stock cubes, chicken	14kJ	✓	YE	Poor
Stock pot, beef	18kJ	✓	YE	Poor
Stock pot, chicken	20kJ	✓	YE	Poor
Stock pot, vegetable	32kJ	✓	YE	Poor

Dolmio

Product Name	Energy	Major Nutrients	Food Additives	Nutritious Rating
Meal base, carbonara	286kJ	↑Salt	✓	Poor
Meal base, chicken alfredo	250kJ	↑Salt	✓	Poor
Meal base, chicken parmagiana	309kJ	↑Salt	✓	Average
Meal base, chicken with tomato & Italian herbs	357kJ	↑Salt	220	Average
Meal base, Italian meatballs	278kJ	↑Salt	220	Average
Meal base, creamy Tuscan chicken	247kJ	↑Salt	223, 220, YE	Average
Meal base, slow cooked Italian beef	345kJ	↑Salt ↑Sugar	220	Average
Meal base, creamy mushroom & bacon	380kJ	↑Salt	223, 220, YE	Average
Meal base, lamb, rosemary & thyme	296kJ	↑Salt	YE	Average

Fountain

Product Name	Energy	Major Nutrients	Food Additives	Nutritious Rating
Marinade, Portuguese chicken	387kJ	↑Salt ↑Sugar	220, 223	Poor
Marinade, red wine & garlic	484kJ	↑Salt ↑Sugar	220	Poor
Marinade, satay	607kJ	↑Salt ↑Sugar	220	Poor
Marinade, soy, honey & garlic	380kJ	↑Salt ↑Sugar	YE, HVP	Poor
Marinade, teriyaki	448kJ	↑Salt ↑Sugar	HVP, 220	Poor

Gravox

Product Name	Energy	Major Nutrients	Food Additives	Nutritious Rating
Gravy mix, brown onion	176kJ	↑Salt	202, 220, 223, YE	Poor
Gravy mix, chicken	175kJ	↑Salt	202, HVP, YE	Poor
Gravy mix, supreme	107kJ	↑Salt	HVP	Poor
Gravy mix supreme lite	118kJ	✓	621, HVP	Poor
Gravy mix, traditional	178kJ	↑Salt	202, YE	Poor
Gravy mix, lamb & rosemary	175kJ	↑Salt	202, YE, 220	Poor
Gravy mix, roast meat gravy	171kJ	↑Salt	202, YE	Poor
Liquid gravy, red wine & garlic	140kJ	✓	YE, 220	Poor
Liquid gravy, brown onion	152kJ	✓	YE	Poor
Liquid gravy, chicken & herb	**177kJ**	**↑Salt**	**✓**	**Poor**
Liquid gravy, roast pork	126kJ	↑Salt	YE	Poor
Liquid gravy, lamb & rosemary	98kJ	✓	YE	Poor
Liquid gravy, traditional	177kJ	↑Salt	YE	Poor
Carvery gravy, chicken, sage & onion	170kJ	↑Salt	202, 220, YE	Poor
Carvery gravy, brown onion & garlic	170kJ	✓	YE, 202, 621, 220, HVP	Poor
Carvery gravy. Lamb & rosemary	169kJ	↑Salt	220, 202, YE	Poor
Cheese sauce	204kJ	✓	202, 220, 223, 635	Poor
Diane sauce	168kJ	↑Salt	202, 220, 223	Poor
Pepper steak sauce liquid	214kJ	↑Salt	YE	Poor

Pepper sauce liquid	176kJ	✓	202, 220, YE, HVP, 621, 627, 631	Poor
Lemon pepper sauce liquid	309kJ	↑Salt	160b, YE, 223	Poor
White parsley sauce	334kJ	↑Salt	YE, 235	Poor
Mushroom & garlic sauce	165kJ	↑Salt	627, HVP, 202, 627, 621, 220, 631, YE	Poor
White sauce powder	218kJ	✓	202, 220, 223	Poor
Hollandaise sauce	411kJ	✓	223, 220, 160b, YE	Poor
Gourmet peppercorn & cream	340kJ	↑Salt	627, 631, 220, YE	Poor

Greens

Product Name	Energy	Major Nutrients	Food Additives	Nutritious Rating
Gravy granules, chicken	202kJ	↑Salt	320, 223, 202, 621, 631, HVP, YE, VP	Poor
Gravy granules, roast meat	248kJ	↑Salt	320, 223, 202, 621, 631, 627, HVP, YE, VP	Poor
Instant gravy, roast meat	175kJ	↑Salt	202, 220, 223, 635, YE	Poor

IGA/Franklins

Product Name	Energy	Major Nutrients	Food Additives	Nutritious Rating
Signature, chicken gravy	179kJ	✓	202, YE	Poor
Signature, brown onion gravy	176kJ	↑Salt	202	Poor
Signature, roast	173kJ	↑Salt	202	Poor

meat gravy				
Signature, traditional gravy	178kJ	↑Salt	202	Poor
Signature, lamb & rosemary liquid gravy	106kJ	✓	YE	Poor
Signature, traditional liquid gravy	142kJ	✓	YE	Poor
Signature, roast chicken liquid gravy	**189kJ**	✓	✓	**Poor**
Signature, red wine & garlic liquid gravy	124kJ	✓	220, HVP	Poor

Kikoman

Product Name	Energy	Major Nutrients	Food Additives	Nutritious Rating
Soy sauce	**411kJ**	↑Salt	✓	Poor
Soy sauce reduced salt	**529kJ**	↑Salt	✓	Poor
Soy sauce, gluten free	**421kJ**	↑Salt	✓	Poor
Marinade, honey soy	1111kJ	↑Salt ↑Sugar	220, 223	Poor
Marinade, teriyaki	490kJ	↑Salt ↑Sugar	220, 223	Poor
Marinade, soy, sweet chilli & ginger	1051kJ	↑Salt ↑Sugar	223, YE	Poor
Marinade, soy, sesame & ginger	904kJ	↑Salt ↑Sugar	YE, 223	Poor

Kraft

Product Name	Energy	Major Nutrients	Food Additives	Nutritious Rating
Bonox	425kJ	↑Salt	YE, HVP, 621, 627, 202	Poor

Leggos

Product Name	Energy	Major Nutrients	Food Additives	Nutritious Rating
Organic tomato paste	282kJ	↑Salt	✓	Average
Tomato paste, jar	272kJ	✓	✓	Average
Tomato paste, no added salt	306kJ	↑Sugar	✓	Average
Tomato paste, tubs	287kJ	✓	✓	Average
Tomato paste, garlic & herb	232kJ	↑Salt	✓	Average
Pizza sauce tubs	224kJ	↑Salt	✓	Average
Pizza sauce sachets	221kJ	↑Salt	✓	Average
Pizza sauce, squeeze bottle	230kJ	↑Salt	202, 234	Average
Pizza sauce, BBQ style squeeze bottle	307kJ	↑Salt	220, HVP, 202, 234	Average

Maggi

Product Name	Energy	Major Nutrients	Food Additives	Nutritious Rating
Marinade, BBQ	845kJ	↑Salt ↑Sugar	220	Poor
Marinade, satay	680kJ	↑Salt ↑Sugar	220	Poor
Marinade, honey soy	870kJ	↑Salt ↑Sugar	220	Poor
Liquid seasoning	175kJ	↑Salt	627, 631, 202	Poor
Recipe mix, gluten free beef stroganoff	1620kJ	↑Salt ↑Fat ↑Sugar	YE, 202, 223	Poor
Pressure cooker, lamb & rosemary casserole	1500kJ	↑Salt ↑Fat ↑Sugar	YE, 202, 223	Poor
Pressure cooker, beef red wine & garlic	1430kJ	↑Salt ↑Sugar	YE, 223	Poor
Pressure cooker, chicken curry	1330kJ	↑Salt ↑Sugar	202, 223, 160b, YE	Poor

Recipe mix, Asian satay chicken	1600kJ	↑Salt ↑Sugar	220, 223	Poor
Recipe mix, butter chicken	1600kJ	↑Salt ↑Sugar	202, 223, 160b, YE	Poor
Recipe mix, mince chow mein	1350kJ	↑Salt	202, 120, 160b	Poor
Recipe mix, tuna & potato pie	1390kJ	↑Salt	202	Poor
Recipe mix, apricot chicken	1470kJ	↑Salt	223, YE	Poor
Recipe mix, beef goulash	1430kJ	↑Salt ↑Sugar	202, 223, YE	Poor
Recipe mix, chicken chasseur	1420kJ	↑Salt	YE, 223, 202	Poor
Recipe mix, chilli con carne	1470kJ	↑Salt ↑Sugar	223, YE, 202	Poor
Recipe mix, lamb ragout	1430kJ	↑Salt	YE	Poor
Recipe mix, mince cottage pie	1330kJ	↑Salt	202	Poor
Recipe mix, sausage casserole	1440kJ	↑Salt	YE, 223, 202	Poor
Recipe mix, Bolognese pasta bake	1370kJ	↑Salt ↑Sugar	YE, 223, 160b, 120	Poor
Recipe mix, devilled sausages	1510kJ	↑Salt ↑Sugar	202, YE	Poor
Recipe mix, lamb casserole	1380kJ	↑Salt ↑Sugar	YE, 223, 202	Poor
Tender Roast, BBQ ribs	1540kJ	↑Salt ↑Sugar	223, 160b	Poor
Tender Roast, chicken tandoori	1520kJ	↑Salt ↑Fat ↑Sugar	223, 120, 160b, 202	Poor
Tender Roast, lamb, mint & roast herbs	1390kJ	↑Salt ↑Sugar	202, YE, 223	Poor
Tender Roast, chicken with garlic	1490kJ	↑Salt ↑Sugar	202	Poor
Tender Roast, Italian chicken	1440kJ	↑Salt ↑Sugar	202	Poor

Tender Roast, Oriental soy chicken	1560kJ	↑Salt ↑Sugar	202	Poor
Tender Roast, mixed herb chicken	1420kJ	↑Salt ↑Sugar	YE, 202	Poor
Tender Roast, lamb & rosemary & garlic	1650kJ	↑Salt ↑Fat	223, 202,	Poor
Vegetable Sensations, cheese & bacon	1430kJ	↑Salt ↑Fat	202. YE, 223, 160b	Poor
Vegetable Sensations, cheese and vegetables	1560kJ	↑Salt ↑Fat	YE, 223, 160b	Poor
Vegetable Sensations, cheesy cauliflower	1530kJ	↑Salt ↑Fat	202. YE, 223	Poor
Vegetable Sensations, creamy potato & garlic bake	1640kJ	↑Salt ↑Fat	202. YE, 223, 160b	Poor
Vegetable Sensations, three cheeses potato bake	1610kJ	↑Salt ↑Fat	202. YE, 223, 160b	Poor
Vegetable Sensations, sour cream & chive potato	1690kJ	↑Salt ↑Fat	202. YE, 223, 160b	Poor
Gravy mix, pork	169kJ	✓	202, 220, YE	Poor
Gravy mix, roast chicken	157kJ	✓	202, 220, YE, 223, 635	Poor
Gravy mix, brown onion	191kJ	✓	635, YE	Poor
Gravy mix, roast meat	177kJ	✓	202, 220, YE, 223	Poor
Sauce mix, hollandaise	530kJ	↑Salt	202, 220, 160b	Poor
Sauce mix, tasty cheese	302kJ	✓	202, 220. 160b	Poor

Massel

Product Name	Energy	Major Nutrients	Food Additives	Nutritious Rating
Gravy powder, supreme	146kJ	✓	202, YE, 160b	Poor
Gravy powder, turkey style	135kJ	✓	202, YE	Poor
Gourmet plus liquid stock, beef	31kJ	✓	202, YE	Poor
Gourmet plus liquid stock, chicken	31kJ	✓	202, YE	Poor
Gourmet plus liquid stock, vegetable	37kJ	✓	202, YE	Poor
Stock powder, chicken	11kJ	✓	202, YE	Poor
Stock powder, beef	11kJ	✓	202, YE	Poor
Stock powder, vegetable	11kJ	✓	202, YE	Poor
Stock powder, chicken salt reduced	13kJ	✓	202, YE	Poor
Stock powder, beef salt reduced	11kJ	✓	202, YE	Poor
Stock powder, vegetable salt reduced	13kJ	✓	202, YE	Poor
Stock cubes, chicken	26kJ	✓	YE, VPE, 631	Poor
Stock cubes, beef	25kJ	✓	202, YE	Poor
Stock cubes, chicken salt reduced	25kJ	✓	202, YE	Poor
Stock cubes, vegetable salt reduced	25kJ	✓	202, YE	Poor

Masterfoods

Product Name	Energy	Major Nutrients	Food Additives	Nutritious Rating
Marinade, honey BBQ	619kJ	↑Salt ↑Sugar	✓	Poor
Marinade, Mustard,	602kJ	↑Salt	223	Poor

honey & herb		↑Sugar		
Marinade, honey soy & garlic	681kJ	↑Salt ↑Sugar	VPE	Poor
Marinade, Moroccan	350kJ	↑Salt ↑Sugar	223	Poor
Marinade, teriyaki	748kJ	↑Salt ↑Sugar	220, VPE	Poor
Marinade, Thai	274kJ	↑Salt	220, 223	Poor
Marinade, plum	689kJ	↑Salt ↑Sugar	120	Poor
Marinade, satay	715kJ	↑Salt ↑Sugar	220	Poor
Marinade, red wine & garlic	519kJ	↑Salt ↑Sugar	220, VPE	Poor
Marinade, Portuguese	281kJ	↑Salt	220, 223	Poor
Marinade, smokey BBQ	**584kJ**	**↑Salt ↑Sugar**	✓	**Poor**
Marinade, Tuscan	276kJ	↑Salt	220	Poor
Recipe base, cheesey potato bake	303kJ	↑Salt	YE	Poor
Recipe base, Chinese beef stir-fry	282kJ	↑Salt	220	Poor
Recipe base, chow mein	288kJ	↑Salt	220, VPE, YE	Poor
Recipe base, country beef casserole	214kJ	↑Salt	220, YE	Poor
Recipe base, beef stroganoff	419kJ	↑Salt	220, 223, VPE	Poor
Recipe base, creamy herb & garlic potato bake	463kJ	↑Salt	YE	Poor
Recipe base, curried sausages	**178kJ**	**↑Salt**	✓	**Poor**
Recipe base, devilled sausages	473kJ	↑Salt ↑Sugar	YE	Poor
Recipe base, honey,	468kJ	↑Salt	VPE	Poor

garlic & soy		↑Sugar		
Recipe base, honey mustard chicken	549kJ	↑Salt ↑Sugar	223	Poor
Recipe base, Italian chicken casserole	310kJ	↑Salt ↑Sugar	223	Poor
Recipe base, lamb casserole	205kJ	↑Salt	223, YE	Poor
Recipe base, Moroccan lamb shanks	372kJ	↑Salt ↑Sugar	YE	Poor
Recipe base, satay chicken	349kJ	↑Salt	220	Poor
Recipe base, teriyaki chicken stir-fry	506kJ	↑Sugar	YE, VPE	Poor
Recipe base, Thai chicken stir-fry	**360kJ**	**↑Salt ↑Sugar**	✓	**Poor**
Recipe base, Thai green curry	391kJ	↑Salt ↑Sugar	223	Poor
Recipe base, Tuscan meatballs	255kJ	↑Salt	220, 223	Poor
Recipe base, apricot chicken	248kJ	↑Salt	YE	Poor
Finishing sauce, béarnaise	561kJ	↑Fat	220, YE, 160b	Poor
Finishing sauce, caramelised onion with red wine	259kJ	↑Salt	YE, 220	Poor
Finishing sauce, cheese sauce	472kJ	↑Salt	YE, 160b	Poor
Finishing sauce, cracked pepper	243kJ	↑Salt	YE, 220	Poor
Finishing sauce, creamy white	599kJ	↑Salt ↑Fat	YE, 220	Poor
Finishing sauce, hollandaise	563kJ	↑Fat	YE, 160b 220	Poor
Finishing sauce, mushroom & white wine	532kJ	↑Salt ↑Fat	220	Poor
Finishing sauce,	546kJ	↑Salt	YE, 220	Poor

roasted garlic & herbs		↑Fat		
Finishing sauce, wholegrain mustard & honey	651kJ	↑Salt	220	Poor
Slow Cooker Recipe base, beef, red wine casserole	272kJ	↑Salt	220, YE	Poor
Slow Cooker Recipe base, chicken curry mild	**386kJ**	**↑Salt**	✓	**Poor**
Slow Cooker Recipe base, garlic herb lamb shanks	**326kJ**	**↑Salt ↑Sugar**	✓	**Poor**
Slow Cooker Recipe base, farmhouse chicken	291kJ	↑Salt ↑Sugar	220, YE	Poor
Slow Cooker Recipe base, sausage hot pot	334kJ	↑Salt ↑Sugar	YE	Poor

McCormick

Product Name	Energy	Major Nutrients	Food Additives	Nutritious Rating
One Pot, beef, potato & herb	1183kJ	↑Salt ↑Sugar	HVP	Poor
One Pot, chicken & leek casserole	1333kJ	↑Salt ↑Sugar	223, 202	Poor
One Pot, Spanish chicken & potato	1255kJ	↑Salt ↑Fat ↑Sugar	HVP, 320, 202	Poor
Produce Partner, cauliflower supreme cheese	1503kJ	↑Salt ↑Fat ↑Sugar	HVP, YE	Poor
Produce Partner, Italian herb potato	1403kJ	↑Salt ↑Fat	320, YE	Poor
Produce Partner, scalloped potatoes	1398kJ	↑Salt ↑Sugar	YE, 320, 202, 223	Poor
Produce Partner, sour cream & chive	1680kJ	↑Salt ↑Sugar	YE, 320, 202	Poor

potatoes				
Produce Partner, country potatoes	1340kJ	↑Salt ↑Fat ↑Sugar	202, 220	Poor
Slow-cooker, beef & mushroom	1188kJ	↑Salt ↑Sugar	220, 223, 320, 202	Poor
Slow-cooker, beef & wine casserole	1195kJ	↑Salt	220, 223, HVP	Poor
Slow-cooker, country chicken casserole	**1142kJ**	**↑Salt**	✓	**Poor**
Slow-cooker, garlic, herb & lamb	1160kJ	↑Salt	202, 220	Poor
Slow-cooker, lamb & vegetable casserole	997kJ	↑Salt ↑Sugar	223	Poor
Slow-cooker, mild chicken curry	**1214kJ**	**↑Salt**	✓	**Poor**
Slow-cooker, mild beef curry	1311kJ	↑Salt ↑Sugar	223	Poor
Slow-cooker, roast beef with onion & gravy	1484kJ	↑Salt ↑Sugar	HVP	Poor
Slow-cooker, tomato & onion	1287kJ	↑Salt ↑Sugar	223, 220, 202	Poor
Slow-cooker, chicken, bacon & potato	1232kJ	↑Salt ↑Sugar	223, HVP	Poor
Slow-cooker, chunky beef stroganoff	1097kJ	↑Salt ↑Sugar	HVP	Poor
Slow-cooker, Moroccan lamb	**1097kJ**	**↑Salt ↑Sugar**	✓	**Poor**
Slow-cooker, osso bucco	1188kJ	↑Salt ↑Sugar	220, 223	Poor
Slow-cooker, Portuguese chicken	**1183kJ**	**↑Salt ↑Sugar**	✓	**Poor**
Rice Cookers, chicken & bacon risotto	1281kJ	↑Salt ↑Sugar	223	Poor
Rice Cookers, Spanish chicken & chorizo	1209kJ	↑Salt ↑Sugar	223, 202, HVP	Poor

Rice Cookers, Chinese special fried rice	1343kJ	↑Salt ↑Sugar	202	Poor

Nandos

Product Name	Energy	Major Nutrients	Food Additives	Nutritious Rating
Marinade, Portuguese BBQ	380kJ	↑Salt ↑Sugar	220, 223, 202, 1520	Average
Marinade, Peri peri hot	484kJ	↑Salt	211, 202, 220, 1520, 223	Average
Marinade, sweet & sticky peri peri	727kJ	↑Salt ↑Sugar	220, 211, 202, 1520, 223	Average

Oxo

Product Name	Energy	Major Nutrients	Food Additives	Nutritious Rating
Stock cubes, beef	28kJ	✓	YE, 621, 627, 223, 320	Poor
Stock cubes, chicken	28kJ	✓	621, 635, 220, 320, YE	Poor

Patkas

Product Name	Energy	Major Nutrients	Food Additives	Nutritious Rating
Paste, vindaloo curry	1132kJ	↑Salt ↑Fat	✓	Average
Paste, korma mild	908kJ	↑Salt ↑Fat	✓	Average
Paste, madras	1196kJ	↑Salt ↑Fat	✓	Average
Paste, tandoori curry	837kJ	↑Salt ↑Fat	120, 223	Average
Paste, tiki marsala	1100kJ	↑Salt ↑Fat	223	Average
Paste, rogan josh	1003kJ	↑Salt ↑Fat	223	Average

Product Name	Energy	Major Nutrients	Food Additives	Nutritious Rating
Paste mild curry	1172kJ	↑Salt ↑Fat	✓	Average
Paste balti curry mild	1083kJ	↑Salt ↑Fat	220, 223	Average
Eggplant pickle	1577kJ	↑Salt ↑Fat	✓	Average
Mango pickle	1070kJ	↑Salt ↑Fat	✓	Average

Podravka

Product Name	Energy	Major Nutrients	Food Additives	Nutritious Rating
Vegeta stock cubes, chicken	9kJ	✓	631	Poor
Vegeta Stock powder, gourmet	6kJ	✓	621, 631	Poor

Sharwoods

Product Name	Energy	Major Nutrients	Food Additives	Nutritious Rating
Paste, tandoori curry medium	929kJ	↑Salt ↑Fat	223	Average
Paste, korma	1540kJ	↑Salt ↑Fat	223	Average
Paste, rogan josh	1740kJ	↑Salt ↑Fat	223	Average

Spencers

Product Name	Energy	Major Nutrients	Food Additives	Nutritious Rating
Paste, butter chicken	801kJ	↑Salt ↑Sugar	✓	Average
Paste, korma	1540kJ	↑Salt ↑Fat	✓	Average
Paste, rogan josh	1740kJ	↑Salt ↑Fat	✓	Average
Paste, tandoori	929kJ	↑Salt ↑Fat	224	Average
Paste, Thai red curry	1019kJ	↑Salt	223	Average

		↑Fat ↑Sugar		
Paste, tiki masala	1201kJ	↑Salt ↑Fat ↑Sugar	220, 223	Average
Paste, vindaloo	1769kJ	↑Salt ↑Fat	223	Average

Taylors

Product Name	Energy	Major Nutrients	Food Additives	Nutritious Rating
Marinade, honey mustard	**559kJ**	**↑Salt ↑Sugar**	✓	**Poor**
Marinade, honey soy	474kJ	↑Salt ↑Sugar	HVP	Poor
Marinade, spicy plum	**763kJ**	**↑Salt ↑Sugar**	✓	**Poor**
Marinade, sweet soy chilli & sesame	140kJ	↑Salt ↑Sugar	220	Poor
Marinade, tandoori	455kJ	↑Salt ↑Sugar	223	Poor

Weight Watchers

Product Name	Energy	Major Nutrients	Food Additives	Nutritious Rating
Gravy, chicken	113kJ	✓	202, HVP, 220, 635, YE	Poor
Gravy, brown onion	112kJ	↑Salt	220, 202, 635	Poor

Woolworths/Safeways

Product Name	Energy	Major Nutrients	Food Additives	Nutritious Rating
Select, Portuguese chicken marinade	483kJ	↑Salt ↑Sugar	YE, 220	Poor
Select, smokey BBQ marinade	601kJ	↑Salt ↑Sugar	YE, 220	Poor
Select, teriyaki marinade	546kJ	↑Salt ↑Sugar	220	Poor

Select, Oriental soy & garlic marinade	676kJ	↑Salt ↑Sugar	220	Poor
Select, gravy powder traditional	180kJ	↑Salt	202	Poor
Select, gravy powder roast meat	113kJ	↑Salt	202	Poor
Select, gravy powder brown onion	180kJ	↑Salt	202	Poor
Select, gravy powder chicken	190kJ	↑Salt	202	Poor
Select, hollandaise liquid sauce	284kJ	↑Salt	223, YE	Poor
Select, béarnaise sauce	327kJ	✓	YE	Poor
Select, caramelised onion & roasted garlic reduction	439kJ	↑Salt	220, YE	Poor
Select, Diane sauce	**210kJ**	**↑Salt**	✓	**Poor**
Select, wholegrain mustard & honey sauce	425kJ	↑Salt ↑Sugar	223, YE	Poor
Select, stock chicken	42kJ	✓	202, VPE, 202	Poor
Select, stock chicken salt reduced	46kJ	✓	202, VPE, 202	Poor
Select, stock beef	35kJ	↑Salt	202, 223, YE	Poor
Select, stock vegetable	46kJ	✓	VP, YE, 202	Poor
Select, taco seasoning	1340kJ	↑Salt	223	Poor
Homebrand, Gravy traditional	**141kJ**	**↑Salt**	✓	**Poor**
Homebrand, cheese sauce powder	1570kJ	↑Salt	202, 220, YE, HVP	Poor
Homebrand, white sauce powder	1460kJ	↑Salt	VP, 220, YE, 202	Poor
Homebrand, recipe	1270kJ	↑Salt	YE, 223	Poor

mix chilli con carne		↑Sugar		
Homebrand, recipe mix beef stroganoff	1380kJ	↑Salt ↑Sugar	223, 202, HVP, 220	Poor
Homebrand, recipe mix devilled sausages	1460kJ	↑Salt ↑Sugar	YE, 223	Poor
Homebrand, recipe mix creamy cheese potato bake	1440kJ	↑Salt ↑Sugar	220, 223, 202, HVP	Poor
Homebrand, taco seasoning	1390kJ	↑Salt	✓	Poor

Pickled Vegetables and Condiments

Always Fresh

Product Name	Energy	Major Nutrients	Food Additives	Nutritious Rating
Mushrooms, marinated	252kJ	✓	223	Average
Peppers, fire roasted strips	219kJ	✓	223	Average
Peppers, piquillo whole	149kJ	✓	✓	Average
Sundried tomatoes, deli style	905kJ	↑Fat	220	Average
Sundried tomatoes, halves	905kJ	↑Fat	220	Average
Sundried tomatoes, strips	905kJ	↑Fat	220	Average
Deli style, olive medley	639kJ	↑Salt ↑Fat	✓	Average
Deli style, olives mixed	758kJ	↑Salt ↑Fat	202, 220	Average
Deli style, colossal kalamata olives	522kJ	↑Salt ↑Fat	✓	Average
Deli style, chilli kalamata olives	680kJ	↑Salt ↑Fat	✓	Average
Stuffed anchovy olives	469kJ	↑Salt ↑Fat	621	Average
Stuffed pimento olives	380kJ	↑Salt	202	Average
Spanish sliced black olives	413kJ	↑Salt	✓	Average
Sliced kalamata olives	794kJ	↑Salt ↑Fat	✓	Average
Pitted kalamata olives	788kJ	↑Salt ↑Fat	✓	Average
Whole kalamata olives	794kJ	↑Salt ↑Fat	✓	Average
Sweet & sour	296kJ	↑Sugar	✓	Average

cucumbers				
Original dill cucumber	54kJ	↑Salt	✓	Average
Roasted sweet potato	852kJ	↑Salt ↑Fat ↑Sugar	220	Average
Eggplant chargrilled	431kJ	↑Salt ↑Fat ↑Sugar	220	Average
Antipasto salsa, caramel onion	702kJ	↑Salt ↑Fat	220	Average
Relish chilli jam	1185kJ	↑Sugar	224, 120	Average
Relish, beetroot	713kJ	↑Sugar ↑Salt	224	Average
Relish, caramelised onion	762kJ	↑Salt ↑Fat	102, 122, 133, 123, 220	Average

Anathoth

Product Name	Energy	Major Nutrients	Food Additives	Nutritious Rating
Pickle, farm style	314kJ	↑Sugar	220	Average
Tomato relish	480kJ	↑Sugar	220, 223	Average
Zucchini pickle	400kJ	↑Sugar	220, 223	Average

Aristocrat

Product Name	Energy	Major Nutrients	Food Additives	Nutritious Rating
Cocktail onions, green	220kJ	↑Sugar ↑Salt	102, 133, 223, 202	Average
Cocktail onions, red	220kJ	↑Sugar ↑Salt	122, 223, 202	Average
Pickled onions, white	220kJ	↑Salt ↑Sugar	223, 202	Average
Capers	120kJ	↑Salt	220	Average
Sweet peppers	618kJ	↑Sugar	223, 211	Average
Corn relish	421kJ	↑Sugar	102, 223, 220	Average

Baxters

Product Name	Energy	Major Nutrients	Food Additives	Nutritious Rating
Tomato chutney with red pepper	644kJ	↑Salt ↑Sugar	✓	Average
Tomato chutney	644kJ	↑Sugar	223	Average
Mango chutney	732kJ	↑Sugar	223	Average
Fruit chutney	853kJ	↑Salt ↑Sugar	223, 220	Average
Sweet chilli chutney	647kJ	↑Sugar	223	Average
Red currant jelly	1105kJ	↑Sugar	✓	Average

Beerenberg

Product Name	Energy	Major Nutrients	Food Additives	Nutritious Rating
Worcestershire sauce chutney	530kJ	↑Salt ↑Sugar	220	Poor
Taka Tala chutney	762kJ	↑Sugar	220	Average
Australian mango chutney	614kJ	↑Sugar	220, 223	Average
Tomato chutney	500kJ	↑Sugar	220	Average
Hot tomato chutney	383kJ	↑Sugar	220	Average
Fruit chutney	845kJ	↑Salt ↑Sugar	220	Average
Sweet chilli relish	1010kJ	↑Sugar	220	Average
Green tomato pickle	420kJ	↑Sugar	220	Average
Caramalised onion	730kJ	↑Sugar	220	Poor
Spicy caramalised onion	890kJ	↑Sugar	220	Poor
Mint jelly	1180kJ	↑Sugar	220	Poor
Red currant jelly	1170kJ	↑Sugar	✓	Poor

Blue Banner

Product Name	Energy	Major Nutrients	Food Additives	Nutritious Rating
Pickled onions	305kJ	↑Salt ↑Sugar	✓	Average
Pickled onions, chilli	305kJ	↑Salt ↑Sugar	✓	Average

Coles

Product Name	Energy	Major Nutrients	Food Additives	Nutritious Rating
Pickled onions	331kJ	↑Salt ↑Sugar	✓	Average
Cocktail onions, white	234kJ	↑Salt	223, 202	Average
Char grilled peppers	324kJ	✓	✓	Average
Olives, mixed green & kalamata	780kJ	↑Salt ↑Sugar ↑Fat	220	Average
Sundried tomatoes, strips	865kJ	↑Salt ↑Fat	✓	Average
Corn relish	476kJ	↑Sugar	223	Poor
Sweet mustard pickles	372kJ	↑Salt ↑Sugar	223	Poor
Fruit chutney	448kJ	↑Sugar	223	Poor
Mint jelly	1120kJ	↑Sugar	220	Poor
Mustard Dijon	448kJ	↑Salt	220, 223	Poor
Hot English mustard	617kJ	↑Salt ↑Fat	223	Poor
Wholegrain mustard	622kJ	↑Salt ↑Fat	220, 223	Poor
Sweet & Sour cucumbers	353kJ	↑Sugar	✓	Average
Smart buy pickled onion, white	306kJ	↑Sugar	224	Average

Crosse & Blackwell

Product Name	Energy	Major Nutrients	Food Additives	Nutritious Rating
Branston pickles	120kJ	✓	223	Average

Fehlbergs

Product Name	Energy	Major Nutrients	Food Additives	Nutritious Rating
Pickled onions, chilli	263kJ	↑Salt ↑Sugar	220	Average
Pickled onions, old	263kJ	↑Salt	220	Average

198

English brown		↑Sugar		

French's

Product Name	Energy	Major Nutrients	Food Additives	Nutritious Rating
Mustard, yellow	435kJ	↑Salt	220	Poor

Hoyts

Product Name	Energy	Major Nutrients	Food Additives	Nutritious Rating
Peppers, mild	229kJ	↑Sugar ↑Salt	223	Average
Peppers, hot	144kJ	↑Salt	223	Average
Luppini beans	474kJ	↑Salt	202	Average
Sundried tomatoes	1260kJ	↑Salt ↑Fat	220	Average

IGA/Franklins

Product Name	Energy	Major Nutrients	Food Additives	Nutritious Rating
Black & Gold, corn relish	439kJ	↑Sugar	102, 220, 223	Average
Black & Gold, fruit chutney	740kJ	↑Salt ↑Sugar	223	Average
Black & Gold, white onions	220kJ	↑Salt ↑Sugar	223, 202	Average
Black & Gold, dill gherkins	83kJ	✓	954	Average
Black & Gold, sweet spiced gherkins	280kJ	↑Sugar	102, 133	Average
Black & Gold, green olives	450kJ	↑Salt	202	Average
Black & Gold, green stuffed olives	470kJ	↑Salt	202	Average

Maille

Product Name	Energy	Major Nutrients	Food Additives	Nutritious Rating
Mustard, Dijon	631kJ	↑Salt	224	Poor

		↑Fat		
Mustard, Dijonnaise	426kJ	↑Salt ↑Fat ↑Sugar	220, 223	Poor
Mustard, mild wholegrain	620kJ	↑Salt ↑Fat	224, 220	Poor
Béarnaise	588kJ	↑Salt ↑Fat	220, 223	Poor
Hollandaise	2000kJ	↑Salt ↑Fat	220, 223	Poor

Masterfoods

Product Name	Energy	Major Nutrients	Food Additives	Nutritious Rating
Café relish, tomato	439kJ	↑Salt ↑Sugar	223	Average
Mango chutney	607kJ	↑Sugar	220	Average
Corn relish	460kJ	↑Sugar	223	Average
Green tomato relish	604kJ	↑Sugar	YE	Average
Honey mustard squeeze bottle	677kJ	↑Salt ↑Sugar	223	Poor
Horseradish cream	758kJ	↑Salt ↑Fat	224	Poor
Mustard, French	501kJ	↑Salt	223	Poor
Mustard, American squeeze	480kJ	↑Salt	223	Poor
Mustard, Australian	483kJ	↑Salt	223	Poor
Mustard, Dijon	490kJ	↑Salt ↑Fat	223	Poor
Mustard, English	673kJ	↑Salt ↑Fat	223	Poor
Mint jelly	1140kJ	↑Sugar	220	Poor

Rosella

Product Name	Energy	Major Nutrients	Food Additives	Nutritious Rating
Fruit chutney	675kJ	↑Salt ↑Sugar	220, 223	Average
Sweet mustard	304kJ	↑Salt	223, 220	Average

pickles		↑Sugar		
Sweet tomato chutney	623kJ	↑Sugar	YE, 220, 223	Average

Sandhurst

Product Name	Energy	Major Nutrients	Food Additives	Nutritious Rating
Sundried tomatoes, fat free	1014kJ	↑Salt	220	Average
Sundried tomatoes, vegetable oil	1326kJ	↑Salt ↑Sugar ↑Fat	220	Average
Semi sundried tomatoes	917kJ	↑Salt ↑Fat	220	Average
Semi sundried tomatoes, lite	950kJ	↑Salt	202	Average
Marinated artichokes, fat free	126kJ	✓	✓	Average
Marinated artichokes, 97% fat free	173kJ	✓	✓	Average

Spring Gully

Product Name	Energy	Major Nutrients	Food Additives	Nutritious Rating
Green tomato pickles	556kJ	↑Sugar	✓	Average
Sweet mustard pickles	419kJ	↑Sugar	102, 223	Average
Sweet white onions	275kJ	↑Sugar	223	Average
Corn relish	375kJ	↑Sugar	✓	Average
Savoury tomato chutney	240kJ	✓	✓	Average
Sundried tomato chutney	367kJ	↑Sugar	220	Average
Mango & chilli chutney	678kJ	↑Sugar	✓	Average

Three Threes

Product Name	Energy	Major Nutrients	Food Additives	Nutritious Rating
Sweet mustard pickles	372kJ	↑Salt ↑Sugar	102, 223	Average
Pickled onions, old style	**110kJ**	✓	✓	**Average**
Pickled onions, Australian	280kJ	↑Salt ↑Sugar	220	Average
Sandwich pickles	372kJ	↑Salt ↑Sugar	102, 223	Average

Woolworths/Safeways

Product Name	Energy	Major Nutrients	Food Additives	Nutritious Rating
Select, Italian cerignola olives	**444kJ**	**↑Salt ↑Fat**	✓	**Average**
Select, Greek kalamata olives whole	872kJ	↑Salt ↑Fat	220	Average
Select, Greek kalamata olives pitted	1162kJ	↑Salt ↑Fat	220	Average
Select, borettane onions	178kJ	↑Salt	220	Average
Select, sundried tomatoes	775kJ	↑Salt	220	Average
Select, char-grilled peppers	376kJ	↑Salt	220	Average
Select, red & yellow peppers	162kJ	↑Salt	220	Average
Select, filleted peppers	68kJ	↑Salt	220	Average
Select, char-grilled eggplant	380kJ	↑Salt	220	Average
Select, traditional dolmades	**658kJ**	**↑Salt ↑Fat**	✓	**Average**
Select, pine nut & raisin dolmades	**678kJ**	**↑Salt ↑Fat**	✓	**Average**
Select, eggplant &	**628kJ**	**↑Salt**	✓	**Average**

green pepper dolmades		↑Fat		
Homebrand, gherkins	466kJ	↑Sugar	✓	Average
Homebrand, green olives	523kJ	↑Salt ↑Fat	✓	Average
Homebrand, green stuffed olives	416kJ	↑Salt ↑Fat	✓	Average
Homebrand, fruit chutney	733kJ	↑Salt ↑Sugar	✓	Average
Homebrand, corn relish	441kJ	↑Sugar	102, 220, 223	Average

Mayonnaise, Sauces & Dressings

Best mayonnaise is *Norganic and SW*, for being additive free and using cage free eggs and non GM oils. Best sauces are from the *Outback spirit range, Rosella, Kikoman, IGA purely organic, Macro organic Spring valet, Ocean spray and Ayum.*

Ayam

Product Name	Energy	Major Nutrients	Food Additives	Nutritious Rating
Thick soya sauce	949kJ	↑Salt ↑Sugar	✓	Poor
Soya sauce	247kJ	↑Salt ↑Sugar	✓	Poor
Oyster sauce	535kJ	↑Salt ↑Sugar	YE	Poor
Fish sauce	21kJ	↑Salt	✓	Poor
Honey soy sauce	598kJ	↑Salt ↑Sugar	YE, 223, 220	Poor
Teriyaki sauce	142kJ	↑Salt	✓	Poor
Sweet & sour sauce	786kJ	↑Salt ↑Sugar	✓	Poor
Hoi sin sauce	782kJ	↑Salt ↑Sugar	✓	Poor
Plum sauce	765kJ	↑Salt ↑Sugar	✓	Poor
Chilli garlic sauce	589kJ	↑Salt ↑Sugar	✓	Average
Chilli sweet sauce	752kJ	↑Salt ↑Sugar	✓	Average
Chilli hot sauce	552kJ	↑Salt ↑Sugar	220	Average
Sweet chilli finger sauce	787kJ	↑Salt ↑Sugar	951, 950	Average
Thai green curry sauce	573kJ	↑Salt ↑Fat	✓	Average
Thai red curry	627kJ	↑Fat	✓	Average

sauce				
Thai massaman curry sauce	794kJ	↑Fat	✓	Average
Rendang curry sauce	752kJ	↑Salt ↑Fat	220	Average
Sambal sauce	698kJ	↑Salt ↑Sugar ↑Fat	✓	Average
Laksa sauce	435kJ	↑Salt	202	Average
Satay sauce	986kJ	↑Fat	223, 202	Average

Beerenberg

Product Name	Energy	Major Nutrients	Food Additives	Nutritious Rating
Huey's Asian plum sauce	425kJ	↑Salt ↑Sugar	220	Poor
Tak tala sauce & marinade	1037kJ	↑Sugar	YE, 220	Poor
Honey & lemon soy sauce marinade	572kJ	↑Salt ↑Sugar	220, 223	Poor
Sweet mustard sauce	460kJ	↑Salt ↑Sugar	200, 223	Poor
Peppercorn sauce	1220kJ	↑Salt ↑Fat	YE, 220, 223	Poor
Garlic sauce	1234kJ	↑Salt ↑Fat	220	Poor
Tartare sauce	1075kJ	↑Salt ↑Sugar ↑Fat	220	Poor
Creamy seafood sauce	1730kJ	↑Salt ↑Sugar ↑Fat	320, 220, 223	Poor
Coopers BBQ sauce	572kJ	↑Sugar	220	Poor
Chilli sauce	595kJ	↑Sugar	220	Average
Tomato sauce	457kJ	↑Sugar	220	Average
Hot tomato sauce	457kJ	↑Sugar	220	Average
Traditional Diane sauce	610kJ	↑Salt ↑Sugar	YE	Poor
Sticky rib sauce	770kJ	↑Salt	220	Poor

		↑Sugar		
Creamy parm Caesar dressing	1020kJ	↑Salt ↑Sugar ↑Fat	220	Poor
Blue cheese dressing	1330kJ	↑Salt ↑Fat	220	Poor
Ranch dressing	1390kJ	↑Salt ↑Sugar ↑Fat	YE, 220	Poor
Creamy parm	1020kJ	↑Salt ↑Sugar ↑Fat	220	Poor

Best Foods

Product Name	Energy	Major Nutrients	Food Additives	Nutritious Rating
Mayonnaise	2960kJ	↑Salt ↑Fat	220, 223	Poor

Café 26

Product Name	Energy	Major Nutrients	Food Additives	Nutritious Rating
Caesar dressing	867kJ	↑Salt ↑Fat	220, 223	Poor
Original dressing	695kJ	↑Salt ↑Sugar	220, 223	Poor
Oriental dressing	852kJ	↑Salt ↑Sugar	220, 223	Poor
Tangy dressing	703kJ	↑Salt ↑Sugar	220, 223	Poor

Cardinis

Product Name	Energy	Major Nutrients	Food Additives	Nutritious Rating
Caesar salad dressing	2265kJ	↑Salt ↑Fat	220, 223	Poor
Caesar salad croutons	1550kJ	↑Salt ↑Fat	YE	Poor

Changs

Product Name	Energy	Major Nutrients	Food Additives	Nutritious Rating
Oyster sauce	324kJ	↑Salt	621	Poor

Classic Asia

Product Name	Energy	Major Nutrients	Food Additives	Nutritious Rating
Stir fry wok sauce	538kJ	↑Salt ↑Sugar	✓	Poor
Cantonese black bean sauce	567kJ	↑Salt ↑Sugar	✓	Poor
Cantonese lemon sauce	601kJ	↑Salt ↑Sugar	223	Poor
Cantonese sweet & sour sauce	567kJ	↑Salt ↑Sugar	220	Poor
Cantonese dim sim sauce	643kJ	↑Salt ↑Sugar	220	Poor

Coles

Product Name	Energy	Major Nutrients	Food Additives	Nutritious Rating
Apple sauce	409kJ	↑Sugar	✓	Average
BBQ sauce	743kJ	↑Salt ↑Sugar	223	Poor
Cranberry sauce	657kJ	↑Sugar	✓	Average
Mayonnaise 97% fat free	520kJ	↑Salt ↑Sugar	160b, 223, 320	Poor
Mayonnaise 97% fat free squeeze bottle	520kJ	↑Salt ↑Sugar	160b, 223, 320	Poor
Whole egg mayonnaise	3030kJ	↑Fat	223, 220	Poor
Oyster sauce	580kJ	↑Salt ↑Sugar	YE	Poor
Tomato sauce	471kJ	↑Salt ↑Sugar	✓	Average
Tomato sauce squeeze bottle	471kJ	↑Salt ↑Sugar	✓	Average

Tomato sauce, organic	540kJ	↑Salt ↑Sugar	✓	Average
Soy sauce	230kJ	↑Salt	202	Poor
Sweet chilli sauce	**1062kJ**	↑Salt ↑Sugar	✓	Average
Worcestershire sauce	417kJ	↑Salt ↑Sugar	VP	Poor
Dressing, caesar	1390kJ	↑Salt ↑Fat	223	Poor
Dressing, coleslaw	1490kJ	↑Salt ↑Fat ↑Sugar	220, 223	Poor
Dijonaise	350kJ	↑Salt ↑Sugar	223	Poor
Smart buy BBQ sauce	**645kJ**	↑Sugar	✓	Poor
Smart buy tomato sauce	**414kJ**	↑Salt ↑Sugar	✓	Average
Smart buy soy sauce	136kJ	↑Salt	HVP	Poor

Colmans

Product Name	Energy	Major Nutrients	Food Additives	Nutritious Rating
Horseradish	468kJ	✓	223, 220	Average

Cornwells

Product Name	Energy	Major Nutrients	Food Additives	Nutritious Rating
Mint sauce	**300kJ**	↑Sugar	✓	Poor
Mint sauce, thick	320kJ	↑Sugar	102, 133, 220	Poor

ETA

Product Name	Energy	Major Nutrients	Food Additives	Nutritious Rating
Barbecue sauce	850kJ	↑Salt ↑Sugar	220	Poor
Potato salad dressing	1040kJ	↑Salt ↑Sugar ↑Fat	320, 220	Poor

Honey BBQ sauce	930kJ	↑Salt ↑Sugar	220	Poor

French's

Product Name	Energy	Major Nutrients	Food Additives	Nutritious Rating
Mustard, yellow	435kJ	↑Salt	220	Poor

Fountains

Product Name	Energy	Major Nutrients	Food Additives	Nutritious Rating
BBQ sauce	715kJ	↑Salt ↑Sugar	✓	Poor
Barbecue classic sauce	738kJ	↑Salt ↑Sugar	✓	Poor
BBQ sauce, reduced salt & sugar	530kJ	↑Sugar	202	Poor
Chilli sauce, mild	315kJ	↑Salt	202, 223	Average
Chilli sauce, hot	720kJ	↑Salt ↑Sugar	220	Average
Sweet chilli sauce	836kJ	↑Salt ↑Sugar	202, 223	Average
Mint sauce	330kJ	↑Sugar	✓	Poor
Mint sauce, thick	628kJ	↑Sugar	202, 223	Poor
Plum sauce	665kJ	↑Salt ↑Sugar	HVP	Poor
Hoisin sauce	728kJ	↑Sugar	HVP	Poor
Spicy red sauce	767kJ	↑Salt ↑Sugar	223	Poor
Steak sauce	884kJ	↑Salt ↑Sugar	223	Poor
Tomato sauce	545kJ	↑Salt ↑Sugar	✓	Average
Tomato sauce, reduced salt & sugar	373kJ	↑Sugar	✓	Average
Worcestershire sauce	363kJ	↑Salt ↑Sugar	223	Poor
Mustard sauce	565kJ	↑Sugar	220, 223	Poor

Satay sauce	965kJ	↑Salt ↑Sugar ↑Fat	220, 223, HVP	Poor
Pepper steak sauce	625kJ	↑Sugar	202, 223	Poor

Heinz

Product Name	Energy	Major Nutrients	Food Additives	Nutritious Rating
Big red tomato sauce, squeezy	470kJ	↑Salt ↑Sugar	✓	Average
Tomato ketchup	515kJ	↑Salt ↑Sugar	✓	Average
Organic ketchup	480kJ	↑Salt ↑Sugar	✓	Average
Mayonnaise	1790kJ	↑Salt ↑Sugar ↑Fat	319	Poor

Hellman's

Product Name	Energy	Major Nutrients	Food Additives	Nutritious Rating
Mayonnaise	2970kJ	↑Salt ↑Fat	223,220	Poor

Holbrook's

Product Name	Energy	Major Nutrients	Food Additives	Nutritious Rating
Worcestershire sauce	330kJ	↑Salt ↑Sugar	220, 223	Poor

HP

Product Name	Energy	Major Nutrients	Food Additives	Nutritious Rating
Original sauce	540kJ	↑Salt ↑Sugar	220	Poor

IGA/Franklins

Product Name	Energy	Major	Food	Nutritious

		Nutrients	Additives	Rating
IGA French dressing	335kJ	↑Salt ↑Sugar	102, 220	Poor
IGA Italian dressing	378kJ	↑Salt ↑Sugar	220	Poor
IGA tomato sauce	455kJ	↑Salt ↑Sugar	✓	Average
IGA Puerly Organic tomato sauce	406kJ	↑Sugar	✓	Average
IGA Puerly Organic sweet chilli sauce	920kJ	↑Salt ↑Sugar	✓	Average
Black & Gold mayonnaise	943kJ	↑Salt ↑Sugar ↑Fat	202, 220, 223	Poor
Black & Gold tomato sauce	455kJ	↑Salt ↑Sugar	✓	Average
Black & Gold BBQ sauce	802kJ	↑Salt ↑Sugar	✓	Average
Black & Gold sweet chilli sauce	820kJ	↑Salt ↑Sugar	220	Average

Kikoman

Product Name	Energy	Major Nutrients	Food Additives	Nutritious Rating
Soy sauce	411kJ	↑Salt	✓	Poor
Soy sauce, salt reduced	529kJ	↑Salt	✓	Poor
Soy sauce, gluten free	421kJ	↑Salt	✓	Poor
Soy sauce, sweet	742kJ	↑Salt	✓	Poor
Soy sauce, organic	392kJ	↑Salt	✓	Poor

Kraft

Product Name	Energy	Major Nutrients	Food Additives	Nutritious Rating
Mayonnaise, classic	973kJ	↑Salt ↑Fat	320, 202, 223	Poor
Mayonnaise, classic squeeze	973kJ	↑Salt ↑Fat	320, 202, 223	Poor
Mayonnaise, 97% fat free	490kJ	↑Salt ↑Sugar	320, 202, 223	Poor
Mayonnaise, egg	2930kJ	↑Fat	223, 320, 200	Poor
Mayonnaise, creamy	2040kJ	↑Salt ↑Sugar ↑Fat	223, 320, 200	Poor
Miracle whip	1592kJ	↑Fat	320, 200	Poor
Salad dressing, Moroccan 99% fat free	343kJ	↑Salt ↑Sugar	220	Poor
Salad dressing, basil & herb pasta	1420kJ	↑Salt ↑Sugar ↑Fat	320, 220	Poor
Salad dressing, Caesar creamy	1320kJ	↑Salt ↑Fat	320, 202	Poor
Salad dressing, Caesar 99% fat free	356kJ	↑Salt ↑Sugar	200, 220	Poor
Salad dressing, coleslaw	1580kJ	↑Salt ↑Sugar ↑Fat	320	Poor
Salad dressing, coleslaw 99% fat free	558kJ	↑Salt ↑Sugar	202, 220	Poor
Salad dressing, French classic	829kJ	↑Salt ↑Sugar ↑Fat	320, 102, 220	Poor
Salad dressing, French 99% fat free	186kJ	↑Salt	102, 220	Poor
Salad dressing, Italian 99% fat free	244kJ	↑Salt ↑Sugar	223, 220	Poor
Salad dressing,	305kJ	↑Salt	223, 220	Poor

Italian balsamic		↑Sugar		
Salad dressing, chilli & lime fat free	279kJ	↑Salt ↑Sugar	220	Poor
Salad dressing, thousand island	1410kJ	↑Salt ↑Sugar ↑Fat	320, 220	Poor
Salad dressing, tangy tomato	1870kJ	↑Salt ↑Sugar ↑Fat	320, 220	Poor

Lea & Perrins

Product Name	Energy	Major Nutrients	Food Additives	Nutritious Rating
Worcestershire sauce	440kJ	↑Salt ↑Sugar	220	Poor

Macro (Woolworths/Safeways)

Product Name	Energy	Major Nutrients	Food Additives	Nutritious Rating
Organic sweet chilli sauce	876kJ	↑Sugar	✓	Average
Organic BBQ sauce	427kJ	↑Salt ↑Sugar	✓	Average
Organic tomato sauce	380kJ	↑Sugar	✓	Average

Maggi

Product Name	Energy	Major Nutrients	Food Additives	Nutritious Rating
Sweet chilli sauce	860kJ	↑Salt ↑Sugar	✓	Average
Hot chilli sauce	750kJ	↑Salt ↑Sugar	220	Average

Masterfoods

Product Name	Energy	Major Nutrients	Food Additives	Nutritious Rating
Barbecue sauce	1074kJ	↑Salt ↑Sugar	YE, 220	Poor
Barbecue sauce, salt reduced	822kJ	↑Salt ↑Sugar	YE, 220	Poor
Tartare sauce	2577kJ	↑Salt ↑Fat	✓	Poor
Tomato ketchup	581kJ	↑Salt ↑Sugar	✓	Average
Tomato sauce, salt reduced	439kJ	↑Salt ↑Sugar	✓	Average
Tomato sauce, sun ripened	475kJ	↑Salt ↑Sugar	223	Average
Seafood sauce	883kJ	↑Salt ↑Sugar ↑Fat	320	Poor
Steak sauce	714kJ	↑Salt ↑Sugar	HVE, 223	Poor
Sweet & sour sauce	642kJ	↑Salt ↑Sugar	220	Average
Sweet chilli sauce	1043kJ	↑Salt ↑Sugar	✓	Average
Hot chilli sauce	399kJ	↑Salt ↑Sugar	223	Average
Smokey BBQ sauce	853kJ	↑Salt ↑Sugar	YE	Poor

McIlhenny

Product Name	Energy	Major Nutrients	Food Additives	Nutritious Rating
Tabasco sauce	60kJ	↑Salt	220	Average

McKenkies

Product Name	Energy	Major Nutrients	Food Additives	Nutritious Rating
BBQ sauce	1380kJ	↑Salt ↑Fat	VPE, 220	Poor

Dijon mustard sauce	1160kJ	↑Salt ↑Sugar	223	Poor
Tomato sauce	510kJ	↑Salt ↑Sugar	✓	Average
Tomato curry sauce	542kJ	↑Salt ↑Sugar	✓	Average

Nandos

Product Name	Energy	Major Nutrients	Food Additives	Nutritious Rating
Peri peri sauce, mild	288kJ	↑Salt	1520, 220	Average
Peri peri sauce, hot	314kJ	↑Salt	1520, 220, 223	Average
Peri peri sauce, extra hot	298kJ	↑Salt	1520, 220, 223	Average
Peri peri sauce, sweet chilli	613kJ	↑Salt ↑Sugar	223	Average
Perinaise	966kJ	↑Salt ↑Fat ↑Sugar	202, 223, 220	Poor

Noganic

Product Name	Energy	Major Nutrients	Food Additives	Nutritious Rating
Golden soya mayonnaise	2760kJ	↑Salt ↑Fat	✓	Poor
Golden soya mayonnaise, organic	962kJ	↑Salt ↑Fat	✓	Poor

Ocean Spray

Product Name	Energy	Major Nutrients	Food Additives	Nutritious Rating
Cranberry sauce	657kJ	↑Sugar	✓	Average
Cranberry sauce, whole berry	657kJ	↑Sugar	✓	Average

Outback Spirit

Product Name	Energy	Major Nutrients	Food Additives	Nutritious Rating
Barbecue sauce	486kJ	↑Sugar	✓	Poor
Tomato chutney	830kJ	↑Sugar ↑Salt	✓	Average
Kakadu plum chilli sauce	927kJ	↑Sugar	✓	Poor
Wild lime, chilli & ginger sauce	954kJ	↑Sugar ↑Salt	✓	Poor
Mango & mint chutney	473kJ	↑Sugar ↑Salt	✓	Average
Tomato sauce	391kJ	↑Sugar ↑Salt	✓	Poor

Paul Newman's Own

Product Name	Energy	Major Nutrients	Food Additives	Nutritious Rating
Egg aioli	2913kJ	↑Fat	220, 223	Poor
Mayonnaise, whole egg	3080kJ	↑Salt ↑Fat	223, 220	Poor
Mayonnaise, whole egg, lime & chilli	2735kJ	↑Fat	223, 220	Poor
Salad dressing, balsamic	1435kJ	↑Salt ↑Fat	220	Poor
Salad dressing, balsamic light	640kJ	↑Salt ↑Fat	220	Poor
Salad dressing, classic	1610kJ	↑Fat	223, 220, 200	Poor
Salad dressing, creamy Caesar	2281kJ	↑Salt ↑Fat	223	Poor
Salad dressing, classic Asian	840kJ	↑Salt ↑Fat ↑Sugar	223, 220	Poor
Salad dressing, parmesan & roasted garlic	1575kJ	↑Salt ↑Fat	223, 220	Poor
Salad dressing, honey mustard light	975kJ	↑Salt ↑Fat	223, 202	Poor

| Salad dressing, ranch | 2480kJ | ↑Salt ↑Fat | 223 | Poor |
| Salad dressing, south west | 2120kJ | ↑Salt ↑Fat | 223 | Poor |

Pearl River Bridge

Product Name	Energy	Major Nutrients	Food Additives	Nutritious Rating
Soy sauce, light	209kJ	↑Salt	202	Poor

Praise

Product Name	Energy	Major Nutrients	Food Additives	Nutritious Rating
Mayonnaise, traditional	2605kJ	↑Salt ↑Fat	320, 220	Poor
Mayonnaise, traditional squeeze bottle	2605kJ	↑Salt ↑Fat	320, 220	Poor
Mayonnaise, whole egg	3100kJ	↑Fat	223 320	Poor
Mayonnaise, whole egg light	1350kJ	↑Salt ↑Fat ↑Sugar	320, 220	Poor
Mayonnaise, whole egg squeeze bottle	1350kJ	↑Salt ↑Fat ↑Sugar	320, 220	Poor
Mayonnaise, 97% fat free	510kJ	↑Salt ↑Sugar	320, 220	Poor
Mayonnaise, 97% fat free squeeze bottle	510kJ	↑Salt ↑Sugar	320, 220	Poor
Dressing, whole egg potato salad	2625kJ	↑Salt ↑Fat	320, 220	Poor
Dressing, seafood	2010kJ	↑Salt ↑Fat ↑Sugar	320, 220	Poor
Dressing, coleslaw	1790kJ	↑Salt ↑Sugar	320, 202, 220, 223	Poor
Dressing, coleslaw 99% fat free	500kJ	↑Salt ↑Sugar	320, 202, 220	Poor

Dressing, seafood lemon & dill	2140kJ	↑Salt ↑Fat ↑Sugar	320, 223	Poor
Dressing, tartare	1914kJ	↑Salt ↑Fat	320, 223	Poor
Dressing, tartare 97% fat free	600kJ	↑Salt ↑Sugar	320, 223	Poor
Dressing, thousand island	1180kJ	↑Salt ↑Fat ↑Sugar	320, 220	Poor
Dressing, thousand island fat free	620kJ	↑Salt ↑Sugar	160b, 320, 202	Poor
Dressing, ranch 99% fat free	360kJ	↑Salt ↑Sugar	202, 220	Poor
Dressing, Caesar	1330kJ	↑Salt ↑Fat ↑Sugar	320, 220	Poor
Dressing, Caesar 99% fat free	500kJ	↑Salt ↑Sugar	202, 223	Poor
Dressing, deli style creamy roasted garlic	2145kJ	↑Salt ↑Fat	320, 220	Poor
Dressing, deli style balsamic & roasted garlic	885kJ	↑Salt ↑Fat ↑Sugar	220, 320	Poor
Dressing, deli style French vinaigrette	830kJ	↑Salt ↑Fat	320, 407	Poor
Dressing, deli style Italian herb vinaigrette	805kJ	↑Salt ↑Fat ↑Sugar	320, 407	Poor
Dressing, balsamic	885kJ	↑Salt ↑Fat ↑Sugar	320, 407	Poor
Dressing, balsamic fat free	205kJ	↑Salt ↑Sugar	223, 220, 407	Poor
Dressing, classic vinaigrette	845kJ	↑Salt ↑Fat	320, 407, 220	Poor
Dressing, French	930kJ	↑Salt ↑Fat	320, 407, 220	Poor

Product Name	Energy	Major Nutrients	Food Additives	Nutritious Rating
		↑Sugar		
Dressing, French fat free	320kJ	↑Sugar ↑Salt	220, 407	Poor
Dressing, Italian	830kJ	↑Salt ↑Fat	320, 407, 223	Poor
Dressing, Italian fat free	180kJ	↑Sugar	223, 407	Poor
Dressing, Italian balsamic	850kJ	↑Salt ↑Fat	320, 407, 223, 220	Poor
Dressing, honey Dijon	1040kJ	↑Salt ↑Fat ↑Sugar	320, 202, 220, 223	Poor

Red Kelly's

Product Name	Energy	Major Nutrients	Food Additives	Nutritious Rating
Dressing, basil & garlic	1610kJ	↑Salt ↑Sugar	223	Poor
Dressing, Italian	1500kJ	↑Sugar ↑Fat	223	Poor
Dressing, lemon myrtle	1520kJ	↑Sugar ↑Fat	223	Poor
Dressing, traditional	1470kJ	↑Sugar ↑Fat	223	Poor

Rosella

Product Name	Energy	Major Nutrients	Food Additives	Nutritious Rating
Tomato sauce	441kJ	↑Salt ↑Sugar	✓	Poor
Tomato sauce, squeeze bottle	441kJ	↑Salt ↑Sugar	✓	Poor
BBQ sauce	668kJ	↑Salt ↑Sugar	✓	Poor

S&W

Product Name	Energy	Major Nutrients	Food Additives	Nutritious Rating
Mayonnaise, whole	3070kJ	↑Salt	220, 223	Poor

		↑Fat		
Mayonnaise, whole egg squeeze bottle	3070kJ	↑Salt ↑Fat	220, 223	Poor
Mayonnaise, light	1710kJ	↑Salt ↑Fat	220, 223	Poor

SPC

Product Name	Energy	Major Nutrients	Food Additives	Nutritious Rating
Apple sauce	**386kJ**	↑Sugar	✓	**Poor**
Plum sauce	1330kJ	↑Sugar	HVP, VP	Poor

Spring Gully

Product Name	Energy	Major Nutrients	Food Additives	Nutritious Rating
Worcestershire sauce	835kJ	↑Sugar	✓	Poor

Thomy

Product Name	Energy	Major Nutrients	Food Additives	Nutritious Rating
Mayonnaise, delikatess	3163kJ	↑Fat	220, 223	Poor

Three Threes

Product Name	Energy	Major Nutrients	Food Additives	Nutritious Rating
BBQ rib sauce	692kJ	↑Sugar ↑Salt	160b, 220	Poor
Mint jelly	1115kJ	↑Sugar	220	Poor
Apple sauce	**409kJ**	↑Sugar	✓	**Poor**
Tomato sauce	433kJ	↑Sugar ↑Salt	220, 223	Poor
Burger & steak sauce	1045kJ	↑Sugar ↑Fat	211, 223, 220	Poor

Trident

Product Name	Energy	Major Nutrients	Food Additives	Nutritious Rating
Sweet chilli & ginger sauce	1280kJ	↑Sugar ↑Salt	220	Poor
Sweet chilli sauce	1280kJ	↑Sugar ↑Salt	220	Poor
Sweet chilli sauce, squeeze bottle	1280kJ	↑Sugar ↑Salt	220	Poor
Thai sweet chilli sauce	1280kJ	↑Sugar ↑Salt	220	Poor

Wilds

Product Name	Energy	Major Nutrients	Food Additives	Nutritious Rating
Ezy sauce	40kJ	✓	✓	Poor

Woolworths/Safeways

Product Name	Energy	Major Nutrients	Food Additives	Nutritious Rating
Select, sweet chilli sauce	882kJ	↑Sugar ↑Salt	223	Poor
Select, steak sauce	906kJ	↑Sugar ↑Salt	220 , 223	Poor
Select, chilli BBQ sauce	995kJ	↑Sugar ↑Salt	✓	Poor
Select, Worcestershire sauce	454kJ	↑Sugar ↑Salt	VP	Poor
Select, ketchup	574kJ	↑Sugar ↑Salt	✓	Poor
Select, barbecue sauce	921kJ	↑Sugar ↑Salt	✓	Poor
Select, burger sauce	477kJ	↑Sugar	223	Poor
Select, tomato sauce	685kJ	↑Sugar ↑Salt	✓	Average
Select, coleslaw dressing	1480kJ	↑Sugar ↑Salt ↑Fat	202, 223, 220	Poor

Select, 97% fat free mayonnaise	640kJ	↑Sugar ↑Salt	VP, 220, 223	Poor
Select, ranch dressing	2470kJ	↑Fat ↑Salt	223, 220	Poor
Select, whole egg mayonnaise	3050kJ	↑Fat ↑Salt	223, 220	Poor
Select, honey mustard dressing	1720kJ	↑Sugar ↑Salt ↑Fat	220, 223, 200, 202	Poor
Select, balsamic dressing	651kJ	↑Sugar ↑Salt ↑Fat	202, 223, 220	Poor
Select, Italian dressing	752kJ	↑Salt	202, 223, 220	Poor
Select, Italian dressing 99% fat free	358kJ	↑Sugar ↑Salt	202, 223, 220	Poor
Select, balsamic dressing 99% fat free	448kJ	↑Sugar ↑Salt	202, 223, 220	Poor
Select, Greek dressing 99% fat free	249kJ	↑Salt	202, 223, 220	Poor
Select, Caeser dressing	1580kJ	↑Sugar ↑Salt ↑Fat	202, 220, 211, 223	Poor
Select, French dressing fat free	374kJ	↑Sugar ↑Salt	220	Poor
Select, zesty Portuguese dressing	1880kJ	↑Sugar ↑Salt ↑Fat	202	Poor
Select, soy sauce	**289kJ**	**↑Salt**	✓	**Poor**
Select, tartare sauce	979kJ	↑Sugar ↑Salt ↑Fat	200, 220	Poor
Select, tartare sauce light	669kJ	↑Sugar ↑Salt	220, 223	Poor
Select, thick mint sauce	665kJ	↑Sugar	220	Poor

Select, cranberry sauce	657kJ	↑Sugar	✓	Average
Select, Apple sauce	180kJ	✓	✓	Average
Fish sauce	183kJ	↑Salt	✓	Poor
Hosin sauce	1436kJ	↑Sugar ↑Salt	✓	Poor
Oyster sauce	717kJ	↑Sugar ↑Salt	211	Poor
Keap manis sauce	781kJ	↑Sugar ↑Salt	220	Poor
Homebrand, thousand island dressing	1110kJ	↑Sugar ↑Salt ↑Fat	220, 320	Poor
Homebrand, French dressing	320kJ	↑Sugar ↑Salt	220	Poor
Homebrand, Italian dressing	380kJ	↑Sugar ↑Salt	220	Poor
Homebrand mayonnaise	691kJ	↑Sugar ↑Salt	220, 200	Poor
Homebrand, mayonnaise 97% fat free	650kJ	↑Sugar ↑Salt	220, 223, 200	Poor
Homebrand, tomato sauce	646kJ	↑Sugar ↑Salt	✓	Average
Homebrand, barbecue sauce	770kJ	↑Sugar ↑Salt	✓	Poor
Homebrand, Worcestershire sauce	398kJ	↑Sugar ↑Salt	VP	Poor
Homebrand, oyster sauce	822kJ	↑Sugar ↑Salt	✓	Poor
Homebrand, soy sauce	150kJ	↑Sugar ↑Salt	202	Poor
Homebrand, taco sauce mild	222kJ	↑Salt	220	Average
Homebrand, taco sauce medium	228kJ	↑Salt	220	Average

Jams & Spreads

My picks for jams and spreads are *Anathoth, Coles, Dick Smiths, Ceres organic,*

Eskal, Macro and Sanitarium.

Anathoth

Product Name	Energy	Major Nutrients	Food Additives	Nutritious Rating
Apricot jam	1130kJ	↑Sugar	✓	Average
Boysenberry jam	1140kJ	↑Sugar	✓	Average
Breakfast marmalade	1130kJ	↑Sugar	✓	Average
Cherry berry jam	1130kJ	↑Sugar	✓	Average
Raspberry jam	1150kJ	↑Sugar	✓	Average
Rhubarb & red cherry jam	1130kJ	↑Sugar	✓	Average
Strawberry jam	1120kJ	↑Sugar	✓	Average
Three berry jam	1150kJ	↑Sugar	✓	Average

Beerenberg

Product Name	Energy	Major Nutrients	Food Additives	Nutritious Rating
Apricot jam	1120kJ	↑Sugar	223	Average
Blackberry jam	1090kJ	↑Sugar	220	Average
Fig & almond jam	**1140kJ**	↑Sugar	✓	**Average**
Fruits of forest jam	1115kJ	↑Sugar	223	Average
Ginger marmalade	1170kJ	↑Sugar	223	Average
Lime & lemon marmalade	1110kJ	↑Sugar	220	
Orange marmalade	**1140kJ**	↑Sugar	✓	**Average**
Raspberry jam	1134kJ	↑Sugar	223	Average

Satsuma plum jam	1130kJ	↑Sugar	223	Average
Strawberry jam	1150kJ	↑Sugar	223	Average

Bonne Maman

Product Name	Energy	Major Nutrients	Food Additives	Nutritious Rating
Apricot jam	1000kJ	↑Sugar	223	Average
Blackberry jam	1000kJ	↑Sugar	223	Average
Blueberry jam	1000kJ	↑Sugar	223	Average
Cherry jam	1000kJ	↑Sugar	223	Average
Peach jam	1000kJ	↑Sugar	223	Average
Raspberry jam	1000kJ	↑Sugar	223	Average
Strawberry jam	1000kJ	↑Sugar	223	Average

Buderim

Product Name	Energy	Major Nutrients	Food Additives	Nutritious Rating
Ginger marmalade	1281kJ	↑Sugar	✓	Average
Ginger, lemon & lime spread	1264kJ	↑Sugar	223	Average

Ceres Organic

Product Name	Energy	Major Nutrients	Food Additives	Nutritious Rating
Peanut butter, crunchy	2380kJ	↑ Fat	✓	Average
Peanut butter, smooth	2380kJ	↑ Fat	✓	Average

Coles

Product Name	Energy	Major Nutrients	Food Additives	Nutritious Rating
Apricot jam	1114kJ	↑Sugar	✓	Average
Blackberry jam	1135kJ	↑Sugar	✓	Average
Blackcurrant jam	1123kJ	↑Sugar	✓	Average
Breakfast	1112kJ	↑Sugar	✓	Average

marmalade				
Plum jam	1112kJ	↑Sugar	✓	Average
Raspberry jam	1118kJ	↑Sugar	✓	Average
Strawberry jam	1118kJ	↑Sugar	✓	Average
Sweet orange marmalade	1156kJ	↑Sugar	✓	Average
Peanut butter, crunchy	2600kJ	↑ Fat	✓	Average
Peanut butter, smooth	2560kJ	↑ Fat	✓	Average
Peanut butter, no added salt	2560kJ	↑ Fat	✓	Average
Peanut butter, super crunchy	2550kJ	↑ Fat	✓	Average
Hazelnut spread	2356kJ	↑Sugar ↑Fat	✓	Average
Smart buy, apricot spread	1110kJ	↑Sugar	220	Average
Smart buy, breakfast marmalade	1110kJ	↑Sugar	220	Average
Smart buy, strawberry jam	1110kJ	↑Sugar	220	Average
Smart buy, crunchy peanut butter	2620kJ	↑ Fat	✓	Average
Smart buy, smooth peanut butter	2600kJ	↑ Fat	✓	Average

Cottees

Product Name	Energy	Major Nutrients	Food Additives	Nutritious Rating
Apricot jam	1140kJ	↑Sugar	220	Average
Blackberry jam	1150kJ	↑Sugar	220	Average
Blackcurrant jam	1110kJ	↑Sugar	220	Average

Breakfast marmalade	1150kJ	↑Sugar	223, 220	Average
Ginger marmalade	1140kJ	↑Sugar	220	Average
Mandarin & orange marmalade	1120kJ	↑Sugar	223, 220	Average
Plum jam	1100kJ	↑Sugar	✓	Average
Raspberry jam	1130kJ	↑Sugar	220	Average
Strawberry conserve	1110kJ	↑Sugar	220	Average

Dick Smiths

Product Name	Energy	Major Nutrients	Food Additives	Nutritious Rating
Peanut butter, crunchy	2570kJ	↑Salt ↑Fat	✓	Average
Peanut butter smooth	2530kJ	↑Salt ↑Fat	✓	Average

Eskal

Product Name	Energy	Major Nutrients	Food Additives	Nutritious Rating
Free nut, smooth	2620kJ	↑ Fat	✓	Average
Free nut, crunchy	2620kJ	↑ Fat	✓	Average

Freedom Foods

Product Name	Energy	Major Nutrients	Food Additives	Nutritious Rating
Vege spread	741kJ	↑Salt	VPE, 202	Poor

IGA/Franklins

Product Name	Energy	Major Nutrients	Food Additives	Nutritious Rating
Signature, hazelnut spread	2400kJ	↑Sugar ↑Fat	202	Average
Signature, peanut butter smooth	2610kJ	↑Fat	✓	Average

Signature, peanut butter smooth light	2040kJ	↑Fat	✓	Average
Signature, peanut butter crunchy	2600kJ	↑Fat	✓	Average
Signature, peanut butter crunchy light	2030kJ	↑Fat	✓	Average
Black & Gold, peanut butter smooth	2560kJ	↑Fat	✓	Average
Black & Gold, peanut butter crunchy	2450kJ	↑Fat	✓	Average
Black & Gold, cream cheese spread	1320kJ	↑Salt ↑Fat	202, 234	Poor
Black & Gold, apricot jam	1114kJ	↑Sugar	✓	Average
Black & Gold, blackberry jam	1119kJ	↑Sugar	✓	Average
Black & Gold, orange marmalade	1111kJ	↑Sugar	✓	Average
Black & Gold, plum jam	1124kJ	↑Sugar	123	Average
Black & Gold, raspberry jam	1113kJ	↑Sugar	✓	Average
Black & Gold, strawberry jam	1114kJ	↑Sugar	✓	Average

IXL

Product Name	Energy	Major Nutrients	Food Additives	Nutritious Rating
All about fruit, apricot spread	873kJ	↑Sugar	223	Average
All about fruit, marmalade spread	886kJ	↑Sugar	223	Average
All about fruit strawberry spread	893kJ	↑Sugar	223	Average
Breakfast marmalade	1130kJ	↑Sugar	✓	Average
Conserve, apricot	1115kJ	↑Sugar	✓	Average

Conserve, blackberry	1128kJ	↑Sugar	✓	Average
Conserve, fruits of the forest	1119kJ	↑Sugar	✓	Average
Conserve, ginger	1109kJ	↑Sugar	220	Average
Conserve, plum, raspberry & cranberry	1120kJ	↑Sugar	✓	Average
Conserve, blueberry, strawberry & cranberry	1112kJ	↑Sugar	✓	Average
Jam, plum	1114kJ	↑Sugar	✓	Average
Jam, grapefruit, lemon & lime	1108kJ	↑Sugar	✓	Average
Jam, raspberry	1116kJ	↑Sugar	✓	Average
Jam, strawberry	1123kJ	↑Sugar	✓	Average
Jam, blackberry 50% less sugar	583kJ	↑Sugar	202	Average
Jam, strawberry 50% less sugar	551kJ	↑Sugar	202	Average
Breakfast marmalade 50% less sugar	561kJ	↑Sugar	202	Average

John West

Product Name	Energy	Major Nutrients	Food Additives	Nutritious Rating
Spreadable, tuna	670kJ	↑Salt ↑Fat	220	Average
Spreadable, tuna tomato & basil	690kJ	↑Salt ↑Fat	220	Average

Kraft

Product Name	Energy	Major Nutrients	Food Additives	Nutritious Rating
Easy cheese spread, cheddar	1190kJ	↑Salt ↑Fat	200, 234, 160b	Poor
Easy cheese spread, cheddar light	1000kJ	↑Salt ↑Fat	200, 234, 160b	Poor
Easy cheese spread, cream cheese	1300kJ	↑Salt ↑Fat	200, 234	Poor
Easy cheese spread, cream cheese light	1150kJ	↑Salt ↑Fat	200, 234	Poor
Peanut butter, crunchy	2642kJ	↑Salt ↑Fat	320	Average
Peanut butter, crunchy light	2334kJ	↑Salt ↑Fat	320	Average
Peanut butter, smooth	2671kJ	↑Salt ↑Fat	320	Average
Peanut butter, smooth light	2532kJ	↑Salt ↑Fat	320	Average
Vegemite	798kJ	↑Salt	YE	Poor
Vegemite, my first	932kJ	↑Salt	YE	Poor
Vegemite, cheesybite	1062kJ	↑Salt ↑Fat	YE, 202, 314	Poor

Marmite

Product Name	Energy	Major Nutrients	Food Additives	Nutritious Rating
Yeast spread	680kJ	↑Sugar ↑Salt	YE, 202	Poor

Macro (Woolworths/Safeways)

Product Name	Energy	Major Nutrients	Food Additives	Nutritious Rating
Organic peanut butter, smooth	2670kJ	↑Fat	✓	Average
Organic peanut butter, crunchy	2660kJ	↑Fat	✓	Average
Organic apricot spread	896kJ	↑Sugar	✓	Average

Organic raspberry spread	900kJ	↑Sugar	✓	Average
Organic strawberry jam	842kJ	↑Sugar	✓	Average

Masterfoods

Product Name	Energy	Major Nutrients	Food Additives	Nutritious Rating
Lemon butter	1250kJ	↑Sugar	220	Poor
Promite	869kJ	↑Sugar ↑Salt	220, VPE, YE, 627, 631, 407	Poor

Melrose

Product Name	Energy	Major Nutrients	Food Additives	Nutritious Rating
ABC spread	2730kJ	↑Fat	✓	Average

Mighty Mite

Product Name	Energy	Major Nutrients	Food Additives	Nutritious Rating
Yeast spread	634kJ	↑Salt	YE, 202, 220	Poor

Nutella

Product Name	Energy	Major Nutrients	Food Additives	Nutritious Rating
Hazelnut spread	2175kJ	↑Sugar ↑Fat	✓	Average

Nutino

Product Name	Energy	Major Nutrients	Food Additives	Nutritious Rating
Hazelnut spread	2210kJ	↑Sugar ↑Fat	✓	Poor

Outback Spirit

Product Name	Energy	Major Nutrients	Food Additives	Nutritious Rating
Native currants &	1068kJ	↑Sugar	407	Average

muntries jam				
Passionfruit & fig jam	1240kJ	↑Sugar	407	Average
Quandong jam	**1023kJ**	**↑Sugar**	✓	**Average**

Pantalica

Product Name	Energy	Major Nutrients	Food Additives	Nutritious Rating
Cheese spread	1320kJ	↑Salt ↑Fat	202, 234	Poor
Milk chocolate ezi spread	1450kJ	↑Sugar ↑Fat	202, 234	Poor

Pecks

Product Name	Energy	Major Nutrients	Food Additives	Nutritious Rating
Anchovette	**488kJ**	**↑Salt**	✓	**Poor**
Chicken & ham spread	969kJ	↑Salt ↑Fat	YE, 250, 621, 627	Poor
Devilled ham spread	759kJ	↑Salt ↑Fat	YE, 250, 621	Poor
Salmon & lobster spread	532kJ	↑Salt	621	Poor

Roses

Product Name	Energy	Major Nutrients	Food Additives	Nutritious Rating
Conserve, apricot	1170kJ	↑Sugar	220	Average
Conserve, raspberry	1140kJ	↑Sugar	220	Average
Conserve, strawberry	1150kJ	↑Sugar	220	Average
Marmalade, English breakfast	1150kJ	↑Sugar	223, 220	Average

Sanatarium

Product Name	Energy	Major Nutrients	Food Additives	Nutritious Rating
Peanut butter, crunchy	2580kJ	↑Salt ↑Fat	✓	Average
Peanut butter, smooth	2580kJ	↑Salt ↑Fat	✓	Average
Peanut butter, super crunchy	2580kJ	↑Salt ↑Fat	✓	Average

St Dalfour

Product Name	Energy	Major Nutrients	Food Additives	Nutritious Rating
Fruit spread, black cherry	882kJ	↑ Sugar	223	Average
Fruit spread, blackberry	884kJ	↑ Sugar	223	Average
Fruit spread, four fruits	884kJ	↑ Sugar	223	Average
Fruit spread, orange marmalade	884kJ	↑ Sugar	223	Average
Fruit spread, raspberry	950kJ	↑ Sugar	223	Average
Fruit spread, royal fig	884kJ	↑ Sugar	223	Average
Fruit spread, strawberry	884kJ	↑ Sugar	223	Average
Fruit spread, thick apricot	884kJ	↑ Sugar	223	Average
Fruit spread, wild blueberry	884kJ	↑ Sugar	223	Average

Sweet William

Product Name	Energy	Major Nutrients	Food Additives	Nutritious Rating
Chocolate spread mud	1980kJ	↑ Fat ↑ Sugar	202	Average

Terra Australis

Product Name	Energy	Major Nutrients	Food Additives	Nutritious Rating
Fig & ginger conserve	966kJ	↑ Sugar	220	Average
Ginger & date conserve	983kJ	↑ Sugar	220	Average
Mango & macadamia conserve	916kJ	↑ Sugar	220	Average
Pineapple & passionfruit conserve	920kJ	↑ Sugar	220	Average
Raspberry & ginger conserve	916kJ	↑ Sugar	220	Average

Weight Watchers

Product Name	Energy	Major Nutrients	Food Additives	Nutritious Rating
Fruit spread, apricot	560kJ	↑ Sugar	202	Average
Fruit spread, fruits of the forest	569kJ	↑ Sugar	202	Average
Fruit spread, strawberry	563kJ	↑ Sugar	124, 202	Average

Woolworths/Safeways

Product Name	Energy	Major Nutrients	Food Additives	Nutritious Rating
Select, apricot jam	1140kJ	↑ Sugar	220	Average
Select, blackberry jam	1140kJ	↑ Sugar	220	Average
Select, blackcurrant jam	1140kJ	↑ Sugar	220	Average
Select, English breakfast	1110kJ	↑ Sugar	220	Average
Select, plum jam	1130kJ	↑ Sugar	220	Average
Select, raspberry jam	1140kJ	↑ Sugar	220	Average
Select, strawberry jam	1090kJ	↑ Sugar	220	Average
Select, peanut butter smooth	**2710kJ**	**↑ Fat**	**✓**	**Average**

Select, peanut butter smooth light	2410kJ	↑ Fat ↑ Sugar	202	Average
Select, peanut butter crunchy	**2680kJ**	**↑ Fat**	✓	**Average**
Select, peanut butter crunchy light	2390kJ	↑ Fat	202	Average
Select, peanut butter super crunchy	**2670kJ**	**↑ Fat**	✓	**Average**
Homebrand, Chocolate spread	**2360kJ**	**↑ Fat ↑ Sugar**	✓	**Average**
Homebrand, apricot jam	1120kJ	↑ Sugar	220	Average
Homebrand, English marmalade	1140kJ	↑ Sugar	220, 223	Average
Homebrand, mixed berry jam	1110kJ	↑ Sugar	220	Average
Homebrand, plum jam	1120kJ	↑ Sugar	220	Average
Homebrand, strawberry jam	1120kJ	↑ Sugar	220	Average
Homebrand, peanut butter smooth	2530kJ	↑ Sugar ↑ Fat ↑ Salt	✓	Average
Homebrand, peanut butter crunchy	2510kJ	↑ Sugar ↑ Fat	✓	Average

Yackandandah

Product Name	Energy	Major Nutrients	Food Additives	Nutritious Rating
Strawberry jam	1127kJ	↑ Sugar	220, 223	Average
Raspberry jam	1147kJ	↑ Sugar	220, 223	Average
Lemon curd	1200kJ	↑ Sugar	220, 223	Average

Nuts, Seeds & Dried Fruits

Nuts are super nutritious and should be an integral part of our diet. Unfortunately, they have been outlawed in schools which make it challenging. It's interesting that shellfish, eggs and dairy allergy affect more people than nuts, yet they are still allowed. It has also been suggested nut allergy has increased with the introduction of sulphite preservative use. Sulphites are a known asthma trigger.

Nuts are energy dense, so it is important not to over indulge, which can be hard as they are just so moorish!

Bibo

Product Name	Energy	Major Nutrients	Food Additives	Nutritious Rating
Polenta	1480kJ	✔	✔	Average

Nu Vit

Product Name	Energy	Major Nutrients	Food Additives	Nutritious Rating
Cashews, roasted	2528kJ	↑ Fat	✔	Excellent
Fruit & nut mix	2042kJ	↑ Fat ↑ Sugar	220, 129	Good
Lecithin	2620kJ	↑ Fat	✔	Good
Pepitas	2264kJ	↑ Fat	✔	Excellent
Polenta	1406kJ	✔	✔	Average
Protein mix	2637kJ	↑ Fat	✔	Good
Psyllium husks	755kJ	✔	✔	Good
Sesame seeds	2397kJ	↑ Fat	✔	Excellent

Olympic Fine Foods

Product Name	Energy	Major Nutrients	Food Additives	Nutritious Rating
Polenta	1480kJ	✔	✔	Average

Sun Sol

Product Name	Energy	Major Nutrients	Food Additives	Nutritious Rating
Almond, blanched	2618kJ	↑ Fat	✓	Good
Almond, flaked	2618kJ	↑ Fat	✓	Good
Almond, meal	2618kJ	↑ Fat	✓	Good
Almond, slithered	2618kJ	↑ Fat	✓	Good
Apricot slice	1710kJ	↑ Fat ↑ Sugar	160b, 220	Average
Bhuja mix	1961kJ	↑ Fat ↑ Sugar	102, 110	Average
Brazil nuts	2743kJ	↑ Fat	✓	Excellent
Fruit & nut mix	1738kJ	↑ Fat ↑ Sugar	220	Good
Hazelneuts	2689kJ	↑ Fat	✓	Excellent
Honey popcorn	1580kJ	↑ Salt ↑ Sugar	220	Poor
Japanese rice crackers	1525kJ	↑ Salt	102, 110, 133	Poor
Macadamias	3068kJ	↑ Fat	✓	Excellent
Paw paw, diced	1470kJ	↑ Sugar	220, 129	Good
Peanuts in shell	2600kJ	↑ Fat	✓	Good
Phyto soy LSA mix	2029kJ	↑ Fat	✓	Good
Pine nuts	2892kJ	↑ Fat	✓	Excellent
Pineapple, diced	1440kJ	↑ Sugar	220	Average
Pistachios	2458kJ	↑ Fat	✓	Excellent
Pretzels	1594kJ	↑ Salt	✓	Average
Psyillium husks	775kJ	✓	✓	Good
Rice crackers, salad mix	1594kJ	↑ Salt	102, 110, 122, 133	Average
Sesame seeds	2397kJ	↑ Fat	✓	Excellent
Soya chips	2090kJ	↑ Salt ↑ Sugar ↑ Fat	✓	Average
Walnuts	2904kJ	↑ Fat	✓	Excellent

Snack Foods

Lunchbox Treats

It's so hard being a mum and wanting to give your child something that is nutritious and something that will also seem a treat. No matter how much you feel like your loving them more with a healthy snack, the kids seem to feel the opposite and just want to be the cool one a packet of chips or chocolate biscuits. If you can't bake your own, I recommend: *Carman's, Nature valley and Uncle Toby's roll ups.*

Be Natural

Product Name	Energy	Major Nutrients	Food Additives	Nutritious Rating
Trail bars, berry	1450kJ	↑ Sugar	420, 220	Good
Trail bars, dark chocolate	1550kJ	↑ Sugar	420, 220	Good
Trail bars, fruit & nut	1490kJ	↑ Sugar	420, 220	Good
Trail bars, honey nut	1510kJ	↑ Sugar	420, 220	Good

Cadbury

Product Name	Energy	Major Nutrients	Food Additives	Nutritious Rating
Brunch bars, hazelnut	1810kJ	↑ Sugar ↑ Fat	160b, 422, 220	Good
Brunch bars, peanut	2100kJ	↑ Sugar ↑ Fat	220	Good
Brunch bars, mixed berry	1820kJ	↑ Sugar ↑ Fat	220, 422	Good
Brunch bars, toasted coconut	1920kJ	↑ Sugar ↑ Fat	220, 422, 160b	Good

Carmans

Product Name	Energy	Major Nutrients	Food Additives	Nutritious Rating
Muesli bars, apricot & almond	1848kJ	↑ Sugar	✓	Good
Muesli bars, classic fruit	1772kJ	↑ Sugar	220	Good
Muesli bars, fruit free	1800kJ	↑ Sugar ↑ Fat	220	Good
Muesli bars, dark chocolate cranberry	1870kJ	↑ Sugar ↑ Fat	✓	Good
Muesli bars, yoghurt & apricot	1850kJ	↑ Sugar ↑ Fat	✓	Good
Muesli rounds, fruit & nut	1799kJ	↑ Sugar ↑ Fat	✓	Good
Muesli rounds, apricot & almond	1799kJ	↑ Sugar ↑ Fat	✓	Good
Muesli bites	1787kJ	↑ Sugar ↑ Fat	✓	Good

Coles

Product Name	Energy	Major Nutrients	Food Additives	Nutritious Rating
Fruit zip ems, grape & apple	985kJ	↑ Sugar	202, 420	Average
Fruit zip ems, strawberry smoothies	1060kJ	↑ Sugar	202, 420	Average
Fruit zip ems, mixed berry smoothies	972kJ	↑ Sugar	420	Average
Rice puff bars, vanilla	1680kJ	↑ Sugar	211, 202, 220, 422	Average
Snack bar, rice puff rainbow choc chip	1700kJ	↑ Sugar	211, 202, 220, 422	Average
Muesli bars, chewy chocolate	1810kJ	↑ Fat ↑ Sugar	220, 422	Average
Muesli bars, yoghurt passionfruit & mango	1850kJ	↑ Fat ↑ Sugar	220	Average

Muesli bars, yoghurt strawberry	1790kJ	↑ Fat ↑ Sugar	220, 422	Average
Muesli bars, chewy mixed berry	1660kJ	↑ Fat ↑ Sugar	220, 422	Average
Muesli bars, chewy apricot & coconut	1630kJ	↑ Fat ↑ Sugar	220	Average
Muesli bars, nut delight	2220kJ	↑ Fat ↑ Sugar	220	Average
Fruit & nut bars	1960kJ	↑ Fat ↑ Sugar	220	Average
Fruit filled bars, apple	1390kJ	↑ Sugar	223, 422, 220	Average
Fruit filled bars, apricot	1390kJ	↑ Sugar	223, 422, 220	Average
Fruit filled bars, mixed berry	1390kJ	↑ Sugar	223, 422, 220	Average
Fruit sticks, assorted	1572kJ	↑ Sugar	220, 202, 223, 160b, 110, 102, 133	Average
Snack packs, cheddar	1630kJ	↑ Fat ↑ Salt	234	Average
Snack packs, bacon	1610kJ	↑ Fat ↑ Salt	621, 234, 129	Average
Snack packs, French onion	1620kJ	↑ Fat ↑ Salt	234	Average
Smart buy, muesli bar chewy chocolate chip	1730kJ	↑ Fat ↑ Sugar	220	Average
Smart buy muesli bars yoghurt strawberry	1860kJ	↑ Fat ↑ Sugar	220	Average
Smart buy cheese & crispbread	1570kJ	↑ Fat ↑ Salt	202, 234	Average
Smart buy fruit filled bars, apple	1480kJ	↑ Sugar	220, 422, 320, 160b	Average
Smart buy fruit filled bars, assorted	1572kJ	↑ Sugar	220, 122	Average

Day Dawn

Product Name	Energy	Major Nutrients	Food Additives	Nutritious Rating
Muesli bars, apricot & yoghurt	1750kJ	↑ Fat ↑ Sugar	220, 422	Average
Muesli bar, honeycomb & peanut	1920kJ	↑ Fat ↑ Sugar	220, 422	Average

Hot Shot

Product Name	Energy	Major Nutrients	Food Additives	Nutritious Rating
Fruit tails	1380kJ	↑ Sugar	220, 120	Average
Scooby doo fruit tails	1380kJ	↑ Sugar	220, 120	Average

IGA/Franklins

Product Name	Energy	Major Nutrients	Food Additives	Nutritious Rating
Signature muesli bars, choc & nut swirls	1820kJ	↑ Fat ↑ Sugar	220, 422	Average
Signature muesli bars, anzac slice	1990kJ	↑ Fat ↑ Sugar	220, 320	Average
Signature muesli bars, strawberry & yoghurt swirl	1610kJ	↑ Fat ↑ Sugar	120, 220, 422	Average
Black & Gold muesli bars, choc coated	1860kJ	↑ Fat ↑ Sugar	220	Average
Black & Gold muesli bars, apricot & coconut	1600kJ	↑ Fat ↑ Sugar	220, 422	Average
Black & Gold muesli bars, three fruits	1610kJ	↑ Fat ↑ Sugar	220, 422	Average
Black & Gold muesli bars, choc peppermint	1840kJ	↑ Fat ↑ Sugar	220, 220, 422	Average
Black & Gold muesli bars, cherry choc	1840kJ	↑ Fat ↑ Sugar	220, 422, 127, 122	Average
Black & Gold muesli	1800kJ	↑ Fat	202, 127,	Average

bars, cherry coconut		↑ Sugar	122, 220	
Black & Gold fruit bars, apricot	1530kJ	↑ Sugar	420, 422, 220, 282	Average
Black & Gold fruit chew bars, strawberry	1594kJ	↑ Sugar	122, 220	Average
Black & Gold fruit chew bars, apricot	1594kJ	↑ Sugar	160b, 220	Average

Kelloggs

Product Name	Energy	Major Nutrients	Food Additives	Nutritious Rating
LCM, 4D choc	1720kJ	↑ Fat ↑ Sugar	220, 320, 422	Average
LCM, split stix yoghurty	1830kJ	↑ Fat ↑ Sugar	220, 320, 422	Average
LCM, rice bubbles	1730kJ	↑ Fat ↑ Sugar	220, 320, 422	Average
LCM, rice bubbles choc chip	1770kJ	↑ Fat ↑ Sugar	220, 320, 422	Average
LCM, rice bubbles kaleidos	1740kJ	↑ Fat ↑ Sugar	220, 320, 422	Average
LCM, choclatey split stix	1780kJ	↑ Fat ↑ Sugar	220, 320, 422	Average
LCM, mashup split stix	1850kJ	↑ Fat ↑ Sugar	220, 320, 422	Average
Special K bar, caramel	1730kJ	↑ Sugar	220, 320, 422	Average
Special K bar, raspberry	1730kJ	↑ Sugar	220, 320, 422	Average
Special K bar, berry cheesecake	1660kJ	↑ Fat ↑ Sugar	220, 320, 422	Average
Special K bar, lemon meringue pie	1700kJ	↑ Fat ↑ Sugar	220, 320, 422, 420	Average
K time twist, strawberry & blueberry	1480kJ	↑ Sugar	160b, 422	Average
K time twist, strawberry &	1430kJ	↑ Sugar	160b, 422	Average

yoghurt				
K time twist, raspberry & apple	1446kJ	↑ Sugar	160b, 422, 221, 120	Average
K time twist, apple & cinnamon	1470kJ	↑ Sugar	160b, 422, 221	Average
Nutri-grain bar	1750kJ	↑ Fat ↑ Sugar	220, 320, 422	Average
Nutrigrain bar, choc malt	1760kJ	↑ Fat ↑ Sugar	320, 422, 420	Average
Crunchynut bars, peanut	2070kJ	↑ Fat ↑ Sugar	320, 422, 420	Average
Crunchynut bars, mixed nuts	2070kJ	↑ Fat ↑ Sugar	320, 422	Average

Kraft

Product Name	Energy	Major Nutrients	Food Additives	Nutritious Rating
Snackabouts, cheese	1650kJ	↑ Fat ↑ Salt	200, 234, 319	Poor
Snackabouts, chicken	1720kJ	↑ Fat ↑ Salt	320, 621, YE, 200, 234	Poor
Snackabouts, vegemite	1527kJ	↑ Fat ↑ Salt	YE, 319, 200, 234	Poor

Nature Valley

Product Name	Energy	Major Nutrients	Food Additives	Nutritious Rating
Bars, chewy choc nut	1744kJ	↑ Fat ↑ Sugar	220, 202	Average
Bars, chewy fruit & nut	1758kJ	↑ Fat ↑ Sugar	220, 202	Average
Bars, oats & honey	**1934kJ**	**↑ Fat ↑ Sugar**	✓	**Average**
Bars, roasted almond	**1926kJ**	**↑ Fat ↑ Sugar**	✓	**Average**
Bars, berry	1722kJ	↑ Fat ↑ Sugar	220, 202	Average

Nestle

Product Name	Energy	Major Nutrients	Food Additives	Nutritious Rating
Milo energy snack bar	1570kJ	↑ Sugar	202, 422, 420	Average
Milo energy snack bar, with milk	1690kJ	↑ Fat ↑ Sugar	202, 220	Average
Dunkaroos	2120kJ	↑ Fat ↑ Sugar	320, 220	Average
Space food sticks, chocolate	1790kJ	↑ Fat ↑ Sugar	220, 110, 123, 124, 133,	Average
Space food sticks, caramel	1800kJ	↑ Fat ↑ Sugar	220, 202, 211	Average

Quakers

Product Name	Energy	Major Nutrients	Food Additives	Nutritious Rating
Fibre bar, golden apricot	1380kJ	↑ Sugar	220, 422	Average
Cereal bar, chewy honey	1500kJ	↑ Sugar	220, 422	Average

SPC

Product Name	Energy	Major Nutrients	Food Additives	Nutritious Rating
Chompies, variety	1580kJ	↑ Sugar	120, 220	Average
Noughts & crosses, raspberry	1580kJ	↑ Sugar	120, 140, 160b, 220	Average
Chewbie fruit bar	1510kJ	↑ Sugar	220, 160b, 120, 220, 202	Average
Drizzly bars	1629kJ	↑ Sugar ↑ Fat	220, 160b	Average
Le snak deli, spicy capsicum	990kJ	↑ Fat ↑ Salt	320, 223, YE	Poor
Le snak deli, tomato	1020kJ	↑ Fat ↑ Salt	YE, 223	Poor

Tasti

Product Name	Energy	Major Nutrients	Food Additives	Nutritious Rating
Muffin bakes, gooey caramel	1380kJ	↑ Sugar ↑ Fat ↑ Salt	202, 282, 420	Poor
Muffin bakes, choc fudge	1500kJ	↑ Sugar ↑ Fat	202, 282, 420	Poor
Milkies, choc vanilla	1400kJ	↑ Sugar ↑ Fat	202, 282, 420	Poor

Uncle Toby's

Product Name	Energy	Major Nutrients	Food Additives	Nutritious Rating
Fruit fix strings, raspberry	1430kJ	↑ Sugar	220	Average
Fruit fix strings, blackcurrant	1460kJ	↑ Sugar	220	Average
Fruit fix strings, strawberry	1460kJ	↑ Sugar	220	Average
Roll ups, strawberry	1380kJ	↑ Sugar	202	Average
Roll ups, rainbow berry	**1390kJ**	**↑ Sugar**	✓	**Average**
Roll ups, fruit salad	**1400kJ**	**↑ Sugar**	✓	**Average**
Muesli bar, chewy apricot	1720kJ	↑ Sugar ↑ Fat	420, 422, 220	Average
Muesli bar, chewy choc chip	1720kJ	↑ Sugar ↑ Fat	420, 422, 220	Average
Muesli bar, chewy fruits of the forest	1720kJ	↑ Sugar ↑ Fat	420, 422, 220	Average
Muesli bar, white choc	1720kJ	↑ Sugar ↑ Fat	420, 422, 220	Average
Muesli bar, crunchy nut crumble	1840kJ	↑ Sugar ↑ Fat	220	Average
Muesli bar, crunchy choc chip	1810kJ	↑ Sugar ↑ Fat	220	Average
Muesli bar, yoghurt top apricot	1810kJ	↑ Sugar ↑ Fat	420, 220	Average

Muesli bar, yoghurt top honeycomb	1850kJ	↑ Sugar ↑ Fat	220, 420	Average
Muesli bar, yoghurt top mango passionfruit	1800kJ	↑ Sugar ↑ Fat	420, 223, 220	Average
Muesli bar, yoghurt top raspberry	1820kJ	↑ Sugar ↑ Fat	420, 422, 220	Average
Muesli bar, yoghurt top strawberry	1800kJ	↑ Sugar ↑ Fat	420, 220	Average
Simply fruit, sultana, apricot, poppy & orange	1390kJ	↑ Sugar	220	Average
Simply fruit, sultana, date, apple & cinnamon	1470kJ	↑ Sugar	220	Average
Le snak, French onion	1660kJ	↑ Fat ↑ Salt	234, 223	Poor
Le snak, cheddar cheese	1700kJ	↑ Fat ↑ Salt	234, 223	Poor
Le snak, tasty cheese	1650kJ	↑ Fat ↑ Salt	234, 223	Poor

Weight Watchers

Product Name	Energy	Major Nutrients	Food Additives	Nutritious Rating
Bar, apricot & almond	1860kJ	↑ Sugar	220, 223, 202, 422	Average
Bar, cranberry & pomegranate	1300kJ	↑ Sugar	422	Average
Bar, strawberry duo	1260kJ	↑ Sugar	220, 422	Average
Bar, macadamia & cranberry	1860kJ	↑ Fat ↑ Sugar	223, 202, 422	Average
Bar, nut deluxe	1860kJ	↑ Fat ↑ Sugar	223, 202, 422	Average
Bar, apple crumble	1270kJ	↑ Sugar	422, 220	Average
Bar, raspberry pie	1270kJ	↑ Sugar	422, 220	Average
Bar, custard & apple	1320kJ	↑ Sugar	220	Average
Bar, hazelnut & orange	1910kJ	↑ Sugar	220, 223, 202, 422	Average

Bar, ginger kiss	1340kJ	↑ Sugar	220, 202, 282, 202	Average

Woolworths/Safeways

Product Name	Energy	Major Nutrients	Food Additives	Nutritious Rating
Select muesli bars, cashew, apricot & coconut	2050kJ	↑ Fat ↑ Sugar	202, 220, 223, 422	Average
Select muesli bars, peanut brittle	1850kJ	↑ Fat ↑ Sugar	220, 202, 422	Average
Select muesli bars, nut & fruit	1900kJ	↑ Fat ↑ Sugar	220, 422, 202	Average
Select muesli bars, cranberry & macadamia	2110kJ	↑ Fat ↑ Sugar	202, 422	Average
Select muesli bars, almond & cinnamon	1860kJ	↑ Fat ↑ Sugar	202, 422	Average
Select muesli bars, cranberry & pomegranate	1720kJ	↑ Fat ↑ Sugar	202, 220	Average
Select fruit bars, strawberry & blueberry	1420kJ	↑ Sugar	422, 223	Average
Select fruit bars, apple & raspberry	1420kJ	↑ Sugar	422, 223	Average
Select fruit bars, apple & cinnamon	1440kJ	↑ Sugar	422, 223	Average
Homebrand fruit bars, assorted	1660kJ	↑ Sugar	220, 160b, 120	Average
Homebrand muesli bars, apricot & apple	1380kJ	↑ Sugar	220, 160b, 422	Average
Homebrand muesli bars, apple	1360kJ	↑ Sugar	220, 160b, 422	Average
Homebrand muesli bars, choc coated honeycomb & nut	1870kJ	↑ Fat ↑ Sugar	220	Average
Homebrand muesli bar, choc swirl	1690kJ	↑ Fat ↑ Sugar	220	Average

Homebrand muesli bars, strawberry & yoghurt	1720kJ	↑ Fat ↑ Sugar	220	Average
Homebrand crispbread & dip, cheese	1620kJ	↑ Fat ↑ Salt	202, 223	Poor
Homebrand crispbread & dip, bacon	1610kJ	↑ Fat ↑ Salt	202, 223	Poor
Homebrand crispbread & dip, French onion	1600kJ	↑ Fat ↑ Salt	202, 223	Poor

Potato/Corn Chips, Popcorn & Salsa

The general rule of thumb is choose the plain varieties and they are most likely to be additive free. A few flavoured varieties include: *Smith's potato chips thin sliced salt and vinegar, The kettle co sea salt and vinegar, and Thomas Chipman cracked pepper.*

Ajitas

Product Name	Energy	Major Nutrients	Food Additives	Nutritious Rating
Vege chips, sweet & sour	1890kJ	↑ Fat ↑ Salt	HVP	Poor
Vege chips, sea salt	1920kJ	↑ Fat ↑ Salt	✓	**Poor**
Vege chips, natural	1950kJ	↑ Fat ↑ Salt	✓	**Poor**
Vege chips, sour cream & chives	1930kJ	↑ Fat ↑ Salt	HVP	Poor
Vege chips, tasty cheese	1960kJ	↑ Fat ↑ Salt	YE, 202, 223	Poor

Coles

Product Name	Energy	Major Nutrients	Food Additives	Nutritious Rating
Potato chips, salt & vinegar crinkle cut	2160kJ	↑ Fat ↑ Salt	YE	Poor
Potato chips, chicken crinkle cut	2180kJ	↑ Fat ↑ Salt	YE, 627, 631, VP, 202	Poor
Potato chips, original crinkle cut	2220kJ	↑ Fat ↑ Salt	✓	**Poor**
Smart buy, potato chips, plain crinkle cut	2240kJ	↑ Fat ↑ Salt	✓	**Poor**
Smart buy, potato chips, plain thin cut	2150kJ	↑ Fat ↑ Salt	✓	**Poor**

Corn chips, cheese supreme	2130kJ	↑ Fat ↑ Salt	202, VP, HVP, YE, 635	Poor
Corn chips, nacho cheese	2170kJ	↑ Fat ↑ Salt	110, 102, VE, 621, 635, VP, 202	Poor
Corn chips, original	2120kJ	↑ Fat ↑ Salt	✓	Poor
RTE popcorn, butter	2032kJ	↑ Fat	✓	Poor
RTE popcorn, caramel	1810kJ	↑ Fat ↑ Sugar	160b, 220	Poor
RTE popcorn, lite	1822kJ	↑ Fat	✓	Poor
Organic popcorn, salted	1895kJ	↑ Fat	✓	Poor
Organic popcorn, sweet & salty	1990kJ	↑ Fat ↑ Sugar	✓	Poor
Salsa dip, mild	183kJ	↑ Salt	✓	Poor
Salsa dip, medium	183kJ	↑ Salt	✓	Poor

Cool Pak

Product Name	Energy	Major Nutrients	Food Additives	Nutritious Rating
Popcorn, butter	19400kJ	↑ Fat ↑ Salt	160b	Poor

Frito-Lay

Product Name	Energy	Major Nutrients	Food Additives	Nutritious Rating
Cheetos cheese & bacon balls	2310kJ	↑ Fat ↑ Salt	621, 110, 102	Poor
Doritos, original	2110kJ	↑ Fat ↑ Salt	✓	Poor
Doritos, nacho cheese	2160kJ	↑ Fat ↑ Salt	621, 160b, YE, 223	Poor
Doritos, supreme cheese	2170kJ	↑ Fat ↑ Salt	110, 621, 627, 631	Poor
Doritos, hot Mexican salsa	2130kJ	↑ Fat ↑ Salt	YE, HVP, 202, 621, 627, 631	Poor
Doritos, Thai sweet chilli	2140kJ	↑ Fat ↑ Salt	YE, HVP, 202, 621, 627, 631	Poor

Doritos salsa dip, mild	187kJ	↑ Salt	220	Poor
Doritos salsa dip, medium	187kJ	↑ Salt	220	Poor
Doritos salsa dip, hot	187kJ	↑ Salt	220	Poor

Greens

Product Name	Energy	Major Nutrients	Food Additives	Nutritious Rating
Microwave popcorn, original	2080kJ	↑ Fat	160b	Poor
Microwave popcorn, lite	1640kJ	↑ Fat ↑ Salt	160b	Poor
Microwave popcorn, triple butter explosion	2080kJ	↑ Fat ↑ Salt	160b	Poor

Old El Paso

Product Name	Energy	Major Nutrients	Food Additives	Nutritious Rating
Chunky tomato dip, mild	155kJ	✓	✓	Good
Chunky tomato dip, medium	144kJ	✓	✓	Good
Chunky roasted capsicum dip,	310kJ	✓	✓	Good

Parkers

Product Name	Energy	Major Nutrients	Food Additives	Nutritious Rating
Pretzels, original	1640kJ	↑ Salt	220	Poor
Pretzels, mini	1660kJ	↑ Salt	220	Poor

Pringles

Product Name	Energy	Major Nutrients	Food Additives	Nutritious Rating
Pringles, classic original	2180kJ	↑ Fat ↑ Salt	202	Poor
Pringles, honey	2173kJ	↑ Fat	621, 627,	Poor

mustard			631, 202, 223	
Pringles, sour cream & onion	2140kJ	↑ Fat ↑ Salt	621, 627, 631, 202, 223	Poor
Pringles, cheddar cheese	2160kJ	↑ Fat ↑ Salt	621, 627, 631, 202, 223	Poor
Pringles, hot & spicy	2140kJ	↑ Fat ↑ Salt	202, 621, 627, 631, HVP, 223	Poor
Pringles, pizza	2140kJ	↑ Fat ↑ Salt	202, 621, 627, 631, YE, 223	Poor
Pringles, tasty bacon	2169kJ	↑ Fat ↑ Salt	202, 621, 627, 631, YE	Poor
Pringles, Texas BBQ	2143kJ	↑ Fat ↑ Salt	202, 621, 627, 631, YE	Poor
Pringles, tomato sauce	2136kJ	↑ Fat ↑ Salt	202, 621, 627, 631, YE	Poor
Pringles multigrain, classic	2076kJ	↑ Fat ↑ Salt	202	Poor
Pringles multigrain, sour cream & onion	2060kJ	↑ Fat ↑ Salt	202, 621, 627, 631	Poor

Rivera

Product Name	Energy	Major Nutrients	Food Additives	Nutritious Rating
Popping corn	1520kJ	✓	✓	Poor

Red Rock

Product Name	Energy	Major Nutrients	Food Additives	Nutritious Rating
Deli chips, chorizo & caramelised onion	2060kJ	↑ Fat ↑ Salt	202, YE, 223	Poor
Deli chips, parmesan, chilli & basil	2060kJ	↑ Fat ↑ Salt	202, YE, 223, HVP	Poor
Deli chips, Dijon mustard & honey	2050kJ	↑ Fat ↑ Salt	202, YE, 223	Poor
Deli chips, honey soy chicken	2060kJ	↑ Fat ↑ Salt	202, YE, 223, HVP	Poor
Deli chips, lime &	2070kJ	↑ Fat	202, YE, 223	Poor

Product Name	Energy	Major Nutrients	Food Additives	Nutritious Rating
pepper		↑ Salt		
Deli chips, sea salt	**2040kJ**	**↑ Fat** **↑ Salt**	✓	**Poor**
Deli chips, sea salt & balsamic	2050kJ	↑ Fat ↑ Salt	202, YE, 223	Poor
Deli chips, sour cream & sweet chilli	2050kJ	↑ Fat ↑ Salt	202, YE, 223, 120	Poor
Deli chips, vintage cheddar & onion	2060kJ	↑ Fat ↑ Salt	202, YE, 223	Poor
Deli rice crisps, sour cream & onion	2232kJ	↑ Fat ↑ Salt	202, YE, 223	Poor

Smiths

Product Name	Energy	Major Nutrients	Food Additives	Nutritious Rating
Burger rings	2200kJ	↑ Fat ↑ Salt	HVP, 621, 102, 110, 155, YE	Poor
Twisties, cheese	2080kJ	↑ Fat ↑ Salt	621, YE, HVP	Poor
Twisties, chicken	2190kJ	↑ Fat ↑ Salt	202, 621, 635, HVP, 223	Poor
Twisties, zig zags wicked cheddar	2430kJ	↑ Fat ↑ Salt	110, 223, 621, 627, 631	Poor
Grain waves, cheddar cheese	1990kJ	↑ Fat ↑ Salt	YE, 202, 160b, 223	Poor
Grain waves, original,	**2030kJ**	**↑ Fat**	✓	**Poor**
Grain waves, sour cream & chives	2030kJ	↑ Fat ↑ Salt	202, 223, YE	Poor
Grain waves, sweet chilli	2010kJ	↑ Fat ↑ Salt	202, VP, 160b, 621, 627, 631, 965	Poor
Potato chips, original	**2180kJ**	**↑ Fat** **↑ Salt**	✓	**Poor**
Potato chips, barbecue	2140kJ	↑ Fat ↑ Salt	YE, 621, 635, 202, 223	Poor
Potato chips, cheese	2150kJ	↑ Fat	621, 223	Poor

& onion		↑ Salt		
Potato chips, chicken	2130kJ	↑ Fat ↑ Salt	621, 620, 635, 202, HVP, YE, 223	Poor
Potato chips, salt & vinegar	2100kJ	↑ Fat ↑ Salt	621	Poor
Potato chips, Heinz big red	2130kJ	↑ Fat ↑ Salt	621, 627, 631, HVP, YE, 223	Poor
Potato chips, vegemite	2130kJ	↑ Fat ↑ Salt	YE, 202	Poor
Potato chips, Sunday roast	2150kJ	↑ Fat ↑ Salt	621, 627, 631, 202, HVP, YE, 223	Poor
Potato chips, meat pie & sauce	2150kJ	↑ Fat ↑ Salt	621, 627, 631, 202, HVP, YE, 223	Poor
Potato chips, thin sliced BBQ ribs	2150kJ	↑ Fat ↑ Salt	621, 627, 631, 202, HVP, YE, 223, 955	Poor
Potato chips, thin sliced sour cream & onion	2140kJ	↑ Fat ↑ Salt	HVP, 621, 635, 223	Poor
Potato chips, thin sliced original	**2180kJ**	**↑ Fat** **↑ Salt**	✓	**Poor**
Potato chips, thin sliced salt & vinegar	**2100kJ**	**↑ Fat** **↑ Salt**	✓	**Poor**
Potato chips thin cut, crispy bacon	2160kJ	↑ Fat	621, 627, 631, 202, HVP, YE	Poor
Thins, Thai sweet chilli	2140kJ	↑ Fat ↑ Salt	951, 631, 621, 627, 120, 160b	Poor
Aussie potato fries	**2181kJ**	**↑ Fat** **↑ Salt**	✓	**Poor**

Skinns Potato Chips

Product Name	Energy	Major Nutrients	Food Additives	Nutritious Rating
Salt & vinegar	1600kJ	↑ Salt	202, 621	Poor
Honey sweet chicken	1610kJ	↑ Salt	YE, 223, HVP	Poor

Snack Foods

Product Name	Energy	Major Nutrients	Food Additives	Nutritious Rating
Cheezels	2220kJ	↑ Fat ↑ Salt	621, 627, 631, YE, VE, 223	Poor
Chickadees chicken	2230kJ	↑ Fat ↑ Salt	621, 631, YE, 223, 202	Poor
CC's, original	**2090kJ**	**↑ Fat** **↑ Salt**	✓	**Poor**
CC's, nacho cheese	2140kJ	↑ Fat ↑ Salt	621, 635, YE, VP	Poor
CC's, tasty cheese	2150kJ	↑ Fat ↑ Salt	621, 627, 631, VP, YE, VE	Poor
CC's, corn smash	2140kJ	↑ Fat ↑ Salt	621, 627, 631, VP, YE, VE	Poor
French fries	**2200kJ**	**↑ Fat** **↑ Salt**	✓	**Poor**
French fries, chicken	2150kJ	↑ Fat ↑ Salt	621, 627, 631, 202, YE, VE,	Poor
French fries, salt & vinegar	2114kJ	↑ Fat ↑ Salt	621	Poor
Samboys, original roast	**2170kJ**	**↑ Fat** **↑ Salt**	✓	**Poor**
Samboys, salt & vinegar	2120kJ	↑ Fat ↑ Salt	621, 202	Poor
Samboys, atomic tomato	2160kJ	↑ Fat ↑ Salt	220, 621, VP	Poor
Samboys, barbecue	2140kJ	↑ Fat	621, VP	Poor

		↑ Salt		
Samboys, cheese & onion	2170kJ	↑ Fat ↑ Salt	621, 635 VE	Poor
Samboys, chicken	2150kJ	↑ Fat ↑ Salt	621, 627, 631, 223, YE, VE,	Poor
Toobs	1960kJ	↑ Fat ↑ Salt	621, 223	Poor
Thins, original	**2150kJ**	**↑ Fat ↑ Salt**	✓	**Poor**
Thins, chicken	2150kJ	↑ Fat ↑ Salt	220, 202, VP,621, 627, 631	Poor
Thins, light & tangy	2100kJ	↑ Fat ↑ Salt	VP, 621, VE	Poor
Thins, salt & vinegar	2060kJ	↑ Fat ↑ Salt	621, 202	Poor
Thins, sweet chilli & sour cream	2080kJ	↑ Fat ↑ Salt	202, 202, VP,635	Poor

Super Pop

Product Name	Energy	Major Nutrients	Food Additives	Nutritious Rating
Movie time coloured popcorn	1740kJ	↑ Sugar	102, 110, 122, 133, 120	Poor

The Kettle Co

Product Name	Energy	Major Nutrients	Food Additives	Nutritious Rating
Potato chips, sea salt	**2090kJ**	**↑ Fat**	✓	**Poor**
Potato chips, chargrilled red pepper & sour cream	2070kJ	↑ Fat	202, YE, 223	Poor
Potato chips, multigrain honey BBQ	1900kJ	↑ Fat ↑ Salt	202, YE, 223	Poor
Potato chips, multigrain sour cream & chives	1920kJ	↑ Fat ↑ Salt	YE, 202	Poor

Potato chips, multigrain sweet chilli & sour cream	1920kJ	↑ Fat ↑ Salt	YE, 202	Poor
Potato chips, peri peri chicken	2060kJ	↑ Fat ↑ Salt	YE, 202	Poor
Potato chips, chilli & lime	2060kJ	↑ Fat	YE	Poor
Potato chips, sea salt & vinegar	2020kJ	↑ Fat ↑ Salt	✓	Poor

Thomas Chipman

Product Name	Energy	Major Nutrients	Food Additives	Nutritious Rating
Corn chips, lightly salted	2047kJ	↑ Fat	✓	Poor
Corn chips, splendid cheese	1960kJ	↑ Fat ↑ Salt	YE	Poor
Potato chips, cracked pepper	2280kJ	↑ Fat	✓	Poor

Uncle Toby's

Product Name	Energy	Major Nutrients	Food Additives	Nutritious Rating
Microwave popcorn, natural	1960kJ	↑ Fat ↑ Salt	✓	Average
Microwave popcorn, butter	1920kJ	↑ Fat ↑ Salt	160b	Average

Woolworths/Safeways

Product Name	Energy	Major Nutrients	Food Additives	Nutritious Rating
Select deli-style, lime & black pepper	2100kJ	↑ Fat ↑ Salt	202, YE, 220	Poor
Select deli-style, sour cream & chilli	2190kJ	↑ Fat ↑ Salt	VE	Poor
Select deli-style, original	2220kJ	↑ Fat ↑ Salt	✓	Poor
Select deli, honey soy chicken	2210kJ	↑ Fat ↑ Salt	202	Poor

Select corn puffs, salt	2250kJ	↑ Fat ↑ Salt	✔	Poor
Select corn puffs, cheese	2220kJ	↑ Fat ↑ Salt	YE, 202	Poor
Select corn chips, supreme cheese	2080kJ	↑ Fat ↑ Salt	202	Poor
Select corn chips, nacho	2090kJ	↑ Fat ↑ Salt	202	Poor
Select rippled wholegrain, original	2010kJ	↑ Fat ↑ Salt	202	Poor
Select rippled wholegrain, sour cream & chives	1960kJ	↑ Fat ↑ Salt	202, YE	Poor
Select rippled wholegrain, sweet chilli	1960kJ	↑ Fat ↑ Salt	YE	Poor
Select rippled wholegrain, roast onion & rosemary	1950kJ	↑ Fat ↑ Salt	202, YE	Poor
Homebrand cheese rings	2170kJ	↑ Fat ↑ Salt	621, 627, 631, VE	Poor
Homebrand thin cut potato chips, original	2310kJ	↑ Fat ↑ Salt	319	Poor
Homebrand thin cut potato chips, salt & vinegar	2220kJ	↑ Fat ↑ Salt	621, 319	Poor
Homebrand thin cut potato chips, chicken	2250kJ	↑ Fat ↑ Salt	YE, 202, 621, 627, 631, HVP	Poor
Homebrand crinkle cut potato chips, original	2370kJ	↑ Fat ↑ Salt	319	Poor
Homebrand crinkle cut potato chips, salt & vinegar	2300kJ	↑ Fat ↑ Salt	319, 621	Poor
Homebrand crinkle cut potato chips, chicken	2320kJ	↑ Fat ↑ Salt	319, 621, 627, 631, 202, YE, HVP	Poor
Homebrand thin cut	2140kJ-	↑ Fat	621, 627,	Poor

potato chips, variety	2250kJ	↑ Salt	631, 160b, YE	
Homebrand crinkle cut potato chips, variety	2160kJ-2260kJ	↑ Fat ↑ Salt	621, 627, 631, 160b, YE	Poor

Biscuits

Biscuits are obviously not nutritious, but there are additive free varieties available.

Butterfingers, Bakers, Borland, Corinthians, D'Lush, Ittal bicotti, Lu, Hotshots and

Orgran.

Arnott's

Product Name	Energy	Major Nutrients	Food Additives	Nutritious Rating
Assorted cream biscuits	1910kJ	↑ Sugar ↑ Fat	220, 129, 132	Poor
Classic assorted	2080kJ	↑ Sugar ↑ Fat	110, 102, 220	Poor
Family assorted	2060kJ	↑ Sugar ↑ Fat	220, 129, 132	Poor
Tim tams, original	2180kJ	↑ Sugar ↑ Fat	129, 110, 102, 133, 220	Poor
Tim tams, dark mint	**2150kJ**	**↑ Sugar ↑ Fat**	✓	**Poor**
Tim tams, dark rum & raisin	2060kJ	↑ Sugar ↑ Fat	220	Poor
Tim tams, chewy caramel	2070kJ	↑ Sugar ↑ Fat	422, 102, 110, 129, 133	Poor
Tim tams, double coat	2200kJ	↑ Sugar ↑ Fat	129, 102, 110, 133	Poor
Tim tams, white	2270kJ	↑ Sugar ↑ Fat	160b	Poor
Tim tams, black forest	2080kJ	↑ Sugar ↑ Fat	422, 120, 129, 110, 102	Poor
Tim tams, honeycomb crush	2180kJ	↑ Sugar ↑ Fat	129, 110, 102	Poor
Caramel crowns	1900kJ	↑ Sugar ↑ Fat	220, 319	Poor
Butter snaps	**2020kJ**	**↑ Sugar ↑ Fat**	✓	**Poor**
Butter snap cookies	2030kJ	↑ Sugar	220	Poor

		↑ Fat ↑ Salt		
Creamy chocolate	**2100kJ**	↑ Sugar ↑ Fat	✓	Poor
Mint slice	**2200kJ**	↑ Sugar ↑ Fat	✓	Poor
Milk chocolate wheatens	2070kJ	↑ Sugar ↑ Fat	160b	Poor
Dark chocolate wheatens	2050kJ	↑ Sugar ↑ Fat	160b	Poor
Gaiety chocolate	**2240kJ**	↑ Sugar ↑ Fat	✓	Poor
Monte chocolate	2090kJ	↑ Sugar ↑ Fat	220	Poor
Chocolate teddy bears	**1990kJ**	↑ Sugar ↑ Fat	✓	Poor
Teddy bears	**1880kJ**	↑ Sugar ↑ Fat	✓	Poor
Tee vee snacks, original	**1970kJ**	↑ Sugar ↑ Fat	✓	Poor
Tee vee snacks, malt	**2030kJ**	↑ Sugar ↑ Fat	✓	Poor
Wagon wheels, mini	1810kJ	↑ Sugar ↑ Fat	220, 122	Poor
Royals, milk	1800kJ	↑ Sugar ↑ Fat	120, 220, 129	Poor
Royals, dark	1780kJ	↑ Sugar ↑ Fat	220	Poor
Scotch finger, chocolate coated	**2090kJ**	↑ Sugar ↑ Fat	✓	Poor
Scotch finger	**2047kJ**	↑ Sugar ↑ Fat	✓	Poor
Gingernuts	**1800kJ**	↑ Sugar ↑ Fat	✓	Poor
Arno shortbread	2090kJ	↑ Sugar ↑ Fat	✓	Poor
Granita	1870kJ	↑ Sugar ↑ Fat	✓	Poor
Honey Jumble	1630kJ	↑ Sugar	422, 129,	Poor

			120, 133	
Hundred & Thousands	1740kJ	↑ Sugar ↑ Fat	102, 110, 129, 133, 120	Poor
Iced vovo	1730kJ	↑ Sugar ↑ Fat	129, 422, 220	Poor
Spicy fruit roll	1550kJ	↑ Sugar ↑ Fat	220	Poor
Yoyo	1924kJ	↑ Sugar ↑ Fat	✓	Poor
Full o fruit	1540kJ	↑ Sugar	220	Poor
Custard cream	2070kJ	↑ Sugar ↑ Fat	102, 110	Poor
Delta cream	**2070kJ**	**↑ Sugar ↑ Fat**	✓	**Poor**
Chocolate ripple	1900kJ	↑ Sugar ↑ Fat	220	Poor
Kingston	**2100kJ**	**↑ Sugar ↑ Fat**	✓	**Poor**
Lattice	**2160kJ**	**↑ Sugar ↑ Fat**	✓	**Poor**
Lemon crisp	2220kJ	↑ Sugar ↑ Fat ↑ Salt	102, 110	Poor
Malt o milk	**1880kJ**	**↑ Sugar ↑ Fat**	✓	**Poor**
Marie	**1860kJ**	**↑ Sugar ↑ Fat**	✓	**Poor**
Milk arrowroot	**1840kJ**	**↑ Sugar ↑ Fat**	✓	**Poor**
Milk coffee	**1780kJ**	**↑ Sugar ↑ Fat**	✓	**Poor**
Monte carlo	2060kJ	↑ Sugar ↑ Fat	129, 132, 220	Poor
Nice	1890kJ	↑ Sugar ↑ Fat	160b	Poor
Orange slice	2050kJ	↑ Sugar ↑ Fat	110, 102	Poor
Premier chocolate chip cookies	2130kJ	↑ Sugar ↑ Fat	220	Poor

Raspberry shortcake	1850kJ	↑ Sugar ↑ Fat	129, 110, 220	Poor
Tic toc	1840kJ	↑ Sugar ↑ Fat	102, 110, 129, 120	Poor
Triple wafer	2190kJ	↑ Sugar ↑ Fat	110, 129, 120	Poor
Tina wafers	2180kJ	↑ Sugar ↑ Fat	110, 129, 120	Poor
Venetian	2160kJ	↑ Sugar ↑ Fat	220	Poor
Rice cookies	2150kJ	↑ Sugar ↑ Fat ↑ Salt	✓	Poor
Shortbread cream	2210kJ	↑ Sugar ↑ Fat	✓	Poor
Shredded wheatmeal	1717kJ	↑ Sugar ↑ Fat	✓	Poor
Snack right fruit pillow, wild berry	1586kJ	↑ Sugar ↑ Fat	120, 202	Poor
Snack right fruit slice sultana choc	1668kJ	↑ Sugar ↑ Fat	220, 202	Poor
Snack right fruit slice, sultana	1490kJ	↑ Sugar ↑ Fat	220, 202	Poor
Tiny teddy, honey	1860kJ	↑ Sugar ↑ Fat	✓	Poor
Tiny teddy, chocolate	1850kJ	↑ Sugar ↑ Fat	✓	Poor
Tiny teddy, half choc	1960kJ	↑ Sugar ↑ Fat	✓	Poor
Tiny teddy, hundreds & thousands	1860kJ	↑ Sugar ↑ Fat	120	Poor
Tiny teddy, choc chip	1860kJ	↑ Sugar ↑ Fat	220	Poor
Farmbake, butter shortbread	2160kJ	↑ Sugar ↑ Fat	✓	Poor
Farmbake, choc chip	2010kJ	↑ Sugar ↑ Fat	✓	Poor
Farmbake, choc chip fudge	1980kJ	↑ Sugar ↑ Fat	✓	Poor

Farmbake, chocolate chip cookies minis	2121kJ	↑ Sugar ↑ Fat	220	Poor
Farmbake, crunchy oat & fruit	1970kJ	↑ Sugar ↑ Fat	220	Poor
Farmbake, pecan brownie	2050kJ	↑ Sugar ↑ Fat	✓	Poor

Aunt Betty's

Product Name	Energy	Major Nutrients	Food Additives	Nutritious Rating
Wheelies	1855kJ	↑ Sugar ↑ Fat	220, 110, 320, 321	Poor

Bakers

Product Name	Energy	Major Nutrients	Food Additives	Nutritious Rating
Choc chip bikkies	1900kJ	↑ Sugar ↑ Fat	✓	Poor
Honey bikkies	1910kJ	↑ Sugar ↑ Fat	✓	Poor

Borland

Product Name	Energy	Major Nutrients	Food Additives	Nutritious Rating
Macadamia shortbread	2244kJ	↑ Sugar ↑ Fat	✓	Poor
Macadamia shortbread, chocolate base	2238kJ	↑ Sugar ↑ Fat	✓	Poor

Butterfingers

Product Name	Energy	Major Nutrients	Food Additives	Nutritious Rating
Macadamia shortbread	2280kJ	↑ Sugar ↑ Fat	✓	Poor
Pure butter shortbread	2180kJ	↑ Sugar ↑ Fat	✓	Poor
Pure butter shortbread, choc	2220kJ	↑ Sugar ↑ Fat	✓	Poor

chip				
Pure butter shortbread, gluten free	2220kJ	↑ Sugar ↑ Fat	✓	Poor

Byron Bay Cookie Co

Product Name	Energy	Major Nutrients	Food Additives	Nutritious Rating
Dark chocolate orange	1770kJ	↑ Sugar ↑ Fat	223	Poor
Dotty	2070kJ	↑ Sugar ↑ Fat	122, 133, 110, 102, 124	Poor
Triple choc fudge	1980kJ	↑ Sugar ↑ Fat	✓	Poor

Coles

Product Name	Energy	Major Nutrients	Food Additives	Nutritious Rating
Assorted creams	1990-2170kJ	↑ Sugar ↑ Fat	220, 160b, 120	Poor
Choc mint supreme	2140kJ	↑ Sugar ↑ Fat	✓	Poor
Mini choc mint	2130kJ	↑ Sugar ↑ Fat	✓	Poor
Mini jaffa toffee	2010kJ	↑ Sugar ↑ Fat	✓	Poor
Mini chocolate honeycomb swirls	2190kJ	↑ Sugar ↑ Fat	160b	Poor
Mini wafers	2081kJ	↑ Sugar ↑ Fat	120	Poor
Butternut creams	2100kJ	↑ Sugar ↑ Fat	220	Poor
Chocolate caramel deluxe	1967kJ	↑ Sugar ↑ Fat	✓	Poor
Chocolate fingers	2038kJ	↑ Sugar ↑ Fat	160b	Poor
Chocolate honeycomb swirls	2122kJ	↑ Sugar ↑ Fat	160b	Poor
Chocolate koalas	2065kJ	↑ Sugar	✓	Poor

		↑ Fat		
Chocolate surrenders	2140kJ	↑ Sugar ↑ Fat	120, 220	Poor
Kids animal shapes, honey	**1171kJ**	↑ Sugar ↑ Fat	✓	**Poor**
Kids animal shapes, chocolate	**1786kJ**	↑ Sugar ↑ Fat	✓	**Poor**
Raspberry & creams	1990kJ	↑ Sugar ↑ Fat	160b, 220, 129	Poor
Raspberry tartlets	1705kJ	↑ Sugar ↑ Fat	124, 122	Poor
Shortbread fingers	**2110kJ**	↑ Sugar ↑ Fat	✓	**Poor**
Ultimate 40% choc chip cookie	2016kJ	↑ Sugar ↑ Fat	220	Poor
Smart buy family assorted	1810-2050kJ	↑ Sugar ↑ Fat	223, 320	Poor
Smart buy gingernuts	1810kJ	↑ Sugar ↑ Fat	320	Poor
Smart buy milk arrowroot	1850kJ	↑ Sugar ↑ Fat	223, 320, 321, 220	Poor
Smart buy scotch finger	**2000kJ**	↑ Sugar ↑ Fat	✓	**Poor**
Smart buy choc chip cookies	2050kJ	↑ Sugar ↑ Fat	160b	Poor
Smart buy, milk coffee	1930kJ	↑ Sugar ↑ Fat	320, 321, 223	Poor
Smart buy nice	1930kJ	↑ Sugar ↑ Fat	223, 320, 321	Poor
Smart buy choc cream wafers	**2038kJ**	↑ Sugar ↑ Fat	✓	**Poor**
Smart buy strawberry cream wafers	2086kJ	↑ Sugar ↑ Fat	124	Poor
Smart buy vanilla cream wafers	**2086kJ**	↑ Sugar ↑ Fat	✓	**Poor**

Corinthians

Product Name	Energy	Major Nutrients	Food Additives	Nutritious Rating
Chocolate straws	1889kJ	↑ Fat ↑ Sugar	✓	Poor

D'Lush

Product Name	Energy	Major Nutrients	Food Additives	Nutritious Rating
Double choc	1930kJ	↑ Fat ↑ Sugar	✓	Poor
Orange	1930kJ	↑ Fat ↑ Sugar	✓	Poor
Peppermint	1930kJ	↑ Fat ↑ Sugar	✓	Poor

Fine Fare

Product Name	Energy	Major Nutrients	Food Additives	Nutritious Rating
Chocolate creams	2000kJ	↑ Sugar ↑ Fat	320, 133	Poor
Custard creams	2070kJ	↑ Sugar ↑ Fat	320, 321	Poor
Nice	1870kJ	↑ Sugar ↑ Fat	320, 321, 220	Poor
Orange creams	2030kJ	↑ Sugar ↑ Fat	320, 321, 110, 102	Poor
Strawberry creams	2060kJ	↑ Sugar ↑ Fat	320, 321, 112	Poor
Tymo, mint	2100kJ	↑ Sugar ↑ Fat	320, 321, 223, 122, 133	Poor
Tymo, original	2120kJ	↑ Sugar ↑ Fat	320, 321, 223, 133, 122	Poor
Vanilla cream	2070kJ	↑ Sugar ↑ Fat	320, 321	Poor

Freedom Foods

Product Name	Energy	Major Nutrients	Food Additives	Nutritious Rating

Blissful berry biscuits	1950kJ	↑ Fat ↑ Sugar	223, HF	Poor
Wild bears, choc coat	1920kJ	↑ Fat ↑ Sugar	HF	Poor

Fresh Bake

Product Name	Energy	Major Nutrients	Food Additives	Nutritious Rating
Almond fingers	1675kJ	↑ Sugar ↑ Fat	420	Poor
Almond rounds	1577kJ	↑ Sugar ↑ Fat	281, 202, 420	Poor

IGA/Franklins

Product Name	Energy	Major Nutrients	Food Additives	Nutritious Rating
Signature, chunky choc chip	2050kJ	↑ Sugar ↑ Fat	220	Poor
Signature, double choc chip	1920kJ	↑ Sugar ↑ Fat	220	Poor
Signature, macadamia & white chocolate	**2250kJ**	**↑ Sugar ↑ Fat**	✓	**Poor**
Black & Gold, choc chip cookies	2050kJ	↑ Sugar ↑ Fat	320, 321, 160b	Poor
Black & Gold, choc cream wafer	**2170kJ**	**↑ Sugar ↑ Fat**	✓	**Poor**
Black & Gold, choc scotch fingers	2060kJ	↑ Sugar ↑ Fat	320, 321, 160b	Poor
Black & Gold, choc wheat	2020kJ	↑ Sugar ↑ Fat	320, 321, 160b	Poor
Black & Gold, crunch choc	2100kJ	↑ Sugar ↑ Fat	320, 321, 160b, 220	Poor
Black & Gold, family assorted	1980kJ	↑ Sugar ↑ Fat	223, 220, 320, 321	Poor
Black & Gold, milk arrowroot	1890kJ	↑ Sugar ↑ Fat	220, 223, 320, 321	Poor
Black & Gold, milk coffee	1910kJ	↑ Sugar ↑ Fat	320, 321, 223	Poor

Black & Gold, scotch finger	2050kJ	↑ Sugar ↑ Fat	320, 321	Poor
Black & Gold, shortbread cookies	2100kJ	↑ Sugar ↑ Fat	320, 321, 160b	Poor
Black & Gold, triple choc	2120kJ	↑ Sugar ↑ Fat	320, 321, 223, 133, 122	Poor
Black & Gold, vanilla cream wafer	2170kJ	↑ Sugar ↑ Fat	✓	Poor

Harvest Kitchen (Unibec)

Product Name	Energy	Major Nutrients	Food Additives	Nutritious Rating
Fruit centres, apple & cinnamon cookies	1920kJ	↑ Sugar ↑ Fat	220, 422	Poor
Fruit centres, apricot & white choc cookies	1900kJ	↑ Sugar ↑ Fat	220, 422	Poor
Soft centres, choc chip cookies	2065kJ	↑ Sugar ↑ Fat	220, 422	Poor
Soft centres, triple choc chip cookies	2025kJ	↑ Sugar ↑ Fat	220, 422	Poor
Oats & choc chip	2070kJ	↑ Sugar ↑ Fat	220	Poor
Original chocolate chip	2020kJ	↑ Sugar ↑ Fat	160b	Poor
Triple choc chip	1820kJ	↑ Sugar ↑ Fat	160b	Poor
White choc chip & macadamia	1870kJ	↑ Sugar ↑ Fat	160b	Poor

Holland House

Product Name	Energy	Major Nutrients	Food Additives	Nutritious Rating
Almond fingers	1790kJ	↑ Sugar ↑ Fat	✓	Average
Spiced cookies	2055kJ	↑ Sugar ↑ Fat ↑ Salt	220	Poor

Hotshots

Product Name	Energy	Major Nutrients	Food Additives	Nutritious Rating
My little pony	1990kJ	↑ Sugar ↑ Fat ↑ Salt	✓	Poor
Scooby Doo	2000kJ	↑ Sugar ↑ Fat	✓	Poor
Simpsons	2000kJ	↑ Sugar ↑ Fat	✓	Poor

Ittal Biscotti

Product Name	Energy	Major Nutrients	Food Additives	Nutritious Rating
Toscani almond	1760kJ	↑ Sugar ↑ Fat	✓	Average

Kambly

Product Name	Energy	Major Nutrients	Food Additives	Nutritious Rating
Coconut chocolate meringue	2450kJ	↑ Sugar ↑ Fat	223	Poor
Florentine	2360kJ	↑ Sugar ↑ Fat	✓	Average

Kez's

Product Name	Energy	Major Nutrients	Food Additives	Nutritious Rating
Florentines	1870kJ	↑ Sugar ↑ Fat	202, 220	Poor
Melting moments	2230kJ	↑ Sugar ↑ Fat	102, 110	Poor

Kookas

Product Name	Energy	Major Nutrients	Food Additives	Nutritious Rating
Choc raspberry cookies	2070kJ	↑ Sugar ↑ Fat	320, 202, 122, 124, 102, 110	Poor

Jam cookies	2000kJ	↑ Sugar ↑ Fat	102, 110, 122, 124, 202	Poor

Kraft

Product Name	Energy	Major Nutrients	Food Additives	Nutritious Rating
Chips ahoy, choc chip cookie	2050kJ	↑ Sugar ↑ Fat	319	Poor
Chips ahoy, choc chip mini cookies	**2090kJ**	**↑ Sugar** **↑ Fat**	✓	**Poor**
Chips ahoy, chunky choc chip cookie	2220kJ	↑ Sugar ↑ Fat	319	Poor
Oreo, original	2030kJ	↑ Sugar ↑ Fat	319	Poor
Oreo, original minis	1964kJ	↑ Sugar ↑ Fat	319, 220	Poor
Oreo, chocolate cream	2070kJ	↑ Sugar ↑ Fat	319	Poor
Oreo, strawberry cream	2010kJ	↑ Sugar ↑ Fat	319, 120	Poor
Oreo, wafer sticks	2130kJ	↑ Sugar ↑ Fat	319	Poor

Lu

Product Name	Energy	Major Nutrients	Food Additives	Nutritious Rating
Petite ecolier, dark	**2070kJ**	**↑ Fat** **↑ Sugar**	✓	**Poor**
Petite ecolier, milk	**2080kJ**	**↑ Fat** **↑ Sugar**	✓	**Poor**
Pims, orange	**1670kJ**	**↑ Fat** **↑ Sugar**	✓	**Poor**
Pims, raspberry	1670kJ	↑ Fat ↑ Sugar	220	Poor

Marcs

Product Name	Energy	Major Nutrients	Food Additives	Nutritious Rating
Choc berry cookie	2160kJ	↑ Fat ↑ Sugar	122, 124	Poor

Choc finger	2220kJ	↑ Fat ↑ Sugar	✓	Poor
Choca jam	2090kJ	↑ Fat ↑ Sugar	122, 124, 202	Poor
Danish style	2090kJ	↑ Fat ↑ Sugar	✓	Poor
Lemon delight cookie	2090kJ	↑ Fat ↑ Sugar	✓	Poor
Macadamia finger	2150kJ	↑ Fat ↑ Sugar	✓	Poor
Sugar & spice	2100kJ	↑ Fat ↑ Sugar	✓	Poor

McVities

Product Name	Energy	Major Nutrients	Food Additives	Nutritious Rating
Chocolate hobnobs	2011kJ	↑ Fat ↑ Sugar	220	Poor
Digestive, original	1990kJ	↑ Fat ↑ Sugar ↑ Salt	220	Poor
Digestive, dark chocolate	2039kJ	↑ Fat ↑ Sugar	220	Poor
Digestive, light	1840kJ	↑ Fat ↑ Sugar ↑ Salt	220	Poor
Digestive, milk chocolate	2044kJ	↑ Fat ↑ Sugar	220	Poor
Dora cookies	2084kJ	↑ Fat ↑ Sugar	220	Poor
Spongebob cookies	2077kJ	↑ Fat ↑ Sugar	220	Poor

Orgran

Product Name	Energy	Major Nutrients	Food Additives	Nutritious Rating
Biscotti amaretti	2011kJ	↑ Fat ↑ Sugar	220	Poor
Itsy bitsy bears	1720kJ	↑ Fat	✓	Poor

		↑ Sugar		
Kids dinosaur cookies	1430kJ	↑ Sugar	✓	Poor
Outback animals	1750kJ	↑ Fat ↑ Sugar	✓	Poor
Rotondo	1670kJ	↑ Fat ↑ Sugar	✓	Poor
Shortbread hearts	2110kJ	↑ Fat ↑ Sugar	✓	Poor

Paradise

Product Name	Energy	Major Nutrients	Food Additives	Nutritious Rating
Choc pinkie fingers	2091kJ	↑ Fat ↑ Sugar	✓	Poor
Cottage cookie, chocolate chip cookies	1994kJ	↑ Fat ↑ Sugar	✓	Poor
Cottage cookie, macadamia cookies	2169kJ	↑ Fat ↑ Sugar	✓	Poor
Family assorted	1954kJ	↑ Fat ↑ Sugar	220	Poor
Jam fancies	1840kJ	↑ Fat ↑ Sugar	160b	Poor
Malt	1850kJ	↑ Fat ↑ Sugar	✓	Poor
Oatmeal highlands	1850kJ	↑ Fat ↑ Sugar	✓	Poor
Rich tea	1880kJ	↑ Fat ↑ Sugar	220	Poor
Strawberry mallows	1590kJ	↑ Fat ↑ Sugar	202, 220	Poor
Triple choc temptation	1935kJ	↑ Fat ↑ Sugar	✓	Poor
Uglies	2000kJ	↑ Fat ↑ Sugar	120	Poor
Vive lites, choc chip	1761kJ	↑ Fat ↑ Sugar	✓	Poor
Vive lites, pecan &	1748kJ	↑ Fat	160b, 422	Poor

caramel		↑ Sugar		

Ritzbury

Product Name	Energy	Major Nutrients	Food Additives	Nutritious Rating
Chocolate fingers	2050kJ	↑ Fat ↑ Sugar	✓	Poor
Chocolate puff	2017kJ	↑ Fat ↑ Sugar ↑ Salt	102, 110, 122, 133	Poor
Coconut crunch	2021kJ	↑ Fat ↑ Sugar	320, 220	Poor
Lemon puff	1978kJ	↑ Fat ↑ Sugar	102, 320	Poor

Sterns

Product Name	Energy	Major Nutrients	Food Additives	Nutritious Rating
Pfeffernusse	1550kJ	↑ Sugar	220	Poor

Unibec

Product Name	Energy	Major Nutrients	Food Additives	Nutritious Rating
Anzac Biscuits	2040kJ	↑ Fat ↑ Sugar	220	Poor
Shortbread finger	2200kJ	↑ Fat ↑ Sugar	✓	Poor
Sponge finger savoiardi	1510kJ	↑ Fat ↑ Sugar	282, 420	Poor

Walkers

Product Name	Energy	Major Nutrients	Food Additives	Nutritious Rating
Shortbread fingers cello	2148kJ	↑ Fat ↑ Sugar	✓	Poor

Weight watchers

Product Name	Energy	Major Nutrients	Food Additives	Nutritious Rating
Chocolate chip cookies	1900kJ	↑ Fat ↑ Sugar	✓	Poor
Fruit slice	1450kJ	↑ Sugar	223, 202, 422	Average
Raspberry tartlets	1720kJ	↑ Sugar	124, 122	Poor

White Wings

Product Name	Energy	Major Nutrients	Food Additives	Nutritious Rating
Chunkies, choc chunk cookies	2020kJ	↑ Fat ↑ Sugar	220	Poor
Chunkies, triple choc cookies	2040kJ	↑ Fat ↑ Sugar	✓	Poor
Chunkies, white chocolate & macadamia cookies	2090kJ	↑ Fat ↑ Sugar	✓	Poor
Creamies, lemon whipped cream	2100kJ	↑ Fat ↑ Sugar	✓	Poor
Creamies, passionfruit	2240kJ	↑ Fat ↑ Sugar	160b	Poor
Creamies, raspberry jam & cream	2060kJ	↑ Fat ↑ Sugar	120	Poor
Creamies, whipped chocolate cream	2300kJ	↑ Fat ↑ Sugar	✓	Poor
Drizzles, choc chunk	2050kJ	↑ Fat ↑ Sugar	220	Poor
Drizzles, white choc chunk	2070kJ	↑ Fat ↑ Sugar	✓	Poor
Splits, choc flakes	2090kJ	↑ Fat ↑ Sugar	220	Poor
Splits homestyle buttery	1915kJ	↑ Fat ↑ Sugar	✓	Poor

Woolworths/Safeways

Product Name	Energy	Major Nutrients	Food Additives	Nutritious Rating
Select, chocolate sandwich	1960kJ	↑ Sugar ↑ Fat	120	Poor
Select, honeycomb crunch	2160kJ	↑ Sugar ↑ Fat	160b	Poor
Select, fruit & nut	2080kJ	↑ Sugar ↑ Fat	220	Poor
Select, toffee caramel	2010kJ	↑ Sugar ↑ Fat	220	Poor
Select, chocolate fingers	2070kJ	↑ Sugar ↑ Fat	160b	Poor
Select, rocky road mallows	1870kJ	↑ Sugar ↑ Fat	120, 224	Poor
Select, mint crème	**2190kJ**	**↑ Sugar ↑ Fat**	**✓**	**Poor**
Select, orange delight	1790kJ	↑ Sugar ↑ Fat	224	Poor
Select, orange creams	2010kJ	↑ Sugar ↑ Fat	319	Poor
Select, chocolate creams	1990kJ	↑ Sugar ↑ Fat	319	Poor
Select, lemon creams	1930kJ	↑ Sugar ↑ Fat ↑ Salt	319	Poor
Select, tiny bears choc	1980kJ	↑ Sugar ↑ Fat	160b	Poor
Select, tiny bears honey	1930kJ	↑ Sugar ↑ Fat	160b	Poor
Select, shortbread creams	2120kJ	↑ Sugar ↑ Fat	160b	Poor
Select, choc chunk cookies	2020kJ	↑ Sugar ↑ Fat	223	Poor
Homebrand, choc mint slice	2240kJ	↑ Sugar ↑ Fat	320, 321	Poor
Homebrand, triple choc	2120kJ	↑ Sugar ↑ Fat	320, 321, 223, 155, 133, 122	Poor

Homebrand, choc scotch finger	**2070kJ**	↑ Sugar ↑ Fat	✓	**Poor**
Homebrand, choc monty	2100kJ	↑ Sugar ↑ Fat	223, 320, 321	Poor
Homebrand, choc macadamia cookie	2020kJ	↑ Sugar ↑ Fat	223	Poor
Homebrand, double choc cookies	**2050kJ**	↑ Sugar ↑ Fat	✓	**Poor**
Homebrand, ginger cookies	1920kJ	↑ Sugar ↑ Fat	220	Poor
Homebrand, scotch finger	2010kJ	↑ Sugar ↑ Fat	220	Poor
Homebrand, assorted creams	2130kJ	↑ Sugar ↑ Fat	220, 120	Poor
Homebrand, family assorted	1980kJ	↑ Sugar ↑ Fat	223, 220, 320, 321	Poor
Homebrand, milk arrowroot	1890kJ	↑ Sugar ↑ Fat	320, 321, 223	Poor
Homebrand, gingernut	1800kJ	↑ Sugar ↑ Fat	320, 321	Poor
Homebrand, raspberry tartlet	1730kJ	↑ Sugar ↑ Fat	202, 123, 110, 320, 160b, 220	Poor
Homebrand, blackberry tartlet	1820kJ	↑ Sugar ↑ Fat	129, 133, 320, 160b, 220	Poor
Homebrand, choc chip cookie	1930kJ	↑ Sugar ↑ Fat	160b	Poor
Homebrand, chocolate chip biscuits	2030kJ	↑ Sugar ↑ Fat	220	Poor

Crackers

The best choices for crackers include: *Abe's real bagels, Albatros, Always fresh, Carrs, Dick Smith, Ecor organic, Kavali, Kurrajong kitchen, Orgran, Ryvita, Pure harvest, Real foods, Tucker's gourmet crackers and Wice crackers.*

Abe's Real Bagels

Product Name	Energy	Major Nutrients	Food Additives	Nutritious Rating
Roasted garlic	1780kJ	↑ Salt	✓	Poor
Sea salt	1810kJ	↑ Salt	✓	Poor

Albatros

Product Name	Energy	Major Nutrients	Food Additives	Nutritious Rating
Mini toast	1780kJ	✓	✓	Poor

Always Fresh

Product Name	Energy	Major Nutrients	Food Additives	Nutritious Rating
Crustini, chives & cheese	1640kJ	↑ Salt ↑ Fat	✓	Poor
Crustini, olive oil & sea salt	1855kJ	↑ Salt ↑ Fat	✓	Poor
Grissini, rosemary & sea salt	1790kJ	↑ Salt ↑ Fat	✓	Poor
Grissini, sesame & sea salt	1810kJ	↑ Salt ↑ Fat	✓	Poor
Wafer crispbread, sesame	1640kJ	↑ Salt	✓	Poor

Arnott's

Product Name	Energy	Major Nutrients	Food Additives	Nutritious Rating
Cheds	2100kJ	↑ Salt ↑ Fat	YE	Poor
Cheeseboard	1898kJ	↑ Salt ↑ Fat	✓	Poor
Counter crackers	1930kJ	↑ Salt ↑ Fat	✓	Poor
Country cheese	1800kJ	↑ Salt ↑ Fat	YE, 160b	Poor
Cruskits, corn	1600kJ	↑ Salt	✓	Poor
Cruskits, light	1570kJ	↑ Salt	✓	Poor
Cruskits, original	1800kJ	↑ Salt ↑ Fat	✓	Poor
Cruskits, rye	1390kJ	↑ Salt	✓	Poor
Lunch slices, soy & linseed	1720kJ	↑ Fat	✓	Average
Lunch slices, sunflower, oats & chia	1700kJ	↑ Fat	✓	Good
Lunch slices, sunflower & pumpkin	1730kJ	↑ Fat	✓	Average
Lunch slices, sunflower & rye	1710kJ	↑ Fat	✓	Average
Jatz, original	1990kJ	↑ Salt ↑ Fat	✓	Poor
Jatz, light	1690kJ	↑ Salt	220	Poor
Jatz, cracked pepper	1940kJ	↑ Salt ↑ Fat	✓	Poor
Jatz, clix	2150kJ	↑ Salt ↑ Fat	✓	Poor
Sensations shapes, balsamic vinegar & sea salt	1830kJ	↑ Salt ↑ Fat	621, 635, 160b, 220	Poor
Sensations shapes, lime & chilli	1830kJ	↑ Salt ↑ Fat	621, 635, VE	Poor
Sensations shapes, roasted garlic &	1870kJ	↑ Salt ↑ Fat	621, 635, 160b, YE	Poor

parmesan				
Sensations shapes, tomato & chilli	1870kJ	↑ Salt ↑ Fat	621, 635, VE YE	Poor
Sensations shapes, honey soy chicken	1870kJ	↑ Salt ↑ Fat	621, 635, 160b, YE, VPE	Poor
Sensations shapes, vintage cheddar	1870kJ	↑ Salt ↑ Fat	621, 635, 160b, VE	Poor
Shapes, barbeque	2030kJ	↑ Salt ↑ Fat	621, 635, VE	Poor
Shapes, cheddar	2000kJ	↑ Salt ↑ Fat	YE, VE	Poor
Shapes, cheese & bacon	1960kJ	↑ Salt ↑ Fat	133, 120, 124, 635, 160b, YE, VE	Poor
Shapes, crimpy chicken	1960kJ	↑ Salt ↑ Fat	621, 635, YE	Poor
Shapes, nacho cheese	1920kJ	↑ Salt ↑ Fat	621, 627, 160b, YE	Poor
Shapes, savoury	2000kJ	↑ Salt ↑ Fat	120, VE	Poor
Shapes, pizza	2070kJ	↑ Salt ↑ Fat	VE	Poor
Shapes, flavours of the world Mediterranean feta & herb	1980kJ	↑ Salt ↑ Fat	621, 635, VE	Poor
Shapes, flavours of the world Texan BBQ	2030kJ	↑ Salt ↑ Fat	621, 635, VE, 160b, YE	Poor
Roadies, peri peri chicken	1860kJ	↑ Salt ↑ Fat	621, 635, YE	Poor
Roadies, sizzling pepper steak	1880kJ	↑ Salt ↑ Fat	621, 635, oil, YE	Poor
Roadies, sea salt & vinegar	1860kJ	↑ Salt ↑ Fat	621, 635, YE	Poor
Roadies, chilli	1870kJ	↑ Salt ↑ Fat	621, 635, YE	Poor
Roadies, crispy potato skins cheddar	1880kJ	↑ Salt ↑ Fat	621, 635, YE	Poor
Roadies, tangy BBQ	1880kJ	↑ Salt	621, 635, YE	Poor

ribs		↑ Fat		
Salada, light	1640kJ	↑ Salt	220	Poor
Salada, original	1790kJ	↑ Salt ↑ Fat	✓	Poor
Salada, wholemeal	1670kJ	↑ Salt	✓	Poor
Sao	1900kJ	↑ Salt ↑ Fat	✓	Poor
Sesame wheat	1930kJ	↑ Salt ↑ Fat	✓	Average
Vita-wheat, 9 grains	1570kJ	↑ Fat	✓	Average
Vita-wheat, original	1630kJ	✓	✓	Average
Vita-wheat, sesame	1650kJ	↑ Fat	✓	Average
Vita-wheat, sesame & poppy crackers	1800kJ	Oil, YE, 160b?	✓	Average
Vita-wheat multigrain crackers	1770kJ	Oil, YE, 160b?	✓	Average
Vita-wheat rice, lime & cracked pepper	1960kJ	↑ Salt ↑ Fat	YE	Poor
Vita-wheat rice, BBQ	1950kJ	↑ Salt ↑ Fat	YE	Poor
Vita-wheat rice, cheddar & chives	1950kJ	↑ Salt ↑ Fat	YE	Poor
Vita-wheat rice, plain	1910kJ	↑ Salt ↑ Fat	✓	Poor

Carrs

Product Name	Energy	Major Nutrients	Food Additives	Nutritious Rating
Table water, original	2000kJ	✓	✓	Poor
Table water, pepper	1740kJ	↑ Salt ↑ Fat	✓	Poor
Table water, sesame	1755kJ	↑ Fat	✓	Poor

Coles

Product Name	Energy	Major Nutrients	Food Additives	Nutritious Rating
Checkers crackers	1925kJ	↑ Salt ↑ Fat	✓	Poor
Rice cakes, thick	1610kJ	✓	✓	Poor
Rice crackers, plain	1690kJ	↑ Salt	627, 631, 320	Poor
Rice crackers, cheese	1740kJ	↑ Salt	627, 631, 320, HVP	Poor
Skipton crackers	1826kJ	↑ Salt ↑ Fat	✓	Poor
Vita bites, rock salt	1700kJ	↑ Salt ↑ Fat	✓	Poor
Water crackers, cracked pepper	1710kJ	↑ Salt	✓	Poor
Water crackers, original	1736kJ	↑ Salt	✓	Poor

Dick Smith's

Product Name	Energy	Major Nutrients	Food Additives	Nutritious Rating
Water crackers	1660kJ	✓	✓	Poor

Ecor Organic

Product Name	Energy	Major Nutrients	Food Additives	Nutritious Rating
Four grain cake	1660kJ	✓	✓	Average
Rice crispbread	16122kJ	✓	✓	Poor
Rice & corn crispbread	1512kJ	✓	✓	Poor
Wholegrain cake with millet	1663kJ	✓	✓	Average
Wholemeal spelt cake	1442kJ	✓	✓	Average

Fantastic

Product Name	Energy	Major Nutrients	Food Additives	Nutritious Rating
Delites, cheese &	1860kJ	↑ Salt	621, 320,	Poor

French onion		↑ Fat	220, 627, 631, HVP, YE	
Delites, flame grill BBQ	1830kJ	↑ Salt ↑ Fat	621, 320, 220, YE	Poor
Delites, lemon Moroccan chicken	1840kJ	↑ Salt ↑ Fat	621, 320, HVP, YE, 627, 631	Poor
Delites, sea salt & balsamic	1820kJ	↑ Salt ↑ Fat	621, 320, 220, 627, 631	Poor
Delites, sea salt & pepper	1800kJ	↑ Salt ↑ Fat	621, 320, 220, 627, 631, 635, HVP, YE	Poor
Delites sour cream & chives	1870kJ	↑ Salt ↑ Fat	621, 320, 220, 627, 631, HVP, YE	Poor
Delites sweet chilli & sour cream	1840kJ	↑ Salt ↑ Fat	320, 220, YE, 631	Poor
Delites, tzatziki	1810kJ	↑ Salt ↑ Fat	621, 320, HVP, YE, 627, 631	Poor
Delites, wood fired pizza	1870kJ	↑ Salt ↑ Fat	621, 320, 220, 627, 631, HVP, YE	Poor
Goodies, 2 seeds	1880kJ	↑ Salt ↑ Fat	320	Average
Goodies 4 grains	1760kJ	↑ Salt	320	Average
Rice crackers, beef & wasabi	1710kJ	↑ Salt	621, 320, HVP, YE, 627, 635	Poor
Rice crackers, barbeque	1680kJ	✓	621, 627, 631, HVP	Poor
Rice crackers, cheddar cheese	1780kJ	↑ Salt ↑ Fat	621, 320, HVP, YE, 627, 631	Poor
Rice crackers, original	1700kJ	✓	627, 631, HVP	Poor
Rice crackers, seaweed	1520kJ	↑ Salt	627, 631, HVP	Poor

Rice crackers, teriyaki	1690kJ	✓	627, 631	Poor
Inspiration rice crackers, French onion & cheese	1740kJ	↑ Salt	YE, HVP, 621, 627, 631, 320, 160b	Poor
Inspiration rice crackers, sweet chilli & sour cream	1760kJ	↑ Salt	YE, 320, 621, 635	Poor
Soho, roast chicken	1760kJ	↑ Salt	320, 621, 627, 631, 220, YE	Poor
Soho, sour cream & chives	1760kJ	↑ Salt	320, 621, 627, 631, 220, YE	Poor

IGA/Franklins

Product Name	Energy	Major Nutrients	Food Additives	Nutritious Rating
Signature cracker bites, cheese supreme	2040kJ	↑ Salt ↑ Fat	102, 110, 621	Poor
Signature cracker bites, sour cream & red onion	2040kJ	↑ Salt ↑ Fat	✓	Poor
Signature, corn cake	1600kJ	✓	✓	Poor
Signature, rice cakes	1680kJ	✓	✓	Poor
Black & Gold crackers, traditional	1870kJ	↑ Salt ↑ Fat	320	Poor
Black & Gold rice crackers, cheese	1650kJ	↑ Salt	627, 631, HVP	Poor
Black & Gold rice crackers, plain	1660kJ	↑ Salt	627, 631	Poor
Black & Gold rice crackers, seaweed	1590kJ	↑ Salt	627, 631, YE	Poor
Black & Gold snax, BBQ	1961kJ	↑ Salt ↑ Fat	319, 223, HVP	Poor
Black & Gold snax,	1967kJ	↑ Salt	319, 223,	Poor

chicken		↑ Fat	HVP	
Black & Gold snax, pizza	1967kJ	↑ Salt ↑ Fat	319, 223, HVP	Poor

Kavali

Product Name	Energy	Major Nutrients	Food Additives	Nutritious Rating
Crispy thin	1320kJ	✓	✓	Poor

Kraft

Product Name	Energy	Major Nutrients	Food Additives	Nutritious Rating
Captain's table, classic	1850kJ	↑ Salt ↑ Fat	319	Poor
Captain's table, cracked pepper	1840kJ	↑ Salt ↑ Fat	319	Poor
Captain's table, sesame	1870kJ	↑ Salt ↑ Fat	319	Poor
Captain's table grissini sticks, rosemary	1640kJ	↑ Salt ↑ Fat	✓	Poor
Captain's table grissini sticks, sesame	1680kJ	↑ Salt ↑ Fat	✓	Poor
In a biscuit, cheese	1970kJ	↑ Salt ↑ Fat	627, 631, 160b, 319, YE	Poor
In a biscuit, chicken	2080kJ	↑ Salt ↑ Fat	319, 320, 627, 631, HVP	Poor
In a biscuit, crispy bacon	2080kJ	↑ Salt ↑ Fat	319, HVP, YE, 621, 635	Poor
In a biscuit, crispy potato	2100kJ	↑ Salt ↑ Fat	YE, 221, 319, 320, 621, 627, 631	Poor
In a biscuit, dixie drumsticks	2010kJ	↑ Salt ↑ Fat	HVP, 160b, 319, 223, 621	Poor
Premium, original	1910kJ	↑ Salt ↑ Fat	319	Poor
Premium, wholemeal	1820kJ	↑ Salt	319	Poor

		↑ Fat		
Premium, 98% fat free	1600kJ	✓	✓	Poor
Ritz, cheese	2090kJ	↑ Salt ↑ Fat	319	Poor
Ritz, original	2120kJ	↑ Salt ↑ Fat	319	Poor

Kurrajong Kitchen

Product Name	Energy	Major Nutrients	Food Additives	Nutritious Rating
Lavosh, bites	1820kJ	↑ Salt ↑ Fat	✓	Poor
Lavosh, original	1760kJ	↑ Salt ↑ Fat	✓	Poor
Lavosh, thins	1820kJ	↑ Salt ↑ Fat	✓	Poor
Shepherd's bread	1691kJ	↑ Salt	✓	Poor

Orgran

Product Name	Energy	Major Nutrients	Food Additives	Nutritious Rating
Crisibread, buckwheat	1490kJ	✓	✓	Average
Crisibread, quinoa	1400kJ	✓	✓	Good
Toasted corndippers	1405kJ	✓	✓	Poor

Peckish

Product Name	Energy	Major Nutrients	Food Additives	Nutritious Rating
Rice crackers, cheddar	1910kJ	↑ Fat	627, 631	Poor
Rice crackers, lime & black pepper	1840kJ	↑ Fat	627, 631	Poor
Rice crackers, original	1870kJ	↑ Fat	627, 631	Poor
Rice crackers, sea salt & vinegar	1870kJ	↑ Fat	627, 631	Poor

Rice crackers, sour cream & chives	1920kJ	↑ Fat	627, 631	Poor
Rice crackers, sweet chilli	1860kJ	↑ Fat	627, 631	Poor
Rice crackers, tangy BBQ	1800kJ	↑ Fat	627, 631	Poor
Rice crackers, wasabi	1860kJ	↑ Fat	627, 631	Poor

Pure Harvest

Product Name	Energy	Major Nutrients	Food Additives	Nutritious Rating
Organic Rice cakes	1610kJ	✓	✓	Poor

Real Foods

Product Name	Energy	Major Nutrients	Food Additives	Nutritious Rating
Corn thins, original	1599kJ	✓	✓	Poor
Corn thins, multigrain	1624kJ	✓	✓	Average
Corn thins, sesame	1606kJ	✓	✓	Average
Corn thins, soy & linseed	1642kJ	✓	✓	Average

Ryvita

Product Name	Energy	Major Nutrients	Food Additives	Nutritious Rating
Cracker bread	1612kJ	✓	✓	Poor
Fruit & seed crunch	1600kJ	✓	220	Good
Multigrain	1500kJ	✓	✓	Average
Original	1460kJ	✓	✓	Average
Pumpkin seed & oats	1570kJ	↑ Fat	✓	Good
Sesame	1600kJ	↑ Fat	✓	Good
Sunflower seeds & oats	1610kJ	↑ Fat	✓	Good

Snakata

Product Name	Energy	Major Nutrients	Food Additives	Nutritious Rating
Rice crackers,	1760kJ	↑ Salt	YE, 202, 220	Poor

cheddar cheese		↑ Fat		
Rice crackers, cheddar & sweet chilli	1750kJ	✓	YE	Poor
Rice crackers, barbecue	1670kJ	✓	YE	Poor
Rice crackers, classic BBQ	1720kJ	↑ Salt	YE, 220	Poor
Rice crackers, Greek fetta & herb	1710kJ	↑ Salt	YE	Poor
Rice crackers, Italian roast & balsamic	1710kJ	↑ Salt	YE, 220	Poor
Rice crackers, honey mustard	1740kJ	✓	YE	Poor
Rice crackers, plain	**1660kJ**	✓	✓	**Poor**
Rice crackers, seaweed	1570kJ	↑ Salt	YE	Poor
Rice crackers, sour cream & chives	1720kJ	↑ Salt	YE	Poor
Rice crackers, wholegrain cheddar & chives	1690kJ	↑ Fat	YE	Poor
Rice crackers wholegrain, original	**1660kJ**	✓	✓	**Poor**
Rice crackers, wholegrain parmesan herb & garlic	1680kJ	↑ Fat	YE	Poor
Rice crackers, wholegrain smokey BBQ	1680kJ	↑ Fat	YE	Poor
Rice crackers, wholegrain lemon & black pepper	1680kJ	↑ Fat	YE	Poor
Rice crackers, wholegrain sweet chilli	1690kJ	↑ Fat	YE	Poor
Gourmet bite snacks, salt & balsamic vinegar	1740kJ	↑ Salt ↑ Fat	YE	Poor

Product Name	Energy	Major Nutrients	Food Additives	Nutritious Rating
Gourmet bite snacks, vintage cheddar & cheese	1750kJ	↑ Salt ↑ Fat	YE	Poor
Gourmet bite snacks, cheddar & sweet chilli	1760kJ	↑ Salt ↑ Fat	YE, HVP	Poor
Gourmet bite snacks, salt & vinegar	1710kJ	↑ Salt	621, 635	Poor
Snakatas, BBQ	1730kJ	↑ Salt	621	Poor
Snakatas, corn cheese supreme	1720kJ	↑ Salt ↑ Fat	621, 635, HVP	Poor
Snakatas, nacho cheese	1730kJ	↑ Salt ↑ Fat	HVP, 621, 635	Poor
Snakatas, roast chicken	1720kJ	↑ Salt	621, 627, 631, 222	Poor
Snakatas, sour cream & chives	1740kJ	↑ Salt	621, 635, YE	Poor

Sunrice

Product Name	Energy	Major Nutrients	Food Additives	Nutritious Rating
Rice cakes, thick original	1630kJ	✓	✓	Poor
Rice cakes, thin original	1630kJ	✓	✓	Poor
Rice cakes, thin rice & corn	1630kJ	✓	✓	Poor
Rice cakes, apple & cinnamon	1720kJ	↑ Sugar	✓	Poor
Rice cakes, caramel	1730kJ	↑ Sugar	160b	Poor
Rice cakes, honey	1670kJ	↑ Sugar	✓	Poor
Rice cakes, thin roast chicken	1690kJ	↑ Salt ↑ Fat	635, HVP	Poor
Rice cakes, thin sea salt & balsamic vinegar	1620kJ	↑ Salt	635, HVP, YE	Poor

Rice cakes, thin sour cream & chives	1690kJ	↑ Salt ↑ Fat	635, HVP, YE	Poor
Rice cakes, thin sundried tomato & basil	1640kJ	↑ Salt	635, HVP, YE	Poor
Rice cakes, thin sweet chilli	1670kJ	↑ Salt ↑ Fat	635, HVP, YE	Poor
Rice cakes, thin vintage cheddar	1690kJ	↑ Salt ↑ Fat	635, HVP, YE	Poor

Tuckers Gourmet Crackers

Product Name	Energy	Major Nutrients	Food Additives	Nutritious Rating
Caramelised onion	1910kJ	↑ Salt ↑ Fat	✓	Poor
Rosemary & rock salt	1860kJ	↑ Salt ↑ Fat	✓	Poor

Water Thins

Product Name	Energy	Major Nutrients	Food Additives	Nutritious Rating
Bagelettes, garlic	1970kJ	↑ Salt ↑ Fat	320	Poor
Bagelettes, original	1911kJ	↑ Salt ↑ Fat	320	Poor
Cheese twists, classic cheddar	1804kJ	↑ Salt ↑ Fat	422	Poor
Cheese twists, parmesan & garlic	1730kJ	↑ Salt ↑ Fat	422	Poor
Cheese twists, triple cheese	1630kJ	↑ Salt ↑ Fat	422	Poor
Corn thins	1780kJ	↑ Salt ↑ Fat	HVP	Poor
Grain thins	1790kJ	↑ Salt ↑ Fat	✓	Poor
Oat thins	1810kJ	↑ Salt ↑ Fat	✓	Poor
Rice thins	1640kJ	↑ Salt	320, HVP	Poor
Wafer crackers,	1679kJ	↑ Salt	220, 202	Poor

natural				
Wafer crackers, pepper & chives	1640kJ	↑ Salt	✓	Poor
Wafer crackers, sesame	1650kJ	↑ Salt	✓	Poor

Wice Crackers

Product Name	Energy	Major Nutrients	Food Additives	Nutritious Rating
Rice crackers	1610kJ	↑ Salt	✓	Poor

Woothworths/Safeways

Product Name	Energy	Major Nutrients	Food Additives	Nutritious Rating
Select, cracker selection	1890kJ	↑ Salt	YE, 223, 319, HVP	Poor
Select, sea salt crackers	2050kJ	↑ Salt ↑ Fat	✓	Poor
Select, wheaten original	2040kJ	↑ Salt ↑ Fat	✓	Poor
Homebrand, crackers	2020kJ	↑ Salt ↑ Fat	✓	Poor
Homebrand, crackers low fat	1620kJ	✓	✓	Poor
Homebrand, crackers traditional	1750kJ	↑ Fat	320, 321, 223	Poor
Homebrand, rice cakes	1710kJ	✓	✓	Poor
Homebrand, rice & corn cakes	1710kJ	✓	✓	Poor
Homebrand, rice cracker BBQ	1690kJ	✓	627, 631, 319	Poor
Homebrand, rice crackers plain	1740kJ	✓	319	Poor
Homebrand, water crackers cracked pepper	1790kJ	✓	320	Poor
Homebrand snack crackers BBQ	2000kJ	↑ Salt ↑ Fat	✓	Poor

Homebrand snack crackers chicken	2070kJ	↑ Salt ↑ Fat	HVP	Poor

Desserts, Cake Mixes & Toppings

As far as packet mixes go, there is none better than Donna Hay. Of course, these items are going to high in fat and sugar and the quantity of consumption needs caution. I love that the Donna Hay mixes contain real ingredients and are not a science experiment. Plus they are packaged ethically and taste great!

Aunty Betty's

Product Name	Energy	Major Nutrients	Food Additives	Nutritious Rating
Pudding, Belgian chocolate	1505kJ	↑Sugar	220, 200, 202, 420	Poor
Pudding, de-lites sticky toffee	1300kJ	↑Sugar	220, 200, 202, 420	Poor
Pudding, golden syrup	1230kJ	↑Sugar	220, 200, 202, 420	Poor
Pudding, gooey caramel	1200kJ	↑Sugar	220, 200, 202, 420	Poor
Pudding, fruit light	1200kJ	↑Sugar	220, 200, 422	Poor

Betty Crocker

Product Name	Energy	Major Nutrients	Food Additives	Nutritious Rating
Devil food cake	1505kJ	↑Fat ↑Sugar ↑Salt	✓	Poor
Chocolate mud cake	1660kJ	↑Fat ↑Sugar	202	Poor
Chocolate swirl cake	1440kJ	↑Fat ↑Sugar	202	Poor
Chocolate fudge cake	1510kJ	↑Fat ↑Sugar ↑Salt	202	Poor
Strawberries &	1602kJ	↑Fat	202	Poor

cream cake		↑Sugar		
Chocolate cupcakes	1445kJ	↑Fat ↑Sugar ↑Salt	202	Poor
Vanilla cupcakes	1486kJ	↑Fat ↑Sugar	202	Poor
Strawberries & cream cupcakes	1515kJ	↑Fat ↑Sugar	202	Poor
Apple & cinnamon muffins	1185kJ	↑Sugar	202	Poor
Triple chocolate muffins	1696kJ	↑Fat ↑Sugar	202	Poor
Mixed berry muffins	1066kJ	↑Sugar	202	Poor
Blueberry muffins	1066kJ	↑Sugar	202	Poor
Cinnamon crumble muffins	1710kJ	↑Fat ↑Sugar	320, 220	Poor
Homestyle scones, fruit & spice	1452kJ	↑Fat ↑Sugar	220	Poor
Homestyle scones, chocolate mud	**1511kJ**	**↑Fat ↑Sugar**	✓	**Poor**
Homestyle scones, berry & white chocolate	1432kJ	↑Fat ↑Sugar	220	Poor
Triple chocolate fudge brownies	1748kJ	↑Fat ↑Sugar	✓	Poor
Chocolate caramel brownies	1602kJ	↑Sugar	202, 420, 422	Poor
Frosted choc brownies	1712kJ	↑Sugar	202	Poor
Reduced fat chocolate brownies	**1474kJ**	**↑Sugar**	✓	**Poor**
Rainbow chocolate brownies	1722kJ	↑Sugar	133, 129, 110, 102, 160b, 220	Poor
Milk chocolate chunk cookies	**1972kJ**	**↑Fat ↑Sugar**	✓	**Poor**
Rainbow cookies	1846kJ	↑Fat ↑Sugar	133, 129, 110, 102, 160b	Poor

Coles

Product Name	Energy	Major Nutrients	Food Additives	Nutritious Rating
Custard, ready made	402kJ	✓	407, 160b	Poor
Pudding, chocolate	**788kJ**	↑Sugar	✓	**Poor**
Pudding, mixed berry	745kJ	↑Sugar	120, 163	Poor
Pudding, sticky date	**671kJ**	↑Sugar	✓	**Poor**
Topping, caramel	937kJ	↑Sugar	202	Poor
Topping, chocolate	933kJ	↑Sugar	202	Poor
Topping, strawberry	864kJ	↑Sugar	120, 202	Poor
Topping, choc top	**2630kJ**	↑Sugar	✓	**Poor**
Smart Buy, choc top	1030kJ	↑Sugar	202	Poor
Smart Buy, custard powder	**375kJ**	↑Sugar	✓	**Poor**
Smart Buy, rice cream	**465kJ**	↑Sugar	✓	**Poor**

Cottees

Product Name	Energy	Major Nutrients	Food Additives	Nutritious Rating
Ice magic, caramel gold	2630kJ	↑Fat ↑Sugar	102, 110, 122, 319	Poor
Ice magic, choc honey	2640kJ	↑Fat ↑Sugar	319	Poor
Ice magic, choc mint	2640kJ	↑Fat ↑Sugar	319	Poor
Instant pudding, chocolate	**435kJ**	↑Sugar	✓	**Poor**
Instant pudding, vanilla	480kJ	↑Sugar	102, 110	Poor
Magic mouse, chocolate	840kJ	↑Fat ↑Sugar	102, 122, 133, 220	Poor
Magic mouse, strawberry	855kJ	↑Fat ↑Sugar	124, 102, 133, 220	Poor
Thick & rich topping, caramel	685kJ	↑Sugar	202, 102, 133	Poor
Thick & rich topping, chocolate	805kJ	↑Sugar	202	Poor
Thick & rich topping,	145kJ	✓	202, 955,	Poor

			954	
Thick & rich topping, strawberry	630kJ	↑Sugar	211, 124, 122	Poor

Donna Hay

Product Name	Energy	Major Nutrients	Food Additives	Nutritious Rating
Almond macaroon with chocolate filling	670kJ	↑Fat ↑Sugar	✓	Poor
Chocolate cupcakes	1530kJ	↑Fat ↑Sugar	✓	Poor
Vanilla cupcakes	1470kJ	↑Fat ↑Sugar	✓	Poor
Brownie choc molten mix		↑Fat ↑Sugar	✓	Poor

Duncan Hines

Product Name	Energy	Major Nutrients	Food Additives	Nutritious Rating
Devils food cake	1800kJ	↑Fat ↑Sugar ↑Salt	✓	Poor

Fosters Clarke

Product Name	Energy	Major Nutrients	Food Additives	Nutritious Rating
Custard ,cups	1250kJ	↑Sugar	202	Poor
Custard, ready made	1080kJ	↑Sugar	202, 133	Poor
Custard, powder	1140kJ	↑Sugar	202	Poor
Snack pack, banana	469kJ	↑Sugar	102, 110	Poor
Snack pack, chocolate	459kJ	↑Sugar	✓	Poor
Snack pack, strawberry	469kJ	↑Sugar	129	Poor

Greens

Product Name	Energy	Major Nutrients	Food Additives	Nutritious Rating
Chocolate mud cake	1390kJ	↑ Fat	160b, 320	Poor

		↑ Sugar		
Chocolate cake	1480kJ	↑ Fat ↑ Sugar	160b, 320	Poor
Classic chocolate	1440kJ	↑ Fat ↑ Sugar	160b, 320	Poor
Smooth coffee cake	1500kJ	↑ Fat ↑ Sugar	160b, 320	Poor
Smooth lemon cake	1460kJ	↑ Fat ↑ Sugar	160b, 320	Poor
Banana cake	1450kJ	↑ Fat ↑ Sugar	160b, 320	Poor
Golden butter cake	1470kJ	↑ Fat ↑ Sugar	160b	Poor
Vanilla cake	1470kJ	↑ Fat ↑ Sugar	160b, 320	Poor
English tea cake	1300kJ	↑ Fat ↑ Sugar	160b, 320	Poor
Date loaf	1180kJ	↑ Fat ↑ Sugar	160b, 320	Poor
Orange cake	1460kJ	↑ Fat ↑ Sugar	160b, 320	Poor
Orange & poppy seed cake	1480kJ	↑ Fat ↑ Sugar	160b, 320	Poor
Sponge cake	**1555kJ**	**↑Fat ↑Sugar**	✓	**Poor**
Vanilla cupcakes	1550kJ	↑Fat ↑Sugar	160b, 320	Poor
Pink cupcakes	1740kJ	↑Fat ↑Sugar ↑Salt	160b, 220	Poor
Chocolate cupcakes	1460kJ	↑Fat ↑Sugar	120, 160b, 320	Poor
Marshmallow delight cupcakes	1400kJ	↑Fat ↑Sugar	160b, 202, 422	Poor
Strawberry dream cupcakes	1420kJ	↑Fat ↑Sugar	160b, 202	Poor
Choc caramel fudge cupcakes	1500kJ	↑Fat ↑Sugar	160b, 202	Poor
Strawberry baby	1540kJ	↑Fat	120, 160b,	Poor

cakes		↑Sugar	320	
Blueberry muffins	1130kJ	↑Salt ↑Sugar	160b, 422	Poor
Choc chip muffins	1070kJ	↑Salt ↑Sugar	160b, 422	Poor
Banana honey muffins	1050kJ	↑Fat ↑Sugar	160b, 422, 223	Poor
Choc profiteroles	**1310kJ**	**↑Fat ↑Sugar**	✓	**Poor**
Gingerbread man cookies	936kJ	↑Fat ↑Sugar	120, 160b	Poor
Racing car cookies	1600kJ	↑Fat ↑Sugar	120, 160b	Poor
Pancake shaker, original	**850kJ**	**↑Sugar**	✓	**Poor**
Pancake shaker, buttermilk	**849kJ**	**↑Sugar**	✓	**Poor**
Pancake shaker, maple	**843kJ**	**↑Sugar**	✓	**Poor**
Pancake shaker, banana	**830kJ**	**↑Sugar**	✓	**Poor**
Pudding, blackberry	685kJ	↑Sugar	160b, 320	Poor
Pudding, butterscotch	678kJ	↑Sugar	160b, 320	Poor
Pudding, caramel fudge	647kJ	↑Sugar	160b, 320	Poor
Pudding, chocolate	675kJ	↑Sugar	223	Poor
Pudding, lemon	685kJ	↑Sugar	160b, 320	Poor
Pudding, sticky date	695kJ	↑Sugar	160b, 320	Poor

IGA/Franklins

Product Name	Energy	Major Nutrients	Food Additives	Nutritious Rating
Signature, golden syrup pudding	1230kJ	↑Sugar	200, 202, 422	Poor
Signature, chocolate pudding	1260kJ	↑Sugar	200, 202, 422	Poor
Signature, ice-cream coating	**2670kJ**	**↑ Fat ↑ Sugar**	✓	**Poor**

Signature, caramel topping	937kJ	↑Sugar	202	Poor
Signature, chocolate topping	933kJ	↑Sugar	202	Poor
Signature, strawberry topping	864kJ	↑Sugar	202, 120	Poor
Black & Gold, custard powder	1520kJ	↑ Salt ↑ Sugar	102, 110	Poor

McKenzies

Product Name	Energy	Major Nutrients	Food Additives	Nutritious Rating
Banana blast topping	1250kJ	↑Sugar	202	Poor
Blue heaven topping	1080kJ	↑Sugar	202, 133	Poor
Choc explosion topping	1140kJ	↑Sugar	202	Poor

The Pancake Parlour

Product Name	Energy	Major Nutrients	Food Additives	Nutritious Rating
Buttermilk pancake mix	1440kJ	↑Salt	✓	Poor

White Wings

Product Name	Energy	Major Nutrients	Food Additives	Nutritious Rating
Choc heaven cake	1115kJ	↑ Fat ↑ Sugar	320	Poor
Dark chocolate mud cake	1505kJ	↑ Fat ↑ Sugar	160b	Poor
White chocolate mud cake	**1820kJ**	**↑ Fat ↑ Sugar**	✓	**Poor**
Milk chocolate cake	1660kJ	↑ Salt ↑ Sugar	220, 320	Poor
Chocolate on chocolate cake	1060kJ	↑Salt ↑Sugar	120, 160b, 220	Poor
Moist chocolate cake	1600kJ	↑ Salt ↑ Sugar	220, 320	Poor
Raspberry swirl cake	1745kJ	↑ Fat	220, 320, 120	Poor

		↑ Sugar ↑ Salt		
Vanilla cake	1040kJ	↑ Sugar	220	Poor
Date loaf	**1630kJ**	**↑ Fat ↑ Sugar**	**✓**	**Poor**
Madeira cake	1300kJ	↑ Fat ↑ Sugar	220	Poor
Golden butter cake	1540kJ	↑ Salt ↑ Sugar	320	Poor
Carrot & walnut cake	1735kJ	↑ Salt ↑ Sugar ↑ Fat	220, 320, HVP	Poor
Banana bread	1740kJ	↑ Fat ↑ Sugar	320	Poor
Angel baby cakes	1740kJ	↑ Sugar	220, 320	Poor
Strawberry baby cakes	1740kJ	↑ Sugar	120, 320	Poor
Double baby cakes	1730kJ	↑ Sugar	220, 320	Poor
Lots a choc chip cupcakes	1720kJ	↑ Salt ↑ Sugar ↑ Fat	220, 320	Poor
Vanilla cupcakes	1670kJ	↑ Fat ↑ Sugar	220, 320	Poor
Chocolate cupcakes	1630kJ	↑ Fat ↑ Sugar ↑ Salt	220, 320	Poor
Banana cupcakes	1740kJ	↑ Fat ↑ Sugar	220, 320	Poor
Choc-vanilla cupcakes	1650kJ	↑ Salt ↑ Sugar	220, 320	Poor
Heavenly banana cupcakes	1020kJ	↑ Fat ↑ Sugar	220, 320	Poor
Triple choc muffins	1610kJ	↑ Fat ↑ Sugar	220, 320	Poor
Blueberry muffins	1435kJ	↑ Sugar	202	Poor
Banana muffins	**1055kJ**	**↑ Sugar**	**✓**	**Poor**
Choc chip muffins	1100kJ	↑ Salt ↑ Sugar	102, 122, 133, 220	Poor
Continental	1290kJ	↑ Fat	202, 223,	Poor

Product Name	Energy	Major Nutrients	Food Additives	Nutritious Rating
cheesecake		↑ Sugar	281, 420	
Lemon cheesecake	1210kJ	↑ Fat ↑ Sugar	202, 223, 281, 420, 220	Poor
Choc chip cookies	1800kJ	↑ Fat ↑ Sugar	220, 320	Poor
Double choc chip cookies	1760kJ	↑ Fat ↑ Sugar	320	Poor
Double choc fudge brownies	1795kJ	↑ Sugar	220, 320	Poor
Choc chunk brownies	1790kJ	↑ Sugar	320	Poor
Pancake shaker, original	780kJ	↑ Sugar	✓	Poor
Pancake shaker, buttermilk	730kJ	✓	✓	Poor
Pancake shaker, golden syrup	780kJ	↑ Sugar	✓	Poor
Pudding, chocolate on chocolate	660kJ	↑ Sugar	✓	Poor
Pudding, golden butter scotch	670kJ	↑ Sugar	✓	Poor
Pudding, vanilla sponge	670kJ	↑ Sugar	160b	Poor
Mousse, chocolate	895kJ	↑ Sugar	220	Poor
Mousse, chocolate craze	1550kJ	↑ Salt ↑ Sugar	✓	Poor
Mousse, chocolate hazelnut	820kJ	↑ Sugar	220	Poor
Lemon meringue pie	1880kJ	↑ Fat ↑ Sugar	223	Poor
Rice cream vanilla	420kJ	✓	✓	Poor
Crème caramel	465kJ	↑ Sugar	160b, 202, 122	Poor
Smoothest vanilla custard	1500kJ	✓	160b	Poor

Woolworths/Safeways

Product Name	Energy	Major Nutrients	Food Additives	Nutritious Rating
Select dessert	1660kJ	↑ Sugar	202, 220	Poor

sauces, chocolate				
Select dessert sauces, mango passionfruit	**880kJ**	↑ Sugar	✓	**Poor**
Select dessert sauces, mixed berry	**800kJ**	↑ Sugar	✓	**Poor**
Select dessert sauces, toffee	1780kJ	↑ Sugar	202, 220	Poor
Select hard top, chocolate	**2630kJ**	↑ Fat ↑ Sugar	✓	**Poor**
Select hard top, choc honeycomb	**2630kJ**	↑ Fat ↑ Sugar	✓	**Poor**
Select hard top, choc mint	**2630kJ**	↑ Fat ↑ Sugar	✓	**Poor**
Select topping, banana	1050kJ	↑ Sugar	202	Poor
Select topping, caramel	998kJ	↑ Sugar	202	Poor
Select topping, chocolate	1160kJ	↑ Sugar	202	Poor
Select topping, strawberry	907kJ	↑ Sugar	202, 120	Poor
Homebrand, custard powder	1580kJ	✓	102, 110	Poor
Homebrand, custard, ready made	417kJ	✓	160b	Poor
Homebrand, chocolate cake	1340kJ	↑ Salt ↑ Sugar	155	Poor
Homebrand, butter cake	**1320kJ**	↑ Salt ↑ Sugar	✓	**Poor**
Homebrand, vanilla cake	**1290kJ**	↑ Salt ↑ Sugar	✓	**Poor**
Homebrand, butter muffins	1630kJ	↑ Salt ↑ Sugar	102, 110	Poor
Homebrand, chocolate muffins	1640kJ	↑ Salt ↑ Sugar	155	Poor
Homebrand, pancake & pikelet mix	1070kJ	↑ Salt ↑ Sugar	320	Poor
Homebrand, pancake	**1090kJ**	↑ Sugar	✓	**Poor**

shaker				
Homebrand topping, caramel	920kJ	↑ Sugar	202, 102, 124	Poor
Homebrand topping, chocolate	1030kJ	↑ Sugar	202	Poor
Homebrand topping, strawberry	1010kJ	↑ Sugar	122, 202, 110	Poor

Beverages

Cordial

Much of the cordial range worries me as most brands contain sodium benzoate (211). When 211 combines with vitamin C it forms benzene – a highly toxic, carcinogenic substance. 211 has been banned in the UK and other countries. In addition, there is a very strong link between 211 and hyperactivity and aggression. The only additive free brand is *Vitafresh*.

Anchor

Product Name	Energy	Major Nutrients	Food Additives	Nutritious Rating
Treehouse, apple & blackcurrant no sugar	12kJ	✓	120, 223, 954, 952	Average
Treehouse, koola	136kJ	✓	211, 223, 133, 102	Average
Treehouse, lemon barley	136kJ	✓	211, 223	Average
Treehouse, lemon barley no sugar	10kJ	✓	223, 954, 952	Average
Treehouse, raspberry	136kJ	✓	120, 223	Average

Bickfords

Product Name	Energy	Major Nutrients	Food Additives	Nutritious Rating
Blackcurrant	184kJ	↑Sugar	202, 223	Average
Cranberry	153kJ	✓	223	Average
Ginger beer	205kJ	↑Sugar	211	Average
Lemon juice	160kJ	✓	223	Average
Lemon juice, diet	8kJ	✓	223, 951	Average

Lemon, lime & bitters	180kJ	✓	211	Average
Lime juice	124kJ	✓	223, 951	Average
Lime juice, diet	10kJ	✓	211, 223	Average
Peach tea	119kJ	✓	202, 211	Average

Bottle Green Cordial

Product Name	Energy	Major Nutrients	Food Additives	Nutritious Rating
Elder flower	1235kJ	↑Sugar	202, 223	Average
Ginger & lemongrass	1226kJ	↑Sugar	202, 223	Average

Cascade

Product Name	Energy	Major Nutrients	Food Additives	Nutritious Rating
Raspberry	172kJ	✓	211	Average
Ultra blackcurrant	160kJ	✓	211	Average

Coles

Product Name	Energy	Major Nutrients	Food Additives	Nutritious Rating
Blackcurrant	218kJ	↑Sugar	202, 223	Average
Lemon	160kJ	✓	211, 223	Average
Lemon barley	173kJ	✓	223	Average
Lime	132kJ	✓	211, 223	Average
Smart buy, fruit cup	132kJ	✓	211, 223	Average
Smart buy, lime	150kJ	✓	211, 223, 102, 133	Average
Smart buy, raspberry	144kJ	✓	211, 223	Average

Cottees

Product Name	Energy	Major Nutrients	Food Additives	Nutritious Rating
Apple & blackcurrant	111kJ	✓	211, 223	Average
Apple & kiwi	106kJ	✓	211, 223, 102, 133	Average
Apple & raspberry	115kJ	✓	211, 223	Average
Apple & raspberry, no sugar	14kJ	✓	211, 223, 950	Average

Cola	105kJ	✓	211, 223	Average
Coola	117kJ	✓	211, 223, 102, 133	Average
Coola, no sugar	4kJ	✓	211, 223, 102, 133, 950	Average
Fruit cup	102kJ	✓	120, 223, 950	Average
Lemon barley	86kJ	✓	223, 950	Average
Lemon crush	89kJ	✓	211, 223, 950	Average
Lemon crush, no sugar	5kJ	✓	223	Average
Orange crush	104kJ	✓	211, 223, 120	Average
Orange & mango	104kJ	✓	211, 223, 120	Average
Orange & mango, no sugar	11kJ	✓	211, 223, 120	Average
Pine lime	104kJ	✓	211, 223, 102, 133	Average
Raspberry	115kJ	✓	211, 223	Average
Tropical crush	104kJ	✓	211, 223, 202, 120	Average

Diet Rite

Product Name	Energy	Major Nutrients	Food Additives	Nutritious Rating
Apple & raspberry	12kJ	✓	211, 223, 952, 950, 955	Average
Cranberry & boysenberry	10kJ	✓	211, 223, 952, 950, 955	Average
Fruit cocktail	10kJ	✓	211, 223, 952, 950, 955	Average
Orange & mango	10kJ	✓	211, 223, 120, 952, 950, 955	Average

Food Zoo

Product Name	Energy	Major Nutrients	Food Additives	Nutritious Rating
Flavour stix, raspberry	12kJ	✓	202, 122, 955	Poor
Flavour stix, lime	15kJ	✓	102, 133, 955, 202	Poor

Golden Circle

Product Name	Energy	Major Nutrients	Food Additives	Nutritious Rating
Apple & raspberry	120kJ	✓	211, 223, 950	Average
Apple & raspberry, light	15kJ	✓	211, 223, 952, 950, 955	Average
Fruit cup	125kJ	✓	211, 223, 120, 950	Average
Fruit cup, light	15kJ	✓	211, 223, 120, 950, 952, 954	Average
Golden pash	125kJ	✓	211, 223, 955	Average
Lime	120kJ	✓	211, 223, 133, 102, 955	Average
Orange crush	125kJ	✓	211, 223, 955	Average
Orange & mango	120kJ	✓	211, 223, 955	Average
Pine orange	125kJ	✓	211, 223, 955	Average
Raspberry	150kJ	✓	211, 223, 122, 955	Average
Raspberry, light	15kJ	✓	211, 223, 122, 952, 954, 950	Average

IGA/Franklins

Product Name	Energy	Major Nutrients	Food Additives	Nutritious Rating
Black & Gold, apple & blackcurrant	185kJ	✓	211, 223, 123	Average
Black & Gold, fruit cup	109kJ	✓	211, 110, 102, 223	Average

Black & Gold, lime	116kJ	✓	102, 133, 223, 211	Average
Black & Gold, orange & mango	109kJ	✓	102, 110, 211, 223	Average
Black & Gold, raspberry	116kJ	✓	122, 211, 223	Average

Ribena

Product Name	Energy	Major Nutrients	Food Additives	Nutritious Rating
Blackcurrant	210kJ	↑Sugar	202, 223	Average
Blackcurrant light	36kJ	✓	202, 223, 955, 950	Average

Schweppes

Product Name	Energy	Major Nutrients	Food Additives	Nutritious Rating
Lime juice	128kJ	✓	223	Average

Soda Stream

Product Name	Energy	Major Nutrients	Food Additives	Nutritious Rating
Cola	55kJ	✓	952, 950	Poor
Cola, diet	1kJ	✓	952, 950	Poor
Cola, sugar free	1.4kJ	✓	952, 950	Poor
Cream soda	62kJ	✓	952, 950, 102, 133, 211	Poor
Ginger beer	42kJ	✓	952, 951, 950	Poor
Lemonade	61kJ	✓	952, 950, 211	Poor
Orange	57kJ	✓	952, 950, 202	Poor
Raspberry	64kJ	✓	952, 950, 122, 211	Poor
Summer lemon	60kJ	✓	952, 950, 211, 104	Poor

The Natural Cordial Company

Product Name	Energy	Major Nutrients	Food Additives	Nutritious Rating
Apple & raspberry	20kJ	✓	223, 960	Average
Fruit cup	21kJ	✓	223, 960	Average
Lime	20kJ	✓	223, 960	Average
Orange	19kJ	✓	223, 960	Average

Vitafresh

Product Name	Energy	Major Nutrients	Food Additives	Nutritious Rating
Jamaican lime	137kJ	✓	✓	Average
Orange & mango	137kJ	✓	✓	Average
Sweet naval orange	137kJ	✓	✓	Average

Woolworths/Safeways

Product Name	Energy	Major Nutrients	Food Additives	Nutritious Rating
Select, apple & raspberry	128kJ	✓	223	Average
Select, blackcurrant	184kJ	✓	223, 202	Average
Select, lemon juice	133kJ	✓	223	Average
Select, lime	118kJ	✓	223, 141, 960	Average
Select, lime juice	133kJ	✓	223	Average
Select, orange	118kJ	✓	223, 960	Average
Select, raspberry	143kJ	✓	223	Average

Fruit Juice

Fresh juice can provide wonderful health benefits to people as it contains many live enzymes, phytochemicals and flavonoids. Unfortunately, this is lost in the bottling process as the enzymes, phytochemicals and flavonoids can be fragile, only surviving up to 20 minutes from juicing. Commercial juice still contains vitamins and not a total loss, but I strongly recommend fresh juice where possible. The best brands are *V8, Berri raw, Golden circle, Just juice, Sunraysia, Ocean spray, Spring Valley, Rosie, Coles, Coles smartbuy, Woolworths select and Homebrand.*

Berri

Product Name	Energy	Major Nutrients	Food Additives	Nutritious Rating
Bottled, apple	187kJ	✓	✓	Good
Bottled, apple & blackcurrant	185kJ	✓	✓	Good
Bottled, apple & cranberry	185kJ	✓	✓	Good
Bottled, apple & mango	190kJ	✓	✓	Good
Bottled, apple, mango & banana	189kJ	↑Sugar	✓	Good
Bottled, apple & pear	187kJ	✓	✓	Good
Bottled, apricot nectar	231kJ	↑Sugar	160b	Good
Bottled grape	238kJ	↑Sugar	223	Good
Bottled, grapefruit	153kJ	✓	✓	Good
Bottled, morning start	177kJ	✓	✓	Good
Bottled, multi V	187kJ	✓	✓	Good
Bottled, orange	189kJ	✓	✓	Good

Bottled, orange no sugar	170kJ	✓	✓	Good
Bottled, pineapple	179kJ	✓	✓	Good
Bottled, tomato	107kJ	✓	✓	Good
Bottled, tropical	182kJ	✓	✓	Good
Can, apricot nectar	248kJ	↑Sugar	160b	Good
Can tomato juice	100kJ	✓	✓	Good
Pop top, apple	187kJ	✓	✓	Average
Pop top, apple & blackcurrant	185kJ	✓	✓	Average
Pop top, orange	170kJ	✓	✓	Average
Multi V tetra, apple	201kJ	✓	✓	Good
Multi V tetra, apple & mango	192kJ	↑Sugar	✓	Good
Multi V tetra, breakfast	187kJ	✓	✓	Good
Multi V tetra, orange	170kJ	✓	✓	Good

Bickfords's

Product Name	Energy	Major Nutrients	Food Additives	Nutritious Rating
Blueberry	219kJ	↑Sugar	✓	Good
Coconut	80kJ	↑Sugar	✓	Good
Pomegranate	269kJ	✓	223	Good
Prune	277kJ	↑Sugar	✓	Good
Super berry	191kJ	↑Sugar	✓	Good

Campbells

Product Name	Energy	Major Nutrients	Food Additives	Nutritious Rating
V8 bottles, apple, carrot & ginger	195kJ	✓	✓	Good
V8 bottles, breakfast	195kJ	✓	✓	Good
V8 bottles, citrus burst	183kJ	✓	✓	Good
V8 bottles, hot & spicy	91kJ	✓	✓	Good

V8 bottles, original	85kJ	✓	✓	Good
V8 bottles, vegetable, low sodium	85kJ	✓	✓	Good
V8 smoothies, mango, peach & pear	207kJ	✓	✓	Good
V8 smoothies, pineapple, passion & banana	220kJ	✓	✓	Good
V8 smoothies, strawberry, raspberry & banana	215kJ	✓	✓	Good
V8 tetra, citrus splash	195kJ	✓	✓	Good
V8 tetra, orange, mango & passion	177kJ	✓	✓	Good
V8 tetra, original	85kJ	✓	✓	Good
V8 tetra, tropical	198kJ	✓	✓	Good

Coles

Product Name	Energy	Major Nutrients	Food Additives	Nutritious Rating
Bottled, apple	190kJ	↑Sugar	✓	Good
Bottled, apple & mango	190kJ	✓	✓	Good
Bottled, orange	170kJ	✓	✓	Good
Bottled, orange & mango	170kJ	✓	✓	Good
Bottled, pineapple	175kJ	✓	✓	Good
Bottled, tomato	105kJ	✓	✓	Good
Bottled, tropical	195kJ	↑Sugar	✓	Good
Bottled, viten	206kJ	↑Sugar	✓	Good
Tetra, apple	180kJ	↑Sugar	✓	Good
Tetra, apple & blackcurrant	189kJ	↑Sugar	✓	Good
Tetra, orange	170kJ	✓	✓	Good
Tetra, orange & mango	182kJ	✓	✓	Good

Product Name	Energy	Major Nutrients	Food Additives	Nutritious Rating
Tetra, tropical	185kJ	✓	✓	Good
Smart Buy tetra, apple	172kJ	✓	✓	Good
Smart buy tetra, orange	170kJ	✓	✓	Good
Smart buy bottled, apple	180kJ	↑Sugar	✓	Good
Smart buy bottled, apple & blackcurrant	185kJ	✓	✓	Good
Smart buy bottled, orange	160kJ	✓	✓	Good

Glo (P&N)

Product Name	Energy	Major Nutrients	Food Additives	Nutritious Rating
Apple	189kJ	↑Sugar	✓	Good
Apple & mango	189kJ	↑Sugar	110, 102	Good
Apple & raspberry	185kJ	↑Sugar	122, 133	Good
Berry blast	190kJ	↑Sugar	122	Good
Orange	189kJ	↑Sugar	110	Good
Orange & mango	194kJ	↑Sugar	110	Good
Pine punch	189kJ	↑Sugar	✓	Good

Golden Circle

Product Name	Energy	Major Nutrients	Food Additives	Nutritious Rating
Bottle, apple, carrot & ginger	196kJ	↑Sugar	✓	Good
Bottle, apple & mango light	80kJ	✓	✓	Good
Bottle, breakfast juice	200kJ	✓	✓	Good
Bottle, forest fruit light	75kJ	✓	✓	Good
Bottle, pineapple unsweetened	216kJ	↑Sugar	✓	Good
Bottle, tomato	80kJ	✓	✓	Good
Bottle, tropical	213kJ	↑Sugar	✓	Good
LOL, apple &	201kJ	↑Sugar	✓	Good

blackcurrant				
LOL, apple, pine & passion	203kJ	↑Sugar	✓	Good
LOL, apple & raspberry	199kJ	↑Sugar	✓	Good
Nectar, guava	210kJ	↑Sugar	✓	Good
Nectar, mango	225kJ	↑Sugar	✓	Good
Popper, apple	204kJ	↑Sugar	✓	Good
Popper, apple & mango	207kJ	↑Sugar	✓	Good
Popper, tropical	205kJ	↑Sugar	✓	Good
Raw, berry blast	**185kJ**	✓	✓	**Good**
Raw, citrus crush	**190kJ**	✓	✓	**Good**
Tetra, apple	**184kJ**	↑Sugar	✓	Good
Tetra, golden pash	**189kJ**	↑Sugar	✓	Good
Tetra, pineapple	**214kJ**	↑Sugar	✓	Good
Tetra, pine mango	**179kJ**	✓	✓	**Good**
Tetra, pine orange	**194kJ**	↑Sugar	✓	Good
Tetra, orange	**185kJ**	↑Sugar	✓	Good
Tetra, sunshine punch	**209kJ**	↑Sugar	✓	Good
Tetra, tropical punch	**192kJ**	↑Sugar	✓	Good

Goulburn Valley

Product Name	Energy	Major Nutrients	Food Additives	Nutritious Rating
Fruity drink, apple & blackcurrant	156kJ	✓	202	**Good**
Quencher, blood orange & passionfruit	**137kJ**	✓	✓	Good
Quencher, mixed berry	142kJ	✓	✓	Good
Quencher, lemon	134kJ	✓	✓	Good

IGA/Franklins

Product Name	Energy	Major Nutrients	Food Additives	Nutritious Rating
Breakfast	185kJ	↑Sugar	✓	Good

Orange	160kJ	✓	✓	Good
Tomato	100kJ	✓	✓	Good
Black & Gold, apple	**165kJ**	✓	✓	**Good**
Black & Gold, orange	162kJ	✓	160b	Good
Black & Gold, orange & mango	162kJ	✓	160b	Good
Black & Gold, tropical	170kJ	✓	160b	Good

Just Juice (Berri)

Product Name	Energy	Major Nutrients	Food Additives	Nutritious Rating
Apple	187kJ	✓	✓	Good
Apple & blackcurrant	185kJ	✓	✓	Good
Orange & mango	170kJ	✓	✓	Good

Langers Juice

Product Name	Energy	Major Nutrients	Food Additives	Nutritious Rating
Cranberry	212kJ	↑Sugar	✓	Good
Cranberry, no sugar	53kJ	✓	950	Good
Cranberry & raspberry	229kJ	↑Sugar	✓	Good

Ocean Spray

Product Name	Energy	Major Nutrients	Food Additives	Nutritious Rating
Cranberry, classic	207kJ	↑Sugar	✓	Good
Cranberry, light	33kJ	✓	950	Good
Cranberry & fruits of forest, grape, apple & pear	192kJ	↑Sugar	✓	Good
Cranberry & pomegranate	200kJ	↑Sugar	✓	Good
Cranberry, pomegranate, apple, pear & grape	205kJ	↑Sugar	✓	Good
Raspberry & cranberry	201kJ	↑Sugar	✓	Good

Ruby red grapefruit	209kJ	↑Sugar	✓	Good

Prima (Berri)

Product Name	Energy	Major Nutrients	Food Additives	Nutritious Rating
Apple	173kJ	↑Sugar	✓	Good
Apple & blackcurrant	184kJ	↑Sugar	✓	Good
Apple & raspberry	**168kJ**	✓	✓	**Good**
Orange & passionfruit	179kJ	↑Sugar	✓	Good
Orange & mango	187kJ	↑Sugar	✓	Good
Tropical	179kJ	↑Sugar	✓	Good

P&N

Product Name	Energy	Major Nutrients	Food Additives	Nutritious Rating
Extra juicy bottle, apple	192kJ	↑Sugar	✓	Good
Extra juicy bottle, apple & blackcurrant	192kJ	↑Sugar	✓	Good
Extra juicy bottle, apple, strawberry & guava	190kJ	↑Sugar	120	Good
Extra juicy bottle, brekky	184kJ	↑Sugar	✓	Good
Extra juicy bottle, grape	260kJ	↑Sugar	✓	Good
Extra juicy bottle, multi fruits	197kJ	↑Sugar	✓	Good
Extra juicy bottle, orange	**175kJ**	✓	✓	**Good**
Extra juicy bottle, veggie	**90kJ**	✓	✓	**Good**
Extra juicy tetra, apple	**192kJ**	✓	✓	**Good**
Extra juice tetra, apple, mango & banana	201kJ	↑Sugar	✓	Good
Extra juice tetra,	204kJ	↑Sugar	✓	Good

apple, mango & coconut				
Extra juicy tetra, apple & raspberry	94kJ	✓	211, 223	Good
Extra juicy tetra, berry blast	92kJ	✓	120, 950, 211, 223	Good
Extra juicy tetra, blackcurrant	**192kJ**	✓	✓	**Good**
Extra juicy tetra, brekky	**184kJ**	✓	✓	**Good**
Extra juicy tetra, fruit cup	114kJ	✓	120, 950, 211, 223	Good
Extra juicy tetra, lime	94kJ	✓	102, 133, 950, 211, 223	Good
Extra juicy tetra, multi fruits	197kJ	↑Sugar	✓	Good
Extra juicy tetra, orange	**175kJ**	✓	✓	**Good**
Extra juicy tetra, orange, mango & banana	92kJ	✓	120, 950, 211, 223	Good
Extra juicy tetra, pine, apple & passion	94kJ	✓	950, 211, 223	Good
Pop tops, apple	189kJ	↑Sugar	211, 223	Good
Pop tops, apple & blackcurrant	184kJ	↑Sugar	211, 223, 120	Good
Pop tops, orange	189kJ	↑Sugar	110, 211, 223	Good
Pop tops, wild berries	189kJ	↑Sugar	211, 223, 120	Good
Toddler pop tops, apple & blackcurrant	**66kJ**	✓	✓	**Good**
Toddler pop tops, apple & pear	**68kJ**	✓	✓	**Good**
Smart juice, brain power	201kJ	↑Sugar	✓	Good
Smart juice, body fuel	182kJ	↑Sugar	✓	Good
Smart juice, energise	201kJ	↑Sugar	✓	Good

Robinson's

Product Name	Energy	Major Nutrients	Food Additives	Nutritious Rating
Fruit shoot, apple	199kJ	↑Sugar	202, 211, 242	Good
Fruit shoot, apple & blackcurrant	195kJ	↑Sugar	202, 211, 242	Good
Fruit shoot, orange	204kJ	↑Sugar	202, 211, 242	Good
Fruit shoot, summer fruits	211kJ	↑Sugar	202, 211, 242	Good

Rosie

Product Name	Energy	Major Nutrients	Food Additives	Nutritious Rating
Apple, blueberry & cranberry	190kJ	✓	✓	Good
Apple, cranberry & raspberry	140kJ	✓	✓	Good
Apple, pomegranate & cranberry	200kJ	↑Sugar	✓	Good
Apple & ruby red grapefruit	210kJ	↑Sugar	✓	Good
Cranberry lite	30kJ	✓	955	Good

Spring Valley

Product Name	Energy	Major Nutrients	Food Additives	Nutritious Rating
Mango & banana	245kJ	↑Sugar	✓	Good

Sunraysia

Product Name	Energy	Major Nutrients	Food Additives	Nutritious Rating
Beetroot & apple	143kJ	✓	✓	Good
Prune	308kJ	✓	✓	Good

Woolworths/Safeways

Product Name	Energy	Major Nutrients	Food Additives	Nutritious Rating
Select, cranberry	199kJ	✓	✓	Good
Select, fruit & veg	179kJ	✓	✓	Good

Select, vegetable	107kJ	✓	✓	Good
Homebrand, apple	195kJ	✓	✓	Good
Homebrand, apple & blackcurrant	194kJ	✓	✓	Good
Homebrand, breakfast juice	193kJ	✓	✓	Good
Homebrand, orange & mango	169kJ	↑Sugar	✓	Good
Homebrand, tetra breakfast	200kJ	✓	✓	Good
Homebrand, tetra orange	179kJ	✓	✓	Good
Homebrand, tetra orange & mango	198kJ	✓	✓	Good
Homebrand, tetra tropical	179kJ	✓	✓	Good

Ya Coya

Product Name	Energy	Major Nutrients	Food Additives	Nutritious Rating
Aloe crush, sugar free	49kJ	✓	955, 420	Good

Soft Drinks, Sports and Energy Drinks

Most fizzy drinks, ice teas and sports drinks contain 211 and a host of colouring agents. My picks are *Appletiser, Cascade, Dilmah* and *V energy drinks*.

Angostura

Product Name	Energy	Major Nutrients	Food Additives	Nutritious Rating
Lemon, lime & bitters	172kJ	✓	211, 122	Poor

Appletiser

Product Name	Energy	Major Nutrients	Food Additives	Nutritious Rating
Sparkling apple juice	182kJ	✓	✓	Average
Sparkling grape juice	218kJ	↑Sugar	✓	Average

Barr

Product Name	Energy	Major Nutrients	Food Additives	Nutritious Rating
Irn bru	182kJ	↑Sugar	110, 211, 124	Average

Buderim

Product Name	Energy	Major Nutrients	Food Additives	Nutritious Rating
Ginger refresher	230kJ	↑Sugar	211	Poor
Lemon, lime & bitters	185kJ	↑Sugar	211	Poor
Lemon, lime & bitters, diet	62kJ	✓	211, 955, 952	Poor

Bundaberg

Product Name	Energy	Major Nutrients	Food Additives	Nutritious Rating
Blood orange	204kJ	↑Sugar	211, 120	Poor
Creaming soda	189kJ	↑Sugar	122, 102, 133, 211	Poor
Ginger beer	184kJ	↑Sugar	202, 211	Poor

Ginger beer, diet	34kJ	✓	211, 223, 951, 950, 955	Poor
Guava mixer	196kJ	↑Sugar	211, 120	Poor
Lemon, lime & bitters	201kJ	↑Sugar	120, 211, 122	Poor
Pink grapefruit	192kJ	↑Sugar	211, 120	Poor
Sarsparella	211kJ	↑Sugar	202, 211	Poor
Sarsparella, diet	34kJ	✓	211, 202, 951, 950, 955	Poor

Cascade

Product Name	Energy	Major Nutrients	Food Additives	Nutritious Rating
Sparkling apple juice	173kJ	✓	✓	Average

Coca Cola Bottlers

Product Name	Energy	Major Nutrients	Food Additives	Nutritious Rating
Coke	180kJ	↑Sugar	✓	Poor
Coke, diet	1.5kJ	✓	211, 950, 951	Poor
Coke, zero	1.4kJ	✓	211, 950, 951	Poor
Coke, vanilla	185kJ	↑Sugar	✓	Poor
Coke, vanilla zero	1.4kJ	✓	211, 950, 951	Poor
Fanta	194kJ	↑Sugar	202	Poor
Lift	194kJ	↑Sugar	202	Poor
Sprite	177kJ	↑Sugar	202	Poor
Sprite, zero	4.2kJ	✓	211, 202, 950, 951	Poor
Powerade, berry ice	129kJ	✓	129, 202	Average
Powerade, blackcurrant	130kJ	✓	122, 133, 202	Average
Powerade, gold rush	129kJ	✓	104, 110, 202	Average
Powerade, lemon/lime	129kJ	✓	102, 202	Average
Powerade, mountain blast	129kJ	✓	133, 202	Average
Mother energy drink	195kJ	↑Sugar	104, 202	Average

Coles

Product Name	Energy	Major	Food	Nutritious

		Nutrients	Additives	Rating
Cola	190kJ	↑Sugar	✓	Poor
Cola, diet	204kJ	✓	211	Poor
Lemonade	204kJ	↑Sugar	211	Poor
Lemonade, diet	2kJ	✓	211, 950, 951	Poor
Lemon	213kJ	↑Sugar	211	Poor
Lemon & mineral water	177kJ	↑Sugar	211	Poor
Lemon, lime & mineral water	177kJ	↑Sugar	211, 141	Poor
Lime	202kJ	↑Sugar	211, 141	Poor
Pineapple, mango & mineral water	194kJ	↑Sugar	211, 141	Poor
Orange	221kJ	↑Sugar	211	Poor
Orange, mango & mineral water	179kJ	↑Sugar	211	Poor
Raspberry	211kJ	↑Sugar	211	Poor
Smart buy, cola	162kJ	✓	211	Poor
Smart buy, lemonade	168kJ	✓	211	Poor

Diet Rite

Product Name	Energy	Major Nutrients	Food Additives	Nutritious Rating
Cranberry & boysenberry	9kJ	✓	211, 952, 950, 955	Poor
Passionfruit	14kJ	✓	211, 123, 952, 950, 955	Poor
Portello	15kJ	✓	211, 123, 952, 950, 955	Poor

Dilmah

Product Name	Energy	Major Nutrients	Food Additives	Nutritious Rating
Iced tea, lemon	138kJ	✓	✓	Average
Iced tea, peach	138kJ	✓	✓	Average

Golden Circle

Product Name	Energy	Major Nutrients	Food Additives	Nutritious Rating
Sports, apple & blackcurrant	110kJ	✓	122, 133, 223, 202	Average
Sports, lime slam	110kJ	✓	102, 133, 223, 202	Average
Sports, orange slam	110kJ	✓	123, 202	Average
Sports, raspberry crush	110kJ	✓	122, 123, 202	Average

IGA/Franklins

Product Name	Energy	Major Nutrients	Food Additives	Nutritious Rating
Black & Gold, cola	196kJ	↑Sugar	✓	Poor
Black & Gold, cola diet	2kJ	✓	211, 952, 950, 955	Poor
Black & Gold, lemon	156kJ	✓	211, 961	Poor
Black & Gold, lemonade	146kJ	✓	211, 961	Poor
Black & Gold, lemonade diet	2kJ	✓	211, 952, 950, 951	Poor
Black & Gold, lime	156kJ	✓	133, 102, 211, 961	Poor
Black & Gold, orange	185kJ	↑Sugar	120, 961, 211	Poor
Black & Gold, red creaming	153kJ	✓	120, 211	Poor

Kirks

Product Name	Energy	Major Nutrients	Food Additives	Nutritious Rating
Club Lemon soda	195kJ	↑Sugar	211, 104	Poor
Club Lemon soda, sugar free	3kJ	✓	104, 211, 952, 950, 961	Poor
Creaming soda	176kJ	↑Sugar	211, 122	Poor
Creaming soda, sugar free	3kJ	✓	122, 211, 950, 952, 961	Poor
Dry ginger ale	139kJ	✓	211, 223	Poor
Ginger ale	214kJ	↑Sugar	211	Poor

Kole beer	186kJ	↑Sugar	211	Poor
Lemonade	190kJ	↑Sugar	211	Poor
Lemonade, sugar free	2kJ	✓	211, 952, 950, 961	Poor
Pastio	196kJ	↑Sugar	102, 110, 211	Poor

Liptons

Product Name	Energy	Major Nutrients	Food Additives	Nutritious Rating
Ice tea, lemon	113kJ	✓	223	Average
Ice tea, peach	**115kJ**	✓	✓	**Average**
Ice tea, peach light	3kJ	✓	950, 951	Average
Ice tea, mango	**118kJ**	✓	✓	**Average**
Ice tea, raspberry	**119kJ**	✓	✓	**Average**
Green tea, citrus	79kJ	✓	960, 223	Average
Green tea, light	4kJ	✓	223, 950, 951	Average
Green tea, original	80kJ	✓	960	Average

Lucozade

Product Name	Energy	Major Nutrients	Food Additives	Nutritious Rating
Original	308kJ	✓	202, 211, 110	Average

Nestle

Product Name	Energy	Major Nutrients	Food Additives	Nutritious Rating
Ice tea, green tea & lemon	123kJ	✓	223	Average
Ice tea, green tea & mango	105kJ	✓	122	Average
Ice tea, green tea, peach & mango	102kJ	✓	122	Average
Ice tea, green tea, pear & honey	**114kJ**	✓	✓	**Average**

No Limit Energy Drink

Product Name	Energy	Major Nutrients	Food Additives	Nutritious Rating
Original	196kJ	↑Sugar	211	Average

Pepsi

Product Name	Energy	Major Nutrients	Food Additives	Nutritious Rating
Pepsi	175kJ	↑Sugar	✓	Poor
Pepsi, diet	2kJ	✓	211, 950, 951	Poor
Pepsi, max	2kJ	✓	211, 950, 951	Poor
Pepsi, light caffeine free	1kJ	✓	211, 950, 951	Poor
7up	162kJ	↑Sugar	211	Poor
Sunkist	222kJ	↑Sugar	211, 110	Poor
Sunkist, sugar free	4kJ	✓	211, 110, 950, 951	Poor

P&N

Product Name	Energy	Major Nutrients	Food Additives	Nutritious Rating
LA ice	201kJ	↑Sugar	211, 110, 102, 122	Poor
LA ice max	204kJ	↑Sugar	211, 110, 122	Poor
Tru Blu, ceda creaming soda	5kJ	✓	211, 242, 122, 961	Poor
Tru Blu, crush lime	155kJ	✓	211, 133, 102, 961	Poor
Tru Blu, crush orange	177kJ	↑Sugar	211, 122, 961	Poor
Tru Blu, crush passion	138kJ	✓	211, 122, 961	Poor
Tru Blu, crush pine	151kJ	✓	211, 961	Poor
Tru Blu, ginger beer	146kJ	✓	211, 961	Poor
Tru Blu, lido	139kJ	✓	211, 961	Poor
Tru Blu, Mc sars	151kJ	✓	211, 961	Poor
Tru Blu, pub squash	148kJ	✓	211, 961	Poor
Tru Blu, pub squash diet	10kJ	✓	211, 952, 950, 955	Poor
Waterfords, apple berry diet	10kJ	✓	211, 123, 950, 955, 952	Poor
Waterfords, blood orange diet	10kJ	✓	211, 129, 110, 950, 955, 952	Poor
Waterfords, lemon,	10kJ	✓	211, 122, 110,	Poor

lime & bitters			950, 955, 952	
Waterfords, lemon, lime & orange	10kJ	✓	211, 102, 110, 950, 955, 952	Poor
Waterfords, portello	10kJ	✓	211, 123, 133, 950, 955, 952	Poor
Wicked energy drink	197kJ	↑Sugar	211, 202	Average

Pink Diet Energy Drink

Product Name	Energy	Major Nutrients	Food Additives	Nutritious Rating
Original	17kJ	✓	211, 950, 955	Average

Red Bull

Product Name	Energy	Major Nutrients	Food Additives	Nutritious Rating
Original	192kJ	↑Sugar	220	Average
Sugar free	14kJ	✓	950, 955	Average

Red Eye

Product Name	Energy	Major Nutrients	Food Additives	Nutritious Rating
Platinum energy drink	192kJ	↑Sugar	211	Average

Rock Star

Product Name	Energy	Major Nutrients	Food Additives	Nutritious Rating
Original	230kJ	↑Sugar	211, 202	Average
Punched guava	285kJ	↑Sugar	129, 110, 202, 211	Average

Schweppes

Product Name	Energy	Major Nutrients	Food Additives	Nutritious Rating
Agrum, blood orange	201kJ	↑Sugar	211, 110, 102, 122	Poor
Agrum, citrus blend	204kJ	↑Sugar	211, 110, 122	Poor

Agrum, citrus blend sugar free	5kJ	✓	211, 110, 122, 950, 951, 952	Poor
Bitter lemon	223kJ	↑Sugar	211	Poor
Dry ginger ale	135kJ	✓	211	Poor
Dry ginger ale, diet	7kJ	✓	211, 950, 951	Poor
Lemon, lime & bitters	176kJ	✓	211	Poor
Lemonade	192kJ	↑Sugar	✓	Poor
Lemonade, sugar free	5kJ	✓	211, 951, 950	Poor
Lime	206kJ	↑Sugar	211, 133, 102	Poor
Mountain dew	200kJ	↑Sugar	211, 202, 102	Poor
Natural mineral, apple & pink grapefruit	125kJ	✓	211, 202, 223, 122	Poor
Natural mineral, lemon	124kJ	✓	211, 202, 223	Poor
Natural mineral, lemon & lime	127kJ	✓	211, 202, 223, 122	Poor
Natural mineral, orange & mango	121kJ	✓	211, 202, 223, 122	Poor
Raspberry	210kJ	↑Sugar	211, 123	Poor
Red creaming soda	227kJ	↑Sugar	211, 123	Poor
Sarsaparilla	192kJ	↑Sugar	211	Poor
Solo	209kJ	↑Sugar	211, 223, 102	Poor
Solo, lemon & lime	194kJ	↑Sugar	211, 223, 102, 133	Poor
Traditional lemonade	182kJ	↑Sugar	211, 223	Poor
Monster energy drink	194kJ	↑Sugar	200, 210, 202, 955	Average
Gatorade, blackberry	108kJ	✓	129, 133	Average
Gatorade, blue bolt	103kJ	✓	133	Average
Gatorade, fierce grape	103kJ	✓	133, 129	Average
Gatorade, lemon ice	103kJ	✓	102, 133	Average
Gatorade, lemon lime	103kJ	✓	129	Average
Gatorade, lime storm	103kJ	✓	102	Average
Gatorade, mango ice	103kJ	✓	110, 102	Average
Gatorade, orange ice	103kJ	✓	110	Average
Gatorade, prime pre-	355kJ	↑Sugar	102, 110	Average

game				
Gatorade, recover post game	109kJ	✓	102, 133, 955	Average
Gatorade, tropical	103kJ	✓	129	Average

V Energy Drinks

Product Name	Energy	Major Nutrients	Food Additives	Nutritious Rating
Call of duty	195kJ	↑Sugar	✓	Good
Double hit	192kJ	↑Sugar	✓	Good
Original	195kJ	↑Sugar	✓	Good
Sugar free	12kJ	✓	955, 950	Good

Woolworths/Safeways

Product Name	Energy	Major Nutrients	Food Additives	Nutritious Rating
Select, apple & blackcurrant	178kJ	↑Sugar	202	Poor
Select, fruit fizz	172kJ	✓	202	Poor
Select, lemonade	200kJ	✓	202	Poor
Select, lemon	210kJ	✓	202	Poor
Select, orange	193kJ	↑Sugar	202	Poor
Select, raspberry	174kJ	✓	202	Poor
Select, tropical	210kJ	✓	202	Poor
Homebrand, cola	209kJ	↑Sugar	✓	Poor
Homebrand, cola diet	10kJ	✓	211, 952, 950, 951	Poor
Homebrand, gingerale	115kJ	✓	211	Poor
Homebrand, lemon diet	10kJ	✓	102, 211, 952, 950, 951	Poor
Homebrand, lemon & lime diet	10kJ	✓	211, 952, 950, 951, 110, 133	Poor
Homebrand, lemon, lime & bitters diet	10kJ	✓	211, 952, 950, 951, 102, 122	Poor
Homebrand, lemonade	181kJ	↑Sugar	211	Poor

Homebrand, lemonade diet	10kJ	✓	211, 952, 950, 951	Poor
Homebrand, lime	196kJ	↑Sugar	211, 102, 133	Poor
Homebrand, orange	231kJ	↑Sugar	211, 110	Poor
Homebrand, orange diet	10kJ	✓	211, 110, 952, 950, 951	Poor
Homebrand, orange & mango diet	12kJ	✓	211, 110, 952, 950, 951	Poor

Frozen Foods

Desserts

Of the desserts, the apple pies and cheesecakes tend to be additive free. But they are all going to be high in fat and sugar; this is why I have included the total grams as an added reference. Personally, I think you just choose your favourite and indulge very occasionally.

Banquet

Product Name	Energy	Major Nutrients	Food Additives	Nutritious Rating
Cheesecake, cookies & cream	1472kJ	20.4g fat 23g sugar	319	Poor
Cheesecake, French cream	**1410kJ**	**19.9g fat 22g sugar**	✓	**Poor**
Cheesecake, passionfruit	1283kJ	16.3g fat 24g sugar	160b	Poor
Chocolate bavarian	**1480kJ**	**22.6g fat 20g sugar**	✓	**Poor**

Bon Gateaux

Product Name	Energy	Major Nutrients	Food Additives	Nutritious Rating
Chocolate Bavarian	1323kJ	18.8g fat 24g sugar	319, 420	Poor
French cream cheesecake	1274kJ	15.8g fat 29g sugar	319, 420	Poor

Borgs

Product Name	Energy	Major Nutrients	Food Additives	Nutritious Rating
Apple & custard desserts	1300kJ	13g fat 8g sugar	102, 110	Average

Vanilla custard dessert	1120kJ	8.1g fat 19g sugar	102, 110	Poor

Coles

Product Name	Energy	Major Nutrients	Food Additives	Nutritious Rating
Apple crumple pie				Average
Apple pie, family	971kJ	9.4g fat 17.1g sugar	160b	Average
Apple light pie, family	969kJ	20.7g sugar	202	Average
Apple pie snacks	1390kJ	14.3g fat 20.1g sugar	160b	Average
Apple snack pies, light	1170kJ	23.1g sugar	202	Average
Apple & blackberry custard strudel	1070kJ	14.9g fat	✓	Average
Apple & caramel lattice pie	967kJ	11.2g fat 16.8g sugar	✓	Average
Apple & mixed berry strudel	1050kJ	12.4g fat 14.1g sugar	✓	Average
Apple & sultana strudel	1020kJ	12g fat 12.3g sugar	✓	Average
Apricot pies, snack	1310kJ	14.1g fat 19.2g sugar	160b	Average
Black forest cake	968kJ	8.7g fat 22g sugar	✓	Poor
Butter croissants	1705kJ	23.5g fat	✓	Poor
Chocolate Bavarian	1350kJ	19.6g fat 22.3g sugar	319	Poor
Cookie melt in the middle chocolate vanilla	1830kJ	20.2g fat 36.8g sugar	✓	Poor
French style cheesecake	1284kJ	15.8g fat 27.1g sugar	319	Average
Lemon tart	1380kJ	14.9g fat 24g sugar	✓	Poor
Melting middle choc chip cookie	1830kJ	20.2g fat 38g sugar	✓	Poor
Peach & mango	1036kJ	12.6g fat	319	Poor

cheesecake		21.7g sugar		
Profiterole cake	**1240kJ**	**20.4g fat 15.9g sugar**	✓	**Poor**
Strawberry cheesecake	1096kJ	12.6g fat 24.7g sugar	120, 319	Poor
Strawberry & cream cake	**1080kJ**	**13.7g fat 17.7g sugar**	✓	**Poor**
Tiramisu	**1120kJ**	**12.5g fat 21.3g sugar**	✓	**Poor**
Triple choc cake	**1180kJ**	**14.6g fat 18.5g sugar**	✓	**Poor**
Smart buy chocolate bavarian	1320kJ	18.8g fat 24.5g sugar	319, 420	Poor
Smart buy apple pie	**1260kJ**	**12.9g fat 17.3g sugar**	✓	**Average**
Smart buy cheesecake, French style	1390kJ	17.3g fat 29.8g sugar	319	Poor

Ernest Adams

Product Name	Energy	Major Nutrients	Food Additives	Nutritious Rating
Chocolate brownie	1830kJ	18.4g fat 45g sugar	320, 202, 422	Poor
Loaf, banana choc chip	1585kJ	10.9g fat 38g sugar	220, 200, 422	Poor
Loaf, date & walnut	1350kJ	35g sugar	200, 202, 211, 1520, 420	Average
Loaf, Jamaican ginger	1490kJ	11.5g fat 34g sugar	200, 422, 220	Poor
Loaf, spiced apple & fruit crumble	1430kJ	11.6g fat 35g sugar	200, 422	Average
Slice, apricot	1650kJ	12g fat 43g sugar	320, 202, 220	Average
Slice, gooey caramel	1895kJ	18.3g fat 43g sugar	320, 202	Poor

IGA/Franklins

Product Name	Energy	Major Nutrients	Food Additives	Nutritious Rating
Signature, chocolate Bavarian	1480kJ	22.6g fat 20g sugar	✓	Poor
Signature, cheesecake dessert	1410kJ	19.9g fat	✓	Poor
Black & Gold, chocolate bavarian	1300kJ	19.4g fat 21g sugar	319	Poor
Black & Gold, croissants	1407kJ	15.6g fat	✓	Poor
Black & Gold, French style cheesecake	1270kJ	15.7g fat 27g sugar	319, 420	Poor
Black & Gold, strawberry cheesecake	1100kJ	12g fat 26g sugar	420, 124, 319	Poor

Master Diermens Master Bakers

Product Name	Energy	Major Nutrients	Food Additives	Nutritious Rating
Cream puffs, chocolate dipped	1639kJ	27.4g fat 20g sugar	✓	Poor
Cream puffs, mini vanilla	1330kJ	23.5g fat 27g sugar	✓	Poor

Nannas

Product Name	Energy	Major Nutrients	Food Additives	Nutritious Rating
Apple crumble pie	865kJ	6.5g fat 20g sugar	320	Average
Apple custard crumble	1018kJ	8g fat 18g sugar	320	Average
Apple pie, family	1000kJ	9.8g fat 16g sugar	220	Average
Apple snack pies	979kJ	11g fat 15g sugar	✓	Average
Apple snack pies, lite	943kJ	5.8g fat 20g sugar	202	Average
Apple mini pies	1260kJ	13.6g fat	✓	Average

		17g sugar		
Apricot snack pies	**991kJ**	**9.6g fat** **5g sugar**	✓	**Average**
Blackberry & apple pie crumble, family	979kJ	6.5g fat 23g sugar	320	Average
Blackberry & apple pie, snack	**1160kJ**	**11g fat** **16g sugar**	✓	**Average**
Mixed berry snack pies, lite	1120kJ	7.6g fat 22g sugar	202	Average
Mixed berry mini pies	**1250kJ**	**13.6g fat** **14g sugar**	✓	**Average**
Premium baked cheesecake tartlets	1500kJ	21g fat 14g sugar	223	Poor
Waffles	**1140kJ**	✓	✓	**Poor**
Waffles, dark choc chips	**901kJ**	**12g sugar**	✓	**Poor**

Pampus

Product Name	Energy	Major Nutrients	Food Additives	Nutritious Rating
Apple lattice puffs	1310kJ	10.3g fat 15g sugar	202, 220, 281, 320	Average
Lemon meringue	1010kJ	10.7g fat 26g sugar	320, 220, 160b	Poor

Patties Gluten Free

Product Name	Energy	Major Nutrients	Food Additives	Nutritious Rating
Lamingtons	1110kJ	↑ Sugar ↑ Fat	✓	Poor
White bread	1010kJ	✓	✓	Average

Sara Lee

Product Name	Energy	Major Nutrients	Food Additives	Nutritious Rating
Apple berry crumble	1170kJ	10.6g fat 22g sugar	120, 320	Average
Apple crumble	1118kJ	8g fat 29g sugar	✓	Average

Apple berry crumble top pie	1388kJ	8.3g fat 42g sugar	120	Average
Apple custard crumble	1018kJ	18g sugar	320	Average
Apple pie	1130kJ	11g fat 20g sugar	320	Average
Apple pie, deep dish	**1080kJ**	**12.6g fat 17g sugar**	✓	**Average**
Apple pies, individual	**1320kJ**	**14g fat 19g sugar**	✓	**Average**
Apple & custard, individual pies	1660kJ	15g fat 18g sugar	120	Average
Apple pie, crumble top	**1290kJ**	**12.4g fat 27g sugar**	✓	**Average**
Apricot apple crumble	1170kJ	10.6g fat 22g sugar	120, 320	Average
Baked cheesecake, original	1528kJ	25.8g fat 20g sugar	319	Poor
Baked cheesecake, premium tartlets	1500kJ	21.2g fat 14g sugar	422, 223	Poor
Bavarian, chocolate	1435kJ	19.4g fat 23g sugar	319	Poor
Bavarian, chocolate swirl	1388kJ	18.9g fat 22g sugar	319	Poor
Bavarian, chocolate caramel	1472kJ	21.3g fat 19g sugar	319	Poor
Bavarian, cookies & cream	1540kJ	22.5g fat 21g sugar	319	Poor
Cake, banana	1184kJ	12.9g fat 43g sugar	420, 160b	Poor
Cake, carrot	**1539kJ**	**20g fat 30g sugar**	✓	**Poor**
Cake, chocolate	1609kJ	16.7g fat 41g sugar	420	Poor
Cheesecake, original minis	1629kJ	22.8g fat 28g sugar	319	Poor
Cheesecake, chocolate	1517kJ	22.6g fat 19g sugar	319, 420	Poor
Cheesecake, mixed	1435kJ	20.3g fat	420, 319	Poor

berry		22g sugar		
Cheesecake, strawberry	1399kJ	20.2g fat 20g sugar	120, 420, 319	Poor
Cheesecake, summer fruits	1362kJ	20.2g fat 18g sugar	420, 319	Poor
Chocolate caramel pie	1590kJ	19.3g fat 24g sugar	320, 220	Poor
Chocolate pie	1710kJ	21g fat 23g sugar	320	Poor
Danish, apple	1186kJ	9.6g fat 22g sugar	920, 420	Average
Danish, apricot	1509kJ	9.7g fat 38g sugar	420, 120, 920	Average
Danish, blueberry	1158kJ	9.8g fat 18g sugar	920, 420	Average
Danish, custard	1232kJ	14.7g fat 14g sugar	120, 920, 420	Poor
French style croissants	**1526kJ**	**16.2g fat**	✓	**Poor**
Mini's, caramel slice	**1680kJ**	**21g fat 33g sugar**	✓	**Poor**
Mini's, choc fudge brownie	**1710kJ**	**18g fat 28g sugar**	✓	**Poor**
Mini's, cookies & cream cheesecake	**1640kJ**	**22.4g fat 29g sugar**	✓	**Poor**
Mini's, rocky road	**1740kJ**	**17.6g fat 33g sugar**	✓	**Poor**
Pudding, butterscotch	1383kJ	20.2g fat 41g sugar	420	Poor
Pudding, Chocolate	1380kJ	15.3g fat 23g sugar	420	Poor
Pudding, sticky date	**1450kJ**	**12.7g fat 39g sugar**	✓	**Poor**
Pudding, sticky date individual	**1260kJ**	**11g fat 33g sugar**	✓	**Poor**
Pudding, triple choc individual	**1360kJ**	**15.3g fat 30g sugar**	✓	**Poor**
Waffles	**1140kJ**	✓	✓	**Poor**
Waffles, dark choc	**901kJ**	**12g sugar**	✓	**Poor**

chips				

Weight Watchers

Product Name	Energy	Major Nutrients	Food Additives	Nutritious Rating
Belgian eclair	1220kJ	11.9g fat 30g sugar	202	Poor
Double chocolate pudding	815kJ	13g sugar	200, 202, 422, 950	Poor

Woolworths/Safeways

Product Name	Energy	Major Nutrients	Food Additives	Nutritious Rating
Homebrand, apple pie	966kJ	9.6g fat 15g sugar	✓	Average
Homebrand, chocolate Bavarian	1270kJ	14.9g fat 26g sugar	319	Poor
Homebrand, French cheesecake	1250kJ	15.8g fat 23g sugar	319	Poor
Homebrand, strawberry cheesecake	1130kJ	12.7g fat 26g sugar	319, 124	Poor

Ice-cream

Generally the chocolate flavoured ice-creams are often additive free. Sorbets however are a much healthier option. My picks are *Fruity fanatics, Gellativo, Sanitarium and Sara Lee.* If you want to buy your kids an ice-cream/icypole at the petrol station that won't lead to a difficult car journey, I suggest: *Magnum sandwich, Magnum temptation fruit, Billabong chocolate, Drumstick choc shock, Choc wedge vanilla, Choc wedge violet crumble,* Larry lemonade, Paddlepop icy twist and Eskimo pie.

Azzura

Product Name	Energy	Major Nutrients	Food Additives	Nutritious Rating
Amore	785kJ	12.4g fat 35g Sugar	102, 142, 407	Poor
Blueberry sorbet	439kJ	20g Sugar	407, 124, 133, 220	Average
Celebrate ice cream cake	870kJ	13g fat 19g sugar	102, 155, 122, 123, 124, 133, 407	Poor
Kisses	1004kJ	13g fat 28g sugar	142, 110, 124, 407, 220	Poor
Lemon sorbet	404kJ	18g sugar	102, 124	Average
Mango sorbet	1185kJ	13g Fat 27.9g Sugar	102, 122	Average
Strawberry sorbet	1470kJ	21.9g fat 27.1g sugar	220, 407	Average
Tartufo	1064kJ	11g fat 33g sugar	407, 155	Poor
Torta gelati	632kJ	9.4g fat	110	Poor

		12g sugar		

Bambino

Product Name	Energy	Major Nutrients	Food Additives	Nutritious Rating
Semi freddo desserts	1191kJ	13.1g Fat 25.9g Sugar	102, 124, 110, 122, 131	Poor
Ferrero desserts	743kJ	13.1g Fat 20g Sugar	407	Poor
Passionfruit sorbet	508kJ	↑ Sugar	102, 110, 150	Poor
Strawberry sorbet	949kJ	↑ Sugar	102, 124	Poor
Piccolo mini cones	1185kJ	13g Fat 27.9g Sugar	102, 122	Poor
Choc coconut mini cones	1470kJ	21.9g Fat 27.1g Sugar	102, 124	Poor
Assorted mini cones	1190kJ	13.7g Fat 29.4g Sugar	102, 124, 132, 420	Poor
Scorched almond mini cones	1520kJ	23g Fat 25.3g Sugar	102, 124, 220	Poor
100's n 1000's mini cones	1280kJ	10.7g Fat 40.7g Sugar	102, 124, 122, 110, 129	Poor
Nut encrusted mini cones	1450kJ	21.7g Fat 21.8g Sugar	✓	Poor

Brownes

Product Name	Energy	Major Nutrients	Food Additives	Nutritious Rating
Chocolate 2L	827kJ	10.5g Fat 19g Sugar	✓	Poor

Bulla

Product Name	Energy	Major Nutrients	Food Additives	Nutritious Rating
Choc bars, vanilla 8pk	1210kJ	19.5g Fat 24.1 Sugar	160b	Poor

Choc bars, variety 10pk	1193-1210kJ	19g Fat 24g Sugar	155, 102, 123, 133, 160b	Poor
Creamy classics sundae, choc mint	1000kJ	10.9g Fat 24.5g Sugar	102, 133, 160b	Poor
Classic chocolate sundae cups	949kJ	10.9g Fat 30.6g Sugar	160b	Poor
Creamy classic ice creams 6pk Neapolitan	1403kJ	22.1g Fat 27.9g Sugar	160b	Poor
Creamy classics chocolate/vanilla 6pk twins	1405kJ	22.2g Fat 27.9g Sugar	160b	Poor
Creamy classic 2L cookies n cream	934kJ	11.7g Fat 20.5g Sugar	160b	Poor
Creamy classic mint choc	1441kJ	22.7g Fat 28.9g Sugar	160b, 102, 133	Poor
Creamy classic vanilla 2L	859kJ	11.4g Fat 20g Sugar	160b	Poor
Creamy classics, toffee crunch 2L	**855kJ**	**10.8g Fat 23g Sugar**	✓	**Poor**
Creamy classics, choc chip	**980kJ**	**12.3g Fat 21g Sugar**	✓	**Poor**
Creamy classics, light vanilla	690kJ	5.6g Fat 19.4g Sugar	160b	Poor
Creamy classics, light boysenberry	678kJ	4g Fat 23.2g Sugar	120, 160b	Poor
Crunch, double choc 8 pk	1258kJ	20g Fat 24g Sugar	155, 123, 133, 102	Poor
Crunch, honeycomb 8pk	1258kJ	20g Fat 24.8g Sugar	110, 160b	Poor
Crunch selection 8pk	1255-1260kJ	20g Fat 24g Sugar	160b, 102, 110, 133	Poor
Crunch variety 8pk	1258-1260kJ	20g Fat 24g Sugar	160b, 102, 110, 133	Poor
Fruit & yoghurt selection 8pk	561	20g sugar	160b	Good
Frozen yoghurt 2L, blueberry	572kJ	20g sugar	160b	Good

Frozen yoghurt, fruit salad 2L	552kJ	19g sugar	160b	Good
Frozen yoghurt 2L, mango	587kJ	22g sugar	160b	Good
Frozen yoghurt 2L, passionfruit	558kJ	19g sugar	160b	Good
Frozen yoghurt 2L, raspberry	563kJ	20g sugar	160b, 162	Good
Frozen yoghurt 2L, strawberry	610kJ	24g sugar	160b, 120	Good
Frozen yoghurt 2L, wildberry	608kJ	23g sugar	160b	Good
Frozen yoghurt 97% Fat Free variety 14pk	483-586kJ	20g sugar	160b, 162	Good
Gourmet frozen yoghurt, mango/passionfruit	644kJ	23g sugar	160b	Good
Gourmet frozen yoghurt, strawberry	664kJ	24g sugar	160b, 120	Good
Real Dairy classic 2L vanilla	819kJ	10.2g Fat 22.1g Sugar	160b	Poor
Real Dairy choc chip	866kJ	11.1g Fat 21.8g Sugar	160b	Poor
Real Dairy Neapolitan	819kJ	10.2g Fat 21.2g Sugar	160b, 124	Poor
Real Dairy chocolate	821kJ	10.2g Fat 21.2g Sugar	✓	**Poor**
Real Dairy choc/vanilla	817kJ	10.2g Fat 21.2g Sugar	160b	Poor

Cadbury

Product Name	Energy	Major Nutrients	Food Additives	Nutritious Rating
2L, caramello	829kJ	10.7g fat 23g sugar	155, 102, 110, 160b	Poor
2L, creamy vanilla	862kJ	11.4g fat 19g sugar	160b	Poor

2L, dairy milk chip	982kJ	13.7g fat 21g sugar	160b	Poor
2L, honeycomb & chocolate	904kJ	11.1g fat 23g sugar	102, 110, 155, 160b	Poor
2L, light vanilla	661kJ	2.5g fat 25g sugar	160b	Poor
2L, triple chocolate	**864kJ**	**11.5g fat 19g sugar**	✓	**Poor**
Caramello 4pk	1370kJ	18.3g fat 31g sugar	155, 102, 110, 202	Poor
Creamy vanilla cone	1416kJ	19.7g fat 27g sugar	160b	Poor
Crunchie mini bars	1500kJ	21.9g fat 37g sugar	102, 110, HVP	Poor
Flake ice creams 4pk	1372kJ	16.3g fat 28g sugar	160b	Poor
Freddo ice cream cake	872kJ	11.1g fat 22g sugar	102, 133, 122, 110, 123, 124	Poor
Fry's Turkish delight bars	1070kJ	13.5g fat 27g sugar	162	Poor
Picnic cones 4pk	1428kJ	17.9g fat 26g sugar	160b, 120	Poor
Rocky road cone 4pk	1272kJ	14.6g fat 26g sugar	122, 155	Poor
Triple choc cone 4pk	1295kJ	15.4g fat 29g sugar	155	Poor

Coles

Product Name	Energy	Major Nutrients	Food Additives	Nutritious Rating
Banana pops 10pk	696kJ	5.2g fat 20g sugar	160b, 320	Poor
Classic vanilla 4pk	1328kJ	20g fat 27g sugar	160b	Poor
Classic vanilla ice cream 2L	952kJ	10.9g fat 26g sugar	160b	Poor
Classic vanilla ice	1378kJ	21.2g fat	160b	Poor

cream, minis		27g sugar		
Classic vanilla ice cream 97% fat free 2L	694kJ	3g fat 20g sugar	160b	Poor
Classic vanilla ice cream, reduced fat 2L	738kJ	6.6g fat 21g sugar	160b	Poor
Chocolate choc chip ice cream 2L	982kJ	12.6g fat 24g sugar	120	Poor
Choc pops 10pk	724kJ	5.4g fat 20g sugar	320	Poor
Cookies & cream ice cream 2L	1021kJ	11.4g fat 26g sugar	160b	Poor
Finest caramel, pecan & date 500ml	1060kJ	16g fat 18g sugar	220	Poor
Finest, caramel & macadamia	1091kJ	16.3g fat 22g sugar	160b	Average
Finest, chocolate fudge	**1010kJ**	**8.4g fat 24g sugar**	✓	**Poor**
Finest, coffee creme	1048kJ	15.2g fat 21g sugar	160b	Poor
Finest, rich & creamy vanilla	1000kJ	14.8g fat 19g sugar	160b	Poor
Finest, fig, ginger & honey	**971kJ**	**12.8g fat 21g sugar**	✓	**Poor**
Fruity yoghurt duos, raspberrry	472kJ	1.6g fat 19g sugar	160b, 220	Average
Fruity yoghurt, mango 2L	584kJ	2.4g fat 20g sugar	160b, 220	Average
Fruity yoghurt sticks 8pk	566kJ	2.8g fat 19g sugar	160b, 220, 162	Average
Fruity yoghurt, wild berry 2 L	576kJ	2.8g fat 20g sugar	120, 160b, 220	Average
Icy pops, raspberry 8pk	**292kJ**	**17g sugar**	✓	**Poor**
Icy pops, tropical	333kJ	18g sugar	162	Poor

8pk				
Raspberry fruity duos 10pk	306kJ	2g fat 12g sugar	162, 160b, 220	Average
Icy pops, raspberry 8pk	**292kJ**	**17g sugar**	✓	**Poor**
Icy pops, tropical 8pk	333kJ	18g sugar	162	Average
Lemonade ice blocks	**289kJ**	**17g sugar**	✓	**Poor**
Lemon sorbet	**456kJ**	**21g sugar**	✓	**Average**
Mango sorbet	**519kJ**	**26g sugar**	✓	**Average**
Neapolitan 2L	825kJ	10.5g fat 19g sugar	122	Poor
Strawberry & cream ice cream 2L	921kJ	9.6g fat 27g sugar	120, 220	Average
Smart buy choc coated ice cream 10pk	1220kJ	19.7g fat 24g sugar	160b	Poor
Smart buy assorted icy pops 20pk	300kJ	17g sugar	160b, 133, 123	Poor

Fruity Fanatics

Product Name	Energy	Major Nutrients	Food Additives	Nutritious Rating
Apple & strawberry	**146kJ**	✓	✓	**Good**
Mango & orange	**209kJ**	✓	✓	**Good**
Orange & passionfruit	**218kJ**	✓	✓	**Good**
Watermelon & apple	**152kJ**	✓	✓	**Good**

Gelati Sky

Product Name	Energy	Major Nutrients	Food Additives	Nutritious Rating
Chocolate	764kJ	↑ Sugar	407	Poor
Death by chocolate	714kJ	↑ Sugar	407	Poor
English toffee crunch	709kJ	↑ Sugar	407	Poor

Hokey pokey	642kJ	↑ Sugar	407	Poor
Honeycomb crunch	695kJ	↑ Sugar	407	Poor
Peanut butter delight	650kJ	↑ Sugar	407	Poor
Super fudge brownie	750kJ	↑ Sugar	407	Poor
Lemon sorbet	339kJ	↑ Sugar	407	Average
Passionfruit sorbet	341kJ	↑ Sugar	407	Average
Very berry sorbet	341kJ	↑ Sugar	407	Average

Gelativo

Product Name	Energy	Major Nutrients	Food Additives	Nutritious Rating
Mango Sorbet	527kJ	↑ Sugar	✓	Average
Lemon lime sorbet	481kJ	↑ Sugar	✓	Average
Strawberry sorbet	472kJ	↑ Sugar	✓	Average
Tropical fruits sorbet	472kJ	↑ Sugar	✓	Average
Chocolate gelato	713kJ	↑ Sugar	✓	Poor
Vanilla bean gelato	785kJ	↑ Sugar	✓	Poor
Hazelnut gelato	848kJ	↑ Sugar	✓	Poor

Golden North

Product Name	Energy	Major Nutrients	Food Additives	Nutritious Rating
Traditional country ice cream, krazy kolors	831kJ	14.6g fat 18g sugar	160b	Poor
Traditional country ice cream, vanilla	934kJ	14.6g fat 18g sugar	160b, 133, 122, 123, 102	Poor

Homer Hudson

Product Name	Energy	Major Nutrients	Food Additives	Nutritious Rating
Chocolate rock	1170kJ	17.5g fat 23g sugar	407	Poor
Choc chunk cookie dough	934kJ	14.6g fat 18g sugar	407	Poor
Cookies & cream	1240kJ	16.2g fat 9.5g	407	Poor

		sugar		
Digger	1240kJ	16.2g fat 27g sugar	407	Poor
Double fudge brownie obsession	1110kJ	15.8g fat 18g sugar	407	Poor
Hoboken crunch	1250kJ	19.2g fat 24g sugar	407	Poor
Vanilla nirvana	110kJ	17.4g fat 20g sugar	407	Poor

IGA/Franklins

Product Name	Energy	Major Nutrients	Food Additives	Nutritious Rating
Signature, boysenberry	835kJ	10.3g fat 25g sugar	122, 133, 407	Poor
Signature, light vanilla	**578kJ**	**2g fat 26g sugar**	✓	**Poor**
Signature, rainbow	835kJ	11.3g fat 23g sugar	102, 110, 132, 120, 407	Poor
Signature, vanilla	864kJ	11.8g fat 22g sugar	407, 160b	Poor
Signature, vanilla fudge ripple	897kJ	11g fat 26g sugar	407, 123, 102, 124, 133, 220	Poor
Black & Gold, chocolate coated ice cream 10pk	**1240kJ**	**22.3g fat 21g sugar**	✓	**Poor**
Black & Gold, milkies 20pk	691kJ	18.5 sugar	155, 102, 124, 122	Poor
Black & Gold, Neapolitan 4L	834kJ	10.2g fat 22g sugar	110, 124, 123, 102, 160b, 407	Poor
Black & Gold, vanilla 4L	849kJ	10.2g fat 24g sugar	160b, 407	Poor
Black & Gold, vanilla choc chip 4L	896kJ	10.8g fat 25g sugar	160b, 407	Poor
Black & Gold, water ice 24pk	300kJ	17g sugar	106b, 133, 123	Poor

Il Gelato

Product Name	Energy	Major Nutrients	Food Additives	Nutritious Rating
Torta chocolat	1160kJ	10g fat 29g sugar	102, 124, 202	Poor
Torta stefania	1160kJ	10g fat 29g sugar	124, 202, 122, 102	Poor

Maggie Beer

Product Name	Energy	Major Nutrients	Food Additives	Nutritious Rating
Dark chocolate & orange ice cream	1062kJ	14.4g fat 24g sugar	407, 220	Poor
Honey comb & caramel ice cream	1062kJ	14g fat 26g sugar	407	Poor
Passionfruit ice cream	1170kJ	18g fat 22g sugar	407, 220	Poor
Quince & bitter almond ice cream	1025kJ	14.9g fat 22g sugar	407, 220, 102, 160b	Poor
Strawberries & cream ice cream	894kJ	13g fat 19g sugar	407, 220	Poor

Nestle

Product Name	Energy	Major Nutrients	Food Additives	Nutritious Rating
Creamy ice cream vanilla slices, light	655kJ	2.7g fat 20g sugar	160b	Poor
Connoisseur, café grande 1L	1150kJ	15.6g fat 21g sugar	160b	Poor
Connoisseur, caramel, honey & macadamia 1L	1140kJ	16.9g fat 19g sugar	160b	Poor
Connoisseur, classic vanilla	1030kJ	14.7g fat 19g sugar	160b	Poor
Connoisseur, chocolate obsession 1L	**1120kJ**	**16.g fat 22g sugar**	✓	**Poor**
Connoisseur,	1080kJ	14.2g fat	160b	Poor

Product Name	Energy	Major Nutrients	Food Additives	Nutritious Rating
chocolate, honey nougat		22g sugar		
Connoisseur, cookies & cream 1L	1160kJ	14.7g fat 20 sugar	319, HVP, 160b	Poor
Connoisseur, strawberry	940kJ	11g fat 23g sugar	120	Poor
Entice, caramel choc mudslide	770kJ	6.7g fat 22g sugar	202, 160b	Poor
Icypole, lemonade 8pk	250kJ	14g sugar	✓	Poor
Maxibon 8pk	1330kJ	15.6g fat 27g sugar	✓	Poor

New Zealand Natural

Product Name	Energy	Major Nutrients	Food Additives	Nutritious Rating
Cookies & cream	1060kJ	13.7g fat 22g sugar	407	Poor

Peters/Nestle

Product Name	Energy	Major Nutrients	Food Additives	Nutritious Rating
Billabong, chocolate 10pk	565kJ	2.5g fat 18g sugar	✓	Poor
Billabong, choc vanilla cups	620kJ	2.6g fat 22g sugar	160b	Poor
Billabong, strawberry & vanilla cups	610kJ	2.6g fat 23g sugar	160b, 120	Poor
Choc wedge choc ripple 8pk	1300kJ	19.5g fat 25g sugar	120	Poor
Choc wedge, vanilla 8pk	1190kJ	17.6g fat 24g sugar	✓	Poor
Choc wedge, violet crumble	1280kJ	19.3g fat 26g sugar	✓	Poor
Drumstick, boysenberry 4pk	1170kJ	11.4g fat 32g sugar	120, 220	Poor
Drumstick, caramel swirl 4pk	1240kJ	13.8g fat 30g sugar	160b	Poor
Drumstick, choc mint	1200kJ	12.5g fat	202	Poor

4pk		26g sugar		
Drumstick, choc shock 4pk	**1260kJ**	**15.4g fat 24g sugar**	✓	**Poor**
Drumstick, super choc 4pk	1460kJ	20g fat 24g sugar	202, 133, 102, 123, 110, 122	Poor
Drumstick, vanilla 4pk	1280kJ	16.3g fat 26g sugar	✓	Poor
Drumstick, vanilla minis	1390kJ	18g fat 23g sugar	✓	Poor
Drumstick, white chocolate & raspberry twister	1095kJ	9.7g fat 25g sugar	133, 120, 129	Poor
Eskimo pie 6pk	**1320kJ**	**21.2g fat 25g sugar**	✓	**Poor**
Frosty fruit, tropical	430kJ	20g sugar	160b	Poor
Frosty fruit, watermelon & pineapple	430kJ	19.5g sugar	120, 160b	Average
Heaven, macadamia 4pk	1510kJ	24.3g fat 27g sugar	160b	Poor
Heaven, rich vanilla	1410kJ	21.9g fat 26g sugar	160b	Poor
Icypoles, larry lemonade	**250kJ**	**14g sugar**	✓	**Poor**
Lifesavers	250kJ	70g fat 14g sugar	120	Poor
Light n creamy, choc caramel swirl	670kJ	2.7g fat 20g sugar	160b	Poor
Light n creamy, classic vanilla	660kJ	2.7g fat 20g sugar	160b	Poor
Light n creamy, classic vanilla no sugar	480kJ	✓	955, 950, 420	Poor
Light n creamy choc vanilla swirl 1.8L	680kJ	2.8g fat 21g sugar	160b	Poor
Light n creamy crème brulee 1.8L	680kJ	2.8g fat 21g sugar	160b	Poor
Light n creamy	650kJ	2.7g fat	160b	Poor

French vanilla 1.8L		20g sugar		
Light n creamy raspberry ripple 1.8L	670kJ	2.6g fat 21g sugar	163, 120, 160b, 220	Poor
Monoco ice cream bar	1140kJ	7.5g fat 22g sugar	223, 160b	Poor
Original neopolitan 2L	740kJ	6.5g fat 21g sugar	120	Poor
Original party cake	755kJ	6.5g fat 22g sugar	120	Poor
Original chocopolitan 2L	**780kJ**	**7.5g fat 21g sugar**	✓	**Poor**
Original triple treat 2L	740kJ	6.5g fat 21g sugar	160b	Poor
Original, vanilla 2L	**750kJ**	**6.4g fat 21g sugar**	✓	**Poor**
Overload, cookie caramel madness 1.2L	980kJ	6.8g fat 29g sugar	160b	Poor
Overload, rolo 1.2L	1010kJ	9.4g fat 30g sugar	160b	Poor

Sanatarium

Product Name	Energy	Major Nutrients	Food Additives	Nutritious Rating
So good, bliss of vanilla 1L	630kJ	2.9g fat 16g sugar	✓	Poor
So good, chocolate bliss 1L	610kJ	2.9g fat 16g sugar	✓	Poor

Sara Lee

Product Name	Energy	Major Nutrients	Food Additives	Nutritious Rating
Cappuccino indulgence ice cream 1L	689kJ	11.3g fat 12g sugar	✓	Poor
Cookies & cream ice cream 1L	789kJ	10.1g fat 17g sugar	✓	Poor
French vanilla ice cream, 1L	688kJ	10.7g fat 16g sugar	✓	Poor
Fruit inspired	683kJ	9.2g fat	✓	Average

raspberry ice cream 1L		17g sugar		
Hazelnut fudge ice cream 1L	784kJ	11.4g fat 17g sugar	✓	Poor
Honeycomb & butterscotch ice cream 1L	792kJ	9.9g fat 17g sugar	✓	Poor
Mango passion swirl ice cream 1L	705kJ	9.1g fat 19g sugar	160b, 120	Average
Mixed berry ice cream 1L	701kJ	9.6g fat 18g sugar	✓	Average
Rocky road overload ice cream 1L	805kJ	10.9g fat 18g sugar	120, 160b	Poor
Ultra choc ice cream 1L	743kJ	10.9g fat 15g sugar	✓	Poor

Skinny Cow

Product Name	Energy	Major Nutrients	Food Additives	Nutritious Rating
Choc mint cup	550kJ	✓	422, 955, 950	Poor
Cookies, coffee	1020kJ	21g sugar	✓	Poor
Cookies, creamy caramel	1020kJ	21g sugar	160b	Poor
Cookies, vanilla	1020kJ	21g sugar	✓	Poor
Old English toffee cup	500kJ	✓	955, 950, 951, 160b	Poor
Vanilla choc cup	530kJ	✓	1520, 160b, 950, 955, 202	Poor
Sundae, double choc	530kJ	✓	1520, 160b, 950, 955, 202, 422	Poor
Sundae, vanilla caramel	500kJ	✓	1520, 160b, 950, 955, 202, 422	Poor

Streets/Homes

Product Name	Energy	Major Nutrients	Food Additives	Nutritious Rating
Blue Ribbon, caramel swirl 2L	729kJ	3.1g fat 22g sugar	102, 160b, 132, 122, 110, 124, 123, 220	Poor
Blue Ribbon, choc banana chip 2L	750kJ	3.7g fat 21g sugar	160b, 120, 220	Poor
Blue Ribbon, choc mint 2L	684kJ	2.7g fat 20g sugar	160b, 120, 220, 102	Poor
Blue Ribbon, double chocolate 2L	862kJ	10.7g fat 19g sugar	160b, 120, 220	Poor
Blue Ribbon, goody drops 2L	717kJ	2.7g fat 22g sugar	160b, 120, 220	Poor
Blue Ribbon, hokey pokey 2L	739kJ	2.6g fat 23g sugar	160b, 120, 220	Poor
Blue Ribbon, Neapolitan twist 2L	684kJ	2.7g fat 20g sugar	160b, 120, 220, 102	Poor
Blue Ribbon, old English toffee 2L	739kJ	2.9g fat 24g sugar	160b, 120, 220	Poor
Blue Ribbon, vanilla 2L	858kJ	10.6g fat 19g sugar	160b, 220	Poor
Blue Ribbon, vanilla light 2L	682kJ	2.7g fat 20g sugar	160b, 220	Poor
Calippo mini poles, lemon 10pk	365kJ	19g sugar	102	Average
Calippo mini poles, orange & lime 10pk	359kJ	19g sugar	102, 110, 133	Poor
Calippo mini poles, raspberry & pineapple 10pk	363kJ	20g sugar	124, 123, 102	Poor
Cornetto, caramel hokey pokey	1329kJ	15.7g fat 30g sugar	102, 132, 122, 110, 124, 123, 120, 160b	Poor
Cornetto, double choc chip	1354kJ	17g fat 29g sugar	129, 102, 133, 122, 120, 160b	Poor
Cornetto, vanilla nut	1385kJ	18.7g fat	122, 102,	Poor

chocolate		25g sugar	160b	
Golden gaytime	1271kJ	19.6g fat 22g sugar	160b, 120	Poor
Magnum, almond	1442kJ	23.7g fat 28g sugar	160b	Poor
Magnum, big choc bikkie	1398kJ	21.1g fat 29g sugar	102, 132, 122, 110, 124, 123, 160b	Poor
Magnum, classic	1302kJ	21g fat 26g sugar	160b	Poor
Magnum, sandwich	**1223kJ**	**16g fat 26g sugar**	✓	**Poor**
Magnum, ego caramel	1460kJ	21.4g fat 34g sugar	220, 160b	Poor
Magnum, equador	1334kJ	22.8g fat 24g sugar	160b	Poor
Magnum, gold	1562kJ	25.4g fat 31g sugar	160b, 120	Poor
Magnum, peppermint	1269kJ	20.1g fat 26g sugar	102, 160b	Poor
Magnum temptation fruit	**1300kJ**	**19g fat 33g sugar**	✓	**Poor**
Magnum, white	1345kJ	21.4g fat 29g sugar	160b	Poor
Magnum minis, almond	1479kJ	24.4g fat 28g sugar	160b	Average
Magnum minis, choc bikkie	1418kJ	21.6g fat 29g sugar	102, 132, 122, 110, 124, 123, 160b	Poor
Magnum minis, classic	1351kJ	21.9g fat 23g sugar	160b	Poor
Magnum minis, ego caramel	1596kJ	24.8g fat 34g sugar	160b, 220	Poor
Magnum minis, equador dark	1386kJ	23.9g fat 24g sugar	160b	Poor
Magnum minis, pure pleasure	1328kJ	21.3g fat 27g sugar	102, 142, 160b	Poor
Magnum minis,	**1400kJ**	**20g fat**	✓	**Poor**

temptation chocolate		**33g sugar**		
Paddle pop, banana	656kJ	4.8g fat 19g sugar	160b	Poor
Paddle pop, chocolate	660kJ	5.1g fat 19g sugar	120, 160b, 220	Poor
Paddle pop, cyclone	409kJ	22g sugar	120	Poor
Paddle pop, icy twist	**374kJ**	**19g sugar**	✓	**Poor**
Paddle pop, fruity stack tutti fruiti	405kJ	21g sugar	162, 160b	Poor
Paddle pop, rainbow	660kJ	4.8g fat 19.8g sugar	120	Poor
Paddle pop, scribbler	370kJ	19g sugar	120	Poor
Paddle pop, solar flare	560kJ	3.1g fat 19g sugar	120, 160b	Poor
Splice, pine lime	527kJ	2.1g fat 19g sugar	160b	Average
Splice, raspberry	541kJ	1.2g fat 20g sugar	160b	Average
Vienetta, chocolate	1090kJ	17.3g fat 20g sugar	160b	Poor
Vienetta, vanilla	1094kJ	17g fat 19g sugar	160b	Poor

The Natural Confectionary Company

Product Name	Energy	Major Nutrients	Food Additives	Nutritious Rating
Fruit Ice, raspberry & pineapple	**390kJ**	**22g sugar**	✓	**Average**
Fruit Ice, tropical	390kJ	22g sugar	160b	Average

Tofutti Cuties

Product Name	Energy	Major Nutrients	Food Additives	Nutritious Rating
Chocolate	1344kJ	15g fat 22g sugar	407	Poor
Marions-nous	1260kJ	11g fat	407	Poor

		22g sugar		
Vanilla	1344kJ	15g fat 22g sugar	407, 160b	Poor

Weight Watchers

Product Name	Energy	Major Nutrients	Food Additives	Nutritious Rating
Berry mudslide 2pk	625kJ	24g sugar	122, 220, 202	Poor
Double choc sundae 2pk	790kJ	26g sugar	220, 202	Poor
Toffee pecan	750kJ	22g sugar	202, 220	Poor
Vanilla 2pk	575kJ	22g sugar	160b, 202, 220	Poor
White chocolate & raspberry	650kJ	22g sugar	160b, 220, 202	Poor

Weis

Product Name	Energy	Major Nutrients	Food Additives	Nutritious Rating
Coffee with cream ice cream	967kJ	14.1g fat 21g sugar	✓	Average
Fruito	598kJ	4.2g fat 22g sugar	✓	Average
Macadamia chunks & mango ice cream	920kJ	13.1g fat 20g sugar	✓	Average
Mango with cream bar	579kJ	4.3g fat 21g sugar	✓	Average
Queensland mango ice cream	748kJ	8.2g fat 23g sugar	✓	Average
Raspberry & cream bar	722kJ	6.4g fat 23g sugar	✓	Average
Sorbet, berry 1L	485kJ	26g sugar	✓	Average
Sorbet, mango 1L	464kJ	25g sugar	✓	Average
Sorbet, lemon	449kJ	24g sugar	✓	Average
Sorbet, passion orange	526kJ	28g sugar	✓	Average
Sorbet bar, mango	480kJ	26g sugar	✓	Average
Sorbet bar, triple berry	443kJ	23g sugar	✓	Average
Vanilla bean ice	983kJ	13.2g fat	✓	Poor

cream		23g sugar		

Woolworths/Safeways

Product Name	Energy	Major Nutrients	Food Additives	Nutritious Rating
Homebrand, choc-coated vanilla 10pk	**1300kJ**	**21.1g fat 23g sugar**	✓	**Poor**
Homebrand, iceblocks	377kJ	15g sugar	160b, 123, 133	Poor
Homebrand, milkies 20pk	643kJ	5.5g fat 17g sugar	155, 133, 102, 124, 122, 102	Poor
Homebrand, Neapolitan ice cream 4L	849kJ	10.5g fat 16g sugar	160b, 155, 122, 133	Poor
Homebrand, vanilla ice cream 4L	849kJ	10.5g fat 16g sugar	160b	Poor

Pastry

Best commercial pastries include: *Careme, Coles puff pastry and Homebrand puff pastry.*

Careme

Product Name	Energy	Major Nutrients	Food Additives	Nutritious Rating
All butter puff pastry	1800kJ	↑Fat ↑Salt	✓	Poor
Sour cream short crust pastry	1980kJ	↑Fat	✓	Poor
Vanilla bean short crust	2060kJ	30.6g fat 17g sugar	✓	Poor

Coles

Product Name	Energy	Major Nutrients	Food Additives	Nutritious Rating
Ready puff pastry	1400kJ	14.9g fat	✓	Poor
Puff pastry, canola	1360kJ	15.6g fat	✓	Poor
Short crust pastry	1580kJ	19.7g fat	320	Poor
Golden eggs frozen egg whites	204kJ	✓	✓	Average

IGA/Franklins

Product Name	Energy	Major Nutrients	Food Additives	Nutritious Rating
Black & Gold, puff pastry	1310kJ	13.2g fat	202, 281, 320	Poor

Pampas

Product Name	Energy	Major Nutrients	Food Additives	Nutritious Rating
Sweet tart cases	1850kJ	22.8g fat	320	Poor
Fillo sheets	1380kJ	✓	223	Poor
Puff pastry, butter	1550kJ	↑Fat	✓	Poor
Puff pastry block	1370kJ	↑Fat	✓	Poor

Puff pastry, reduced fat	1260kJ	↑Fat	✓	Poor
Short crust sheets	1650kJ	↑Fat ↑Salt	320	Poor
Short crust sheets, reduced fat	1480kJ	↑Fat ↑Salt	320	Poor
Pastry spring roll	**1440kJ**	✓	✓	**Poor**
Savoury pie flan	1880kJ	↑Fat	320	Poor
Sweet flan case	1850kJ	↑Fat ↑Sugar	320	Poor

Woolworths/Safeways

Product Name	Energy	Major Nutrients	Food Additives	Nutritious Rating
Homebrand, puff pastry	1300kJ	↑Salt	✓	Poor

Meat pies, Sausage rolls & Canapes

Best brands for canapés are *Borgs, Colonial farm and Nabil.*

Best brand for pies and sausage rolls is *Patties.*

Asiana

Product Name	Energy	Major Nutrients	Food Additives	Nutritious Rating
Cocktail spring rolls	810kJ	✓	631, 627	Poor
Yum cha selection	937kJ	✓	631, 627	Poor

Authentic Asia

Product Name	Energy	Major Nutrients	Food Additives	Nutritious Rating
Bangkok firecracker prawns	876kJ	↑Fat ↑Salt	✓	Poor
Prawn wonton soup noodles	452kJ	↑Salt	621, 631, YE	Poor

Balfour

Product Name	Energy	Major Nutrients	Food Additives	Nutritious Rating
Party pasties	1070kJ	↑Fat ↑Salt	320, 160b	Poor
Party pies	1280kJ	↑Fat	621, 627, 631, 202, HVP, 211, 102, 110	Poor
Party pizza pies	962kJ	↑Fat ↑Salt	202, 234, HVP, 250, 251, 320	Poor
Party sausage rolls	1010kJ	↑Fat ↑Salt	202, 211, 110, 102	Poor

Big Ben

Product Name	Energy	Major Nutrients	Food Additives	Nutritious Rating
Traditional meat pie	1010kJ	↑Fat	160b, YE, HVP, 320	Poor

Extra tasty meat pies	1100kJ	↑Fat ↑Salt	HVP, 160b, 320	Poor

Bocastle

Product Name	Energy	Major Nutrients	Food Additives	Nutritious Rating
Meat pies, Moroccan lamb	1020kJ	↑Fat	320, 223, 282, 202, 102, 124	Average
Meat pies, Korma curry vegetable	995kJ	↑Fat	320, 223, 282, YE, 202, 102, 124	Average
Meat pies, beef burgundy	1014kJ	↑Fat	320, 223, 282, 202, 102, 124	Poor
Sausage rolls, gourmet beef	1060kJ	↑Fat	223, 282, YE, 621, 635, 202, 102, 124	Poor

Borgs

Product Name	Energy	Major Nutrients	Food Additives	Nutritious Rating
Pastizzi spinach & ricotta	1029kJ	↑Fat	✓	Average
Pastizzi spinach & cheese triangles	1139kJ	↑Fat	✓	Average
Spinach & feta pastries	1170kJ	↑Fat	✓	Average
Chicken & vegetable triangles	996kJ	↑Fat	HVP, 223	Average
Ricotta & cheese pastries	1074kJ	↑Fat	635	Average
Spinach & ricotta triangles	1170kJ	↑Fat	✓	Average

Cheese Buddy

Product Name	Energy	Major Nutrients	Food Additives	Nutritious Rating
Cheese buns	1420kJ	↑Fat	319	Poor

Coles

Product Name	Energy	Major Nutrients	Food Additives	Nutritious Rating
Oriental snack selection	953-1890kJ	↑Fat	211	Average
Dim sum selection	529-571kJ	↑Salt	✓	Average
Jumbo tempura prawns	745kJ	↑Fat ↑Salt	✓	Average
Oriental prawn platter	971-1890kJ	↑Fat ↑Salt	YE, 211	Average
Oriental vegetable platter	813-1120kJ	↑Fat ↑Salt	✓	Average
Prawn gyoza	930kJ	↑Fat	✓	Average
Vegetable gyoza	856kJ	↑Fat	1520, 141	Average
Meat pies, chunky beef	923kJ	↑Fat	160b, HVP	Average
Meat pies, beef	950kJ	↑Fat	HVP, 160b	Poor
Meat pies, chicken & vegetable	910kJ	↑Fat	320, 160b, HVP	Poor
Party pie, beef steak	1030kJ	↑Fat ↑Salt	160b, HVP	Poor
Party sausage rolls	1110kJ	↑Fat ↑Salt	223, 635, HVP, 160b, 329	Poor
Smart buy, individual pies	1050kJ	↑Fat	160b, 621	Poor
Smart buy, family pie	1020kJ	↑Fat	160b, 920	Poor
Smart buy, party pies	926kJ	↑Fat	160b, 621	Poor
Smart buy dim sims	790kJ	↑Fat ↑Salt	202	Poor
Smart buy spring rolls	904kJ	↑Fat	✓	Average

Colonial Farm

Product Name	Energy	Major Nutrients	Food Additives	Nutritious Rating
Spring rolls, cocktail	1082kJ	↑Fat	✓	Average

Darshan

Product Name	Energy	Major Nutrients	Food Additives	Nutritious Rating

	706-1058kJ	↑Fat	320, 211, 223	Average
Entertainers pack	706-1058kJ	↑Fat	320, 211, 223	Average
Vegetable curry puffs	918kJ	✓	320, 211, 223	Average

Edgell

Product Name	Energy	Major Nutrients	Food Additives	Nutritious Rating
Chikko rolls	769kJ	↑Fat	HVP, 635, 102, 110	Poor

Four N Twenty Pies

Product Name	Energy	Major Nutrients	Food Additives	Nutritious Rating
Beef & cheese pies	988kJ	↑Fat ↑Salt	HVP, 160b, 202, 234	Poor
Chicken & Vegetable pies	969kJ	↑Fat ↑Salt	HVP, 160b, 320	Average
Traditional meat pies	959kJ	↑Fat ↑Salt	HVP, 160b	Poor
Microwave pies	959kJ	↑Fat ↑Salt	HVP, 160b, 320	Poor
Angus beef pies	1060kJ	↑Fat ↑Salt	HVP	Poor
Angus beef pies, cheese & bacon	1110kJ	↑Fat ↑Salt	HVP, 250, 621, 635	Poor
Angus beef pies, pepper	1090kJ	↑Fat ↑Salt	HVP	Poor
Gold label, chunky steak pies	932kJ	↑Fat ↑Salt	HVP, 160b	Poor
Gold label, shepherds pies	856kJ	↑Fat	222, HVP, 320	Poor
Sausage rolls, jumbo	1080kJ	↑Fat ↑Salt	223, HVP, 635	Poor

Golden Wok

Product Name	Energy	Major Nutrients	Food Additives	Nutritious Rating
Dim sims, mini chicken & veg	708kJ	↑Fat ↑Salt	621	Poor

Dim sims, mini beef	844kJ	↑Fat ↑Salt	621	Poor
Dim sims	1078kJ	↑Fat ↑Salt	621	Poor

Herbert Adams

Product Name	Energy	Major Nutrients	Food Additives	Nutritious Rating
Mixed vegetable pastie	901kJ	↑Fat ↑Salt	223, 320, 160b	Average
Gourmet beef pies, king island	1010kJ	↑Fat ↑Salt	234, 204, HVP	Poor
Gourmet beef pies, pepper steak	930kJ	↑Fat	HVP	Poor
Gourmet beef pies, chilli con carne	989kJ	↑Fat	HVP, 160b	Average
Gourmet beef pies, beef & mushroom	914kJ	↑Fat	HVP, 635	Average
Party pies	1030kJ	↑Fat ↑Salt	HVP, 160b	Poor
Sausage rolls	1090kJ	↑Fat ↑Salt	223, 320, 160b	Poor
Cheese & spinach rolls	1100kJ	↑Fat ↑Salt	222, 160b	Average
Cheese & cauliflower rolls	1010kJ	↑Fat	YE, 202, 222, 631, 627, 635, HVP, 160b	Average
Vol au vents savoury	1130kJ	↑Fat ↑Salt	223, 320, 160b	Poor
Quiche Lorraine tartlets	1090kJ	↑Fat ↑Salt	250	Poor
Spinach & ricotta finger foods	1310kJ	↑Fat ↑Salt	320, 202, 621, 635, HVP	Average

Homai

Product Name	Energy	Major Nutrients	Food Additives	Nutritious Rating
Appetiser entertainer pack	860-927kJ	↑Fat ↑Salt	✓	Average

Spring rolls	1030kJ	↑Fat ↑Salt	621	Average
Yum cha cocktail spring rolls	927kJ	↑Fat ↑Salt	621	Average
Yum cha dim sims	**844kJ**	**↑Fat**	✓	**Poor**
Yum Cha party pack	844-966kJ	↑Fat ↑Salt	621	Poor
Pork & chive dumplings	1105kJ	↑Fat	✓	Poor

Hong Kong Kitchen

Product Name	Energy	Major Nutrients	Food Additives	Nutritious Rating
BBQ pork buns	848kJ	↑Fat ↑Salt	627, 635, 202, YE	Poor

IGA/Franklins

Product Name	Energy	Major Nutrients	Food Additives	Nutritious Rating
Black & Gold, meat pies	1050kJ	↑Fat	621, 320, 160b	Poor
Black & Gold, chicken & vegetable family pie	830kJ	✓	621, 320, 160b, HVP	Average
Black & Gold, party sausage rolls	1110kJ	↑Fat ↑Salt	621, 320, 160b	Poor
Black & Gold, garlic bread	1220kJ	↑Fat ↑Salt	281, 320	Poor
Signature, garlic loaf	1260kJ	↑Fat ↑Salt	281, 320	Poor

Interfrost

Product Name	Energy	Major Nutrients	Food Additives	Nutritious Rating
Herb & pepper fish strips	1396kJ	↑Fat ↑Salt	160b	Average
Samosas	1220kJ	↑Fat	621	Average
Spring rolls, cocktail	**1420kJ**	**↑Fat**	✓	**Average**

Marathon

Product Name	Energy	Major Nutrients	Food Additives	Nutritious Rating
Dim sims	802kJ	↑Salt	621	Poor
Hotdogs, puffy cocktails	1190kJ	↑Fat ↑Salt	250, 320, 110, YE, HVP	Poor
Spring rolls	631kJ	↑Salt	102, 621, 123	Average

Marios

Product Name	Energy	Major Nutrients	Food Additives	Nutritious Rating
Pastizzi, apple	1140kJ	↑Fat	202, 223, 320	Average
Pastizzi, beef & peas	1220kJ	↑Fat ↑Salt	202, 635, 621, HVP	Average
Pastizzi, curry chicken	1280kJ	↑Fat ↑Salt	202, 621, 320	Average
Pastizzi, jam & apple	1310kJ	↑Fat	202, 129	Average
Pastizzi, peas	1300kJ	↑Fat	202, 621, 320	Average
Pastizzi, pizza	1190kJ	↑Fat ↑Salt	202, 221, 250, 320	Average
Pastizzi, ricotta, cheese & spinach	1400kJ	↑Fat	320, 202	Average
Pastizzi, ricotta & fetta	1400kJ	↑Fat ↑Salt	320, 202	Average
Pastizzi, ricotta, cheese & bacon	1380kJ	↑Fat	202, 221, 250, 320, 635	Average
Pastizzi, ricotta & cheese	1300kJ	↑Fat	202, 320	Average
Pastizzi, seafood	1270kJ	↑Fat	621, 320, 202, 120, 160b	Average
Pastizzi, vegetarian	1170kJ	↑Fat	202, 621, 320	Average

Misori

Product Name	Energy	Major Nutrients	Food Additives	Nutritious Rating
Gyoja dumplings	712kJ	✓	621	Average
Vegetable dumplings	736kJ	✓	621	Average

Mrs Macs

Product Name	Energy	Major Nutrients	Food Additives	Nutritious Rating
Microwave sausage roll	1150kJ	↑Fat ↑Salt	HVP, 635, 621, 320	Poor
Microwave pasties	1070kJ	↑Fat ↑Salt	320	Average
Microwave pie	1080kJ	↑Fat ↑Salt	HVP, 621, 320	Poor
Beef & mushroom pie	1000kJ	↑Fat ↑Salt	HVP, 635, 621, 320	Average
Chicken curry pie	859kJ	↑Fat ↑Salt	635	Average
Beef & pepper pie	1070kJ	↑Fat ↑Salt	HVP, 635, 621, 320	Poor

Mrs Quick

Product Name	Energy	Major Nutrients	Food Additives	Nutritious Rating
Sausage rolls	1190kJ	↑Fat	320, HVP	Poor

Nabil

Product Name	Energy	Major Nutrients	Food Additives	Nutritious Rating
Spinach pastry	933kJ	✓	✓	Average
Vegetarian potato balls	1469kJ	✓	✓	Average
Vegetarian samosas	875kJ	✓	✓	Average
Vegetarian spring rolls	423kJ	↑Fat	✓	Average

Pacific West

Product Name	Energy	Major Nutrients	Food Additives	Nutritious Rating
Banquet Asian	883kJ	↑Fat	627, 631	Average
Money bags	908kJ	↑Fat	627, 631	Average
Indian samosas	879kJ	↑Fat	627, 631	Average
Seafood dumplings	679kJ	✓	627, 631	Average
Thai spring rolls	810kJ	✓	627, 631	Average

Cocktail spring rolls	810kJ	↑Fat	627, 631	Average

Patties Gluten Free

Product Name	Energy	Major Nutrients	Food Additives	Nutritious Rating
Party pack quiches	1000kJ	↑Fat ↑Salt	220, HVP	Average
Pasties	970kJ	↑Fat ↑Salt	621, 160b, 223	Average
Meat pie	914kJ	↑Fat	✓	Poor
Pizza rolls	955kJ	↑Fat ↑Salt	250	Average
Vegie rolls	675kJ	✓	✓	Average
Sausage rolls	1070kJ	↑Fat	✓	Poor
Party sausage rolls	988kJ	↑Fat ↑Salt	✓	Poor

Petite Cuisine

Product Name	Energy	Major Nutrients	Food Additives	Nutritious Rating
Hungarian beef rolls	829kJ	✓	320, HVP, YE, 282	Poor
Chicken & mushroom rolls	891kJ	↑Fat	320, HVP, YE, 282	Average
Meat balls	996kJ	↑Fat ↑Salt	320, HVP	Poor

Quorn

Product Name	Energy	Major Nutrients	Food Additives	Nutritious Rating
Dippers	696kJ	↑Fat	✓	Poor
Pasties	1080kJ	↑Fat	✓	Poor
Sausage rolls	1310kJ	↑Fat ↑Salt	✓	Poor
Soy pieces	411kJ	✓	✓	Poor

Sara Lee

Product Name	Energy	Major Nutrients	Food Additives	Nutritious Rating

Quiche lorraine	1150kJ	↑Fat ↑Salt	250, 627, 631, YE	Average
Quiche lorraine snack size	1220kJ	↑Fat ↑Salt	250, 627, 631, YE	Average
Quiche, tomato, feta & spinach	**1160kJ**	**↑Fat** **↑Salt**	✓	**Average**

Sargents

Product Name	Energy	Major Nutrients	Food Additives	Nutritious Rating
Party pack	1113-1285kJ	↑Fat ↑Salt	160b, YE, 627, 631, HVP	Poor
Chunky chicken pie	977kJ	↑Fat	160b, YE, 627, 631	Poor
Extra special angus beef & vegetable pie	920kJ	↑Fat	160b, YE, 627, 631, 320	Average
Traditional meat pie	1043kJ	↑Fat	160b, HVP, 627, 631, 320	Poor
Steak slices pie	1065kJ	↑Fat	160b, 627, 631, HVP, 320	Poor
Beef royale pie	938kJ	↑Fat	160b, 320, HVP	Poor
Vegetable pie	896kJ	↑Fat	160b, 320, 627, 631, HVP,	Average

Simply Special

Product Name	Energy	Major Nutrients	Food Additives	Nutritious Rating
Mini felafels	915kJ	↑Fat	222	Good
Mixed vegetable pakoras	918kJ	↑Fat ↑Salt ↑Sugar	222	Good
Thai selection	838-1220kJ	↑Fat ↑Salt	319, 320, 211, 222	Average

Snowy River

Product Name	Energy	Major Nutrients	Food Additives	Nutritious Rating
Meat pies	1050kJ	↑Fat	621, 160b, 320	Poor
Party sausage rolls	929kJ	↑Fat	200, 211, 110,	Poor

			102, 202	
Heat in bag sausage roll	1070kJ	↑Fat ↑Salt	320, 621, 160b	Poor

Stones

Product Name	Energy	Major Nutrients	Food Additives	Nutritious Rating
Quiche, lorraine	821kJ	↑Fat	250	Average
Quiche, spinach	803kJ	↑Fat	✓	Average

Temptation

Product Name	Energy	Major Nutrients	Food Additives	Nutritious Rating
Quiche petites, salmon & dill	1180kJ	↑Fat ↑Salt	YE, 223, 920, 320	Average
Quiche petites, lorraine	1190kJ	↑Fat ↑Salt	YE, 223, 320	Average
Quiche petites, cheese & spinach	1150kJ	↑Fat ↑Salt	YE, 223, 320	Average

Wedgewood

Product Name	Energy	Major Nutrients	Food Additives	Nutritious Rating
Party pies	912kJ	↑Fat	621	Poor

Woolworths/Safeways

Product Name	Energy	Major Nutrients	Food Additives	Nutritious Rating
Party pies	930kJ	↑Fat	HVP	Poor
Jumbo sausage rolls	1200kJ	↑Fat ↑Salt	160b, HVP, 627, 631, 282	Poor
Meat pies	855kJ	↑Fat	627, 631, 160b, 320	Poor
Dim Sims	**797kJ**	**↑Salt**	✓	**Poor**
Mini spring rolls, beef	961kJ	↑Fat	320, HVP	Average

Pizzas

The best brand for frozen pizzas is *Vics*.

Australian Garlic Bread

Product Name	Energy	Major Nutrients	Food Additives	Nutritious Rating
Garlic bread	1360kJ	↑Fat ↑Salt	282	Poor

Coles

Product Name	Energy	Major Nutrients	Food Additives	Nutritious Rating
Smart buy, Hawaiian	979kJ	✓	223, 250,635	Average
Smart buy, supreme	1000kJ	✓	223, 250	Average

Creative Foods

Product Name	Energy	Major Nutrients	Food Additives	Nutritious Rating
Cheese & bacon ciabatta	1360kJ	↑Salt	250, YE, 202	Poor

Dr Oetker Pizza

Product Name	Energy	Major Nutrients	Food Additives	Nutritious Rating
Ristorate, four cheese	1120kJ	↑Fat	HVP	Average
Ristorate, funghi	980kJ	↑Fat ↑Salt	HVP	Average
Ristorate, mozzerella	1100kJ	↑Fat	HVP	Average

IGA/Franklins

Product Name	Energy	Major Nutrients	Food Additives	Nutritious Rating
Pizza, supreme	1020kJ	↑Fat	621, 250, HVP, 223	Average
Pizza, bellini	1020kJ	↑Fat ↑Salt	HVP, 250	Average

Pizza, ham & pineapple	1020kJ	↑Fat	HVP, 250, 223, 621	Average
Pizza, bellini bbq chicken	1020kJ	↑Fat	HVP, oil, 250, 223, 621	Average
Pizza bases	**1140kJ**	✓	✓	**Poor**
Black & Gold, ham & pineapple pizza	956kJ	✓	223, 250, HVP	Average
Black & Gold, margherita pizza	**962kJ**	✓	✓	**Average**
Black & Gold, cheese & ham pizza	990kJ	✓	223, 250, HVP	Poor
Black & Gold, supreme pizza	907kJ	✓	223, 250, HVP	Average

Le Moulin

Product Name	Energy	Major Nutrients	Food Additives	Nutritious Rating
Pizza base	1070kJ	✓	✓	Poor

McCain

Product Name	Energy	Major Nutrients	Food Additives	Nutritious Rating
Perfection, thin crust speciale pizza	1060kJ	↑Fat	250, 251, HVP	Average
Perfection thin crust tandoori chicken pizza	**926kJ**	✓	✓	**Average**
Pizza bases	1012kJ	✓	320	Poor
Family cheese & bacon pizza	934kJ	✓	250, HVP	Poor
Family ham & pineapple pizza	963kJ	✓	250, HVP	Average
Family marghertia	**1100kJ**	↑Fat	✓	**Average**
Family meat lovers	934kJ	↑Fat	250, HVP	-
Family supreme	955kJ	↑Fat	250, HVP	Average
Garlic pizza	955kJ	✓	320, HVP, VP	Average
Perfection bites bruschetta	990kJ	↑Sugar	320	Average
Perfection bites	1030kJ	↑Sugar	320, VP	Poor

pepperoni				
Pizza perfection house special	978kJ	↑Fat	HVP, 250, 635, 627, 631	Average
Pockets, ham & pineapple	990kJ	✓	250, HVP	Average
Pockets, ham & pineapple	990kJ	✓	250, HVP	Average
Pockets, supreme	993kJ	✓	250, HVP	Average
Pizza subs ham & pineapple	902kJ	↑Salt	320, 250, HVP	Average
Pizza subs, house special	890kJ	↑Salt	320, 250, HVP	Average
Pizza subs, BBQ chicken	867kJ	✓	HVP	Average
Pizza subs, meat lovers	1040kJ	✓	HVP, 250, 251, 220	Poor
Pizza singles, cheese & bacon	974kJ	✓	320, YE, HVP, 250	Poor
Pizza singles, meat lovers	967kJ	✓	320, 250, HVP, YE	Poor
Pizza slices, ham & pineapple	827kJ	✓	320, 250, HVP	Average
Pizza slices, supreme	934kJ	✓	320, 250, HVP	Average
Pizza slices, margherita	1137kJ	↑Fat	320	Average

Papa Giuseppis

Product Name	Energy	Major Nutrients	Food Additives	Nutritious Rating
BBQ chicken pizza	970kJ	✓	250, 223, 635	Average
Hawaiian pizza	904kJ	✓	250, 223, 635, 120	Average
Hot special pizza	956kJ	↑Fat	250, 223, 635, 120	Average
Supreme pizza	942kJ	✓	250, 223, 635, 120	Average
Bacon & beef pizza	942kJ	↑Fat ↑Salt	250, 223, 635	Poor

Pieros

Product Name	Energy	Major Nutrients	Food Additives	Nutritious Rating
Pizza base	1020kJ	✓	✓	Poor

Rosettas

Product Name	Energy	Major Nutrients	Food Additives	Nutritious Rating
Pizza base	1070kJ	✓	320	Poor

Stones

Product Name	Energy	Major Nutrients	Food Additives	Nutritious Rating
Pizza slices, ham & pineapple	880kJ	✓	223, HVP, 250	Average
Pizza slices, supreme	856kJ	✓	223, HVP, 250	Average

Vics

Product Name	Energy	Major Nutrients	Food Additives	Nutritious Rating
Sliced Italian mozzarella pizza	887kJ	↑Salt	✓	Average
Spinach & pesto pizza	862kJ	↑Salt	✓	Average
Four cheeses pizza	1010kJ	↑Salt	✓	Average
Roasted vegetable pizza	746kJ	↑Salt	✓	Average

Woolworths/Safeways

Product Name	Energy	Major Nutrients	Food Additives	Nutritious Rating
Homebrand, supreme pizza	920kJ	✓	250, 635	Average
Homebrand, Hawaiian pizza	920kJ	✓	223, 250	Average
Homebrand, BBQ meat lovers pizza	900kJ	✓	223, 250	Poor

Ready made meals

There are a lot of scattered varieties that are ok frozen dinners, the best overall brands are *Coles, Fry's vegetarian, Rang Mahal, Red pepper, Royal orchard, Tukka tubz and Wang wang.*

Attack a Snack (McCains)

Product Name	Energy	Major Nutrients	Food Additives	Nutritious Rating
Beef chow mein	548kJ	✓	HVP	Poor
Macaroni cheese	599kJ	✓	HVP, YE, 160b, 200	Poor
Creamy bacon & mushroom spirals	522kJ	✓	YE, 250	Poor
Sausage & herb potato	453kJ	✓	223, YE	Poor

Coles

Product Name	Energy	Major Nutrients	Food Additives	Nutritious Rating
Canneloni, spinach & ricotta	358kJ	✓	✓	Good
Butter chicken	624kJ	✓	122, 124	Average
Thai green curry	634kJ	✓	✓	Average
Bechamel beef lasagne	608kJ	✓	✓	Average
Vegetable lasagne	481kJ	✓	✓	Good
Lite Beef lasagne	431kJ	✓	✓	Average
Lite chicken rissotto	401kJ	✓	✓	Average
Chicken korma	576kJ	✓	✓	Average
Tuna bake	640kJ	↑Fat	✓	Average
Veal cordon bleu	893kJ	↑Salt ↑Fat	HVP, 200, 320, 250	Average
Shepherds pie	321kJ	✓	222, 635	Average
Smart buy, beef lasagne	522kJ	✓	220	Average
Smart buy, light beef hot pot	268kJ	✓	222	Average

Smart buy, light chicken fettucine	378kJ	✓	✓	Average
Smart buy, creamy mushroom angolotti	461kJ	✓	✓	Average

Enricos

Product Name	Energy	Major Nutrients	Food Additives	Nutritious Rating
Beef lasagne	1037kJ	↑Salt	HVP, 635	Average
Lasagne, vegetable	1169kJ	✓	HVP, 635, YE	Good
Macaroni cheese	1213kJ	✓	282, 102, 635, HVP	Average

Fry's Vegetarian

Product Name	Energy	Major Nutrients	Food Additives	Nutritious Rating
Crumbed snitzel	880kJ	↑Salt ↑Fat	✓	Average
Hotdogs	1036kJ	↑Salt	✓	Average
Chicken style burgers	713kJ	↑Salt	✓	Average

Gourmet Cuisine

Product Name	Energy	Major Nutrients	Food Additives	Nutritious Rating
Beef stroganoff	982kJ	↑Salt ↑Fat	223, 320, HVP, YE, 631, 627	Average
Veal with mushroom sauce	939kJ	↑Salt ↑Fat	320, VP, HVP, YE	Average
Beef with tomato relish	956kJ	↑Salt ↑Fat	YE, HVP, 320, 223	Average
Chicken honey mustard	816kJ	↑Fat	320, HVP, YE	Average
Veal parmigiana	897kJ	↑Salt ↑Fat	250, 320, 200, HVP	Average
Aranchi spinach & cheese	802kJ	↑Salt	202, 200, HVP, YE, 627, 631	Average

Hormel

Product Name	Energy	Major Nutrients	Food Additives	Nutritious Rating
Main meats lamb shanks, rosemary & mint sauce	672kJ	✓	YE	Average
Main meats lamb shanks, classic red wine sauce	640kJ	↑Fat	YE, 220	Average

IGA/Franklins

Product Name	Energy	Major Nutrients	Food Additives	Nutritious Rating
Signature, spaghetti bolognese	355kJ	✓	220	Average
Signature, fried rice	682kJ	↑Salt	211, YE	Average
Signature, Thai green curry & chicken	**430kJ**	✓	✓	**Average**
Black & Gold, beef lasagne	427kJ	✓	635	Average

Lean Cuisine

Product Name	Energy	Major Nutrients	Food Additives	Nutritious Rating
Beef, red wine & garlic mash	370kJ	✓	160b, YE	Average
Beef stroganoff & pasta	400kJ	✓	160b, 120	Average
Chicken & vegetable risotto	400kJ	✓	160b, YE	Average
Creamy salmon & dill linguine	445kJ	✓	160b, YE	Average
Honey soy beef & noodles	385kJ	✓	YE	Average
Lamb & rosemary hot pot	365kJ	✓	YE	Average
Spaghetti bolognaise	470kJ	✓	YE, 120	Average
Chicken Thai green curry	405kJ	✓	YE	Average
Vegetable cannelloni	405kJ	✓	YE, 120, 160b	Good
Chicken satay noodles	410kJ	✓	YE, 160b	Average
Chilli con carne & rice	357kJ	✓	YE	Good

Moroccan lamb & cous cous	485kJ	✓	YE	Average
Pumpkin, spinach & ricotta lasagne	440kJ	✓	YE, 160b	Good
Rich beef lasagne	425kJ	✓	YE, 160b	Average
Butter chicken & rice	410kJ	✓	120, 160b	Average
Meatball arrabbiata	340kJ	✓	YE, 120, 160b	Average
Sundried tomato & chicken pasta	455kJ	✓	120, YE, 160b	Average
Thai red chicken curry & rice	375kJ	✓	YE	Average
Pasta ravioli with beef	438kJ	✓	120, 160b, YE	Average
Chicken & spinach risotto	375kJ	✓	YE	Good

Mamalinas

Product Name	Energy	Major Nutrients	Food Additives	Nutritious Rating
Spaghetti meatballs	**468kJ**	✓	✓	**Average**
Tortellini carbonara	715kJ	↑Fat	282, 102, 635, HVP	Average
Canneloni, cheese & spinach	518kJ	✓	200	Average

McCain Healthy Choice 97% Fat Free

Product Name	Energy	Major Nutrients	Food Additives	Nutritious Rating
Beef stroganoff	439kJ	✓	HVP	Average
Beef stir fry with hokkein noodles	**404kJ**	✓	✓	**Average**
Chicken carbonara	432kJ	✓	HVP	Average
Honey chicken stir fry	377kJ	✓	HVP	Average
Stir fry chicken with hokkein noodles	404kJ	✓	HVP	Average
Apricot chicken	401kJ	✓	HVP, YE	Average
Chicken casserole	**304kJ**	✓	✓	**Average**
Beef Florentine	372kJ	✓	HVP, VP	Average
Beef lasagne	476kJ	✓	YE	Average
Honey sesame chicken	399kJ	✓	✓	Average

Lemon chicken	526kJ	✓	✓	Average
Spinach & ricotta ravioli	455kJ	✓	✓	Good
Hot pot beef	266kJ	✓	HVP	Average
Honey stir fry chicken	377kJ	✓	✓	Average
Tender beef & mustard	389kJ	✓	HVP, YE	Average
Fillet of lamb	350kJ	✓	HVP	Average
Honey mustard chicken	432kJ	✓	HVP	Average
Cottage pie	369kJ	✓	✓	Good
Creamy chicken pasta	416kJ	✓	✓	Average
Pumpkin ravioli	477kJ	✓	✓	Average

McCains Red box

Product Name	Energy	Major Nutrients	Food Additives	Nutritious Rating
Chicken parmagana	635kJ	✓	200, VP	Average
Turkey dinner	389kJ	✓	HVP, YE, 627, 631, 160b	Average
Bangers n mash	593kJ	✓	223, 222, VP	Average
Lasagne	685kJ	✓	320, HVP, 635	Average
Beef & bacon pasta	592kJ	✓	250, HVP, 635	Average
Shepherds pie	410kJ	✓	222, YE, 631, 627	Average
Tuna mornay	670kJ	✓	✓	Average
Pork riblet meal	507kJ	✓	635	Average
Cordon bleu veal	655kJ	↑Fat	200, 234, 102, 110, 250, 282, HVP	Average

Michelinas

Product Name	Energy	Major Nutrients	Food Additives	Nutritious Rating
Spaghetti bolognaise	476kJ	✓	HVP, YE	Average
Pasta tortellini cheese	615kJ	✓	✓	Average
Fettucine alfredo	485kJ	✓	✓	Average
Beef teriyaki	496kJ	✓	✓	Average
Beef burgundy	376kJ	✓	YE, 321, 320, 223	Average

Prawn & vegetable alfredo	485kJ	✓	627, 631, HVP	Average

On the Menu

Product Name	Energy	Major Nutrients	Food Additives	Nutritious Rating
Angus roast beef & vegetable pie	350kJ	✓	✓	Average
Chicken parmagana	486kJ	✓	HVP, 282	Average
Roast chicken	360kJ	✓	✓	Average
Angus roast beef	340kJ	✓	220	Average
Bangers & mash	637kJ	↑Fat	223	Average

Quorn

Product Name	Energy	Major Nutrients	Food Additives	Nutritious Rating
Lasagne	449kJ	✓	160b	Average
Sausages	407kJ	↑Salt	✓	Average
Mince	434kJ	✓	✓	Average

Rang Mahal

Product Name	Energy	Major Nutrients	Food Additives	Nutritious Rating
Biryani Chicken	732kJ	↑Fat	✓	Average
Lamb rogan josh & cumin rice	607kJ	✓	✓	Average

Ready Go Eat

Product Name	Energy	Major Nutrients	Food Additives	Nutritious Rating
Egg & bacon muffin	810kJ	✓	250, YE, 120, 282	Poor
Roast chicken rolls	486kJ	↑Fat ↑Salt	202, 160b, 282	Poor
Double cheeseburger	1040kJ	↑Fat ↑Salt	202, HVP, 282	Poor
Italian meatball	1130kJ	↑Fat	282, YE, 635,	Poor
Chicken fillet burger	983kJ	↑Fat ↑Salt	102, 110, HVP, 282, 220, 621,	Poor

			635, 631, 627, 202, 160b, YE	

Red Pepper

Product Name	Energy	Major Nutrients	Food Additives	Nutritious Rating
Chicken green curry & rice	450kJ	✓	✓	Good
Chicken red curry & rice	450kJ	✓	✓	Good
Prawn panaeng & rice	470kJ	✓	✓	Good
Chicken laksa & noodles	517kJ	✓	✓	Good

Royal Orchard

Product Name	Energy	Major Nutrients	Food Additives	Nutritious Rating
Mango chicken curry & rice	584kJ	✓	✓	Good
Green curry with vegetables & rice	552kJ	✓	✓	Good

Savoia

Product Name	Energy	Major Nutrients	Food Additives	Nutritious Rating
Potato gnocchi	852kJ	✓	222	Average
Beef tortellini	1020kJ	✓	282	Average
Beef ravioli	1070kJ	✓	282	Average
Ricotta & spinach ravioli	1140kJ	✓	282, 222	Average
Chicken & leek agnolotti	1040kJ	✓	282, 320, 635, 621, 631	Average
Spaghetti & meatballs	**559kJ**	✓	✓	**Average**
Spinach & four cheese tortellini	710kJ	✓	282	Average
Chicken lasagne	469kJ	✓	320	Average

The Biggest Loser

Product Name	Energy	Major Nutrients	Food Additives	Nutritious Rating
Lamb korma	370kJ	✓	✓	Average
Flame grilled meatballs	345kJ	✓	YE, 120	Average
Sweet & sour chicken	365kJ	✓	160b, 120	Average
Satay beef sausages	400kJ	✓	YE	Average
Beef ragu	350kJ	✓	YE	Average

The Good Meal

Product Name	Energy	Major Nutrients	Food Additives	Nutritious Rating
Cottage pie	321kJ	✓	635, 250	Average
Butter chicken	558kJ	✓	120	Average
Chicken satay & rice	607kJ	✓	✓	Average
Beef stroganoff & rice	531kJ	✓	635	Average

Tukka Tubz

Product Name	Energy	Major Nutrients	Food Additives	Nutritious Rating
Kicken chicken	4131kJ	✓	✓	Average
BBQ fried rice	542kJ	✓	✓	Average
Italian chicken & pasta	415kJ	✓	✓	Average

Wang Wang

Product Name	Energy	Major Nutrients	Food Additives	Nutritious Rating
Prawn in szechaun chilli & rice	519kJ	✓	✓	Average
Fried rice & prawns	561kJ	✓	✓	Average

Weight Watchers

Product Name	Energy	Major Nutrients	Food Additives	Nutritious Rating
Beef lasagne	400kJ	✓	627, 631	Average
Beef cannelloni	400kJ	✓	627, 631	Average

Product Name	Energy	Major Nutrients	Food Additives	Nutritious Rating
Chicken & mushroom fettuccine	415kJ	✓	YE	Average
Creamy mushroom agnolotti	420kJ	✓	YE	Average
Thai chicken curry	**440kJ**	✓	✓	**Average**
Tomato gnocchi	**425kJ**	✓	✓	**Average**
Chicken risotto	410kJ	✓	620, YE	Average
Tuna bake	405kJ	✓	YE	Average
Beef & tomato Bolognese	420kJ	✓	YE	Average
Mushroom & spinach penne	435kJ	✓	YE, 220	Good
Chicken parmagana	**380kJ**	✓	✓	**Average**
Spaghetti meatballs	360kJ	✓	YE	Average
Peppered beef	270kJ	✓	YE	Average
Mushroom & pumpkin risotto	430kJ	✓	YE, HVP, 620	Good
Tuna mornay	440kJ	✓	YE	Average
Sweet potato & pumpkin risotto	365kJ	✓	627, 631	Good
Chicken fettuccine	**425kJ**	✓	✓	**Average**
Pesto spaghetti	455kJ	✓	223, YE	Average
Satay chicken	**465kJ**	✓	✓	**Average**
Honey soy chicken	420kJ	✓	YE	Average

Woolworths/Safeways

Product Name	Energy	Major Nutrients	Food Additives	Nutritious Rating
Homebrand, beef lasagne	**580kJ**	✓	✓	Average

Oven Bake Chips

Best choices are *Birds eye golden crunch, McCains and Woolworths select.*

Birds Eye

Product Name	Energy	Major Nutrients	Food Additives	Nutritious Rating
Golden crunch, original	526kJ	✓	✓	Poor
Golden crunch, beer batter	450kJ	✓	✓	Poor
Golden crunch, crinkles	643kJ	✓	✓	Poor
Golden crunch, steakhouse	475kJ	✓	✓	Poor
Golden crunch, monster chips beer batter	437kJ	✓	✓	Poor
Golden crunch, wedges	564kJ	✓	✓	Poor
Golden crunch, wedges in beer batter	474kJ	✓	✓	Poor
Crunchy potato bites	791kJ	↑Fat ↑Salt	320, VE, 220, 223	Poor
Golden crunch, curly fries	845kJ	✓	YE	Poor
Golden crunch, super crunch chips	572kJ	✓	✓	Poor
Golden crunch, super crunch	560kJ	✓	✓	Poor
Golden crunch, hashbrowns	733kJ	↑Fat	223, 320	Poor
Golden crunch, potato gems	639kJ	✓	✓	Poor
Hashbrowns	733kJ	✓	✓	Poor
Potato swirls	676kJ	✓	✓	Poor
Oven bake chips, steakhouse	491kJ	✓	160b	Poor
Oven bake chips, straight	491kJ	✓	160b	Poor
Oven bake chips chunky steakhouse	491kJ	✓	160b	Poor

Oven bake chips, crinkle cut	519kJ	✓	160b	Poor
Oven bake chips, , homestyle	491kJ	✓	160b	Poor
Oven bake chips French fries	522kJ	✓	160b	Poor
Oven bake chips, seasoned straight cut	**638kJ**	✓	✓	**Poor**
Oven bake chips, light n tasty, lightly seasoned wedges	**744kJ**	✓	✓	**Poor**
Oven roast, country style	565kJ	✓	YE	Poor
Oven roast, rosemary & garlic	**597kJ**	✓	✓	**Poor**
Oven roast, potato, carrot & pumpkin	**321kJ**	✓	✓	**Average**
Pommies	744kJ	✓	319	Poor

Coles

Product Name	Energy	Major Nutrients	Food Additives	Nutritious Rating
Oven fries, crinkle cut	519kJ	✓	160b	Poor
Hash browns	737kJ	↑Fat	223, 320	Poor
French fries	522kJ	✓	160b	Poor
Steakhouse	491kJ	✓	160b	Poor
Straighthouse	491kJ	✓	160b,	Poor
Potato mash	**427kJ**	✓	✓	**Poor**
Potato royals	**613kJ**	✓	✓	**Poor**
Potato wedges	**730kJ**	✓	✓	**Poor**
Smart buy straight chips	**574kJ**	✓	✓	**Poor**

IGA/Franklins

Product Name	Energy	Major Nutrients	Food Additives	Nutritious Rating
Signature, steakhouse chips	**569kJ**	✓	✓	**Poor**
Signature, straight cut	**737kJ**	✓	✓	**Poor**

chips				
Signature, potato jewels	522kJ	✓	220	Poor
Black & Gold, hash browns	491kJ	↑Fat	✓	Poor
Black & Gold, French fries	491kJ	✓	320	Poor

McCain

Product Name	Energy	Major Nutrients	Food Additives	Nutritious Rating
Healthy choice, chunky cut	517kJ	✓	✓	Poor
Healthy choice, straight cut	519kJ	✓	✓	Poor
Potato cake scallops	807kJ	✓	✓	Poor
Fries beer battered thin n crispy	738kJ	✓	✓	Poor
Fries, crunchy original	627kJ	✓	✓	Poor
Fries, beer battered steakhouse	636kJ	✓	✓	Poor
Fries, crunchy beer battered thick n chunky	620kJ	✓	✓	Poor
Smiles	740kJ	↑Fat	✓	Poor
Cross trax	826kJ	↑Fat ↑Salt	160b	Poor
Curly fries	782kJ	↑Fat	160b	Poor
Seasoned mini hash browns	933kJ	↑Fat ↑Salt	✓	Poor
Super fries, shoestring	717kJ	✓	✓	Poor
Super fries, crinkle cut	642kJ	✓	✓	Poor
Super fries, mum's cut	500kJ	✓	✓	Poor
Super fries, straight cut	648kJ	✓	✓	Poor
Super fries, chunky cut	565kJ	✓	✓	Poor
Sweet potato crinkle cut	729kJ	✓	160b	Poor
Sweet potato straight cut	682kJ	✓	✓	Poor

Sweet potato thin cut	780kJ	✓	160b	Poor
Potato wedges, crunchy	627kJ	✓	✓	Poor
Potato wedges, original	627kJ	✓	✓	Poor
Potato wedges, hot bandito	627kJ	✓	✓	Poor
Potato wedges, beer battered	653kJ	✓	✓	Poor
Potato nuggets	735kJ	✓	✓	Poor
Mini roasts, Italian herb	592kJ	✓	✓	Poor
Mini roasts, sea salt & garlic	592kJ	✓	✓	Poor
Purely potato	361kJ	✓	✓	Poor

Woolworths/Safeways

Product Name	Energy	Major Nutrients	Food Additives	Nutritious Rating
Mashed potato, traditional	581kJ	✓	✓	Poor
Mashed potato, cracked pepper	581kJ	✓	✓	Poor
Select, straight cut	569kJ	✓	✓	Poor
Select, crinkle cut	569kJ	✓	✓	Poor
Select, chunky steakhouse	548kJ	✓	✓	Poor
Select, potato wedges	4565kJ	✓	✓	Poor

Patties & Fritters

The best choices are *Syndian gluten free and Nabil.*

Aunty Betty's

Product Name	Energy	Major Nutrients	Food Additives	Nutritious Rating
Yorkshire puddings	1221kJ	↑Fat ↑Salt	✓	Poor

Birdseye

Product Name	Energy	Major Nutrients	Food Additives	Nutritious Rating
Bubble n squeak	867kJ	↑Fat	160b	Average
Chicken & vegetable patties	810kJ	✓	✓	Average
Corn fritters	880kJ	↑Fat	✓	Average
Vegetable fingers	813kJ	↑Fat	HVP	Average

Colonial Farm

Product Name	Energy	Major Nutrients	Food Additives	Nutritious Rating
Meat balls	865kJ	↑Fat ↑Salt	320, 223	Poor

IGA/Franklins

Product Name	Energy	Major Nutrients	Food Additives	Nutritious Rating
Black & Gold beef burgers	1510kJ	↑Fat ↑Salt	621, 251	Poor

I&J

Product Name	Energy	Major Nutrients	Food Additives	Nutritious Rating
Big beef patties	1122kJ	↑Fat	HVP	Poor
Microwave beef n bacon burger	1070kJ	↑Fat ↑Salt	250, 202, VPE	Poor
Cheeseburger	1100kJ	↑Fat	HVP, 202	Poor

		↑Salt		
Bacon & cheese burger	1070kJ	↑Fat ↑Salt	250, 202, VPE	Poor
Lean beefers	618kJ	✓	407	Poor

Macro

Product Name	Energy	Major Nutrients	Food Additives	Nutritious Rating
Meat balls	940kJ	↑Fat	HVP	Poor

Nabil

Product Name	Energy	Major Nutrients	Food Additives	Nutritious Rating
Falafel burger	1016kJ	↑Fat	✓	Good
Falafel with hummos	963kJ	↑Fat	✓	Good
Falafel	963kJ	↑Fat	✓	Good
Kubbe	724kJ	✓	✓	Good
Vegetarian potato balls	1469kJ	✓	✓	Good

Pacific Valley

Product Name	Energy	Major Nutrients	Food Additives	Nutritious Rating
Tatter patties	762kJ	↑Fat	✓	Poor

Sanitarium

Product Name	Energy	Major Nutrients	Food Additives	Nutritious Rating
Veggie delight snitzel	790kJ	↑Salt	635, HVP	Good
Veggie delight not burgers	790kJ	✓	YE	Good
Lentil patties	740kJ	✓	407, YE	Good

Syndian Gluten Free & Vegan

Product Name	Energy	Major Nutrients	Food Additives	Nutritious Rating
Asian bean & kumara	605kJ	↑Fat	✓	Good

Curry pumpkin bite	670kJ	↑Fat ↑Salt	✓	Good
Felafels	740kJ	↑Fat ↑Salt	✓	Good
Lentil burgers	805kJ	↑Fat ↑Salt	✓	Good
Veggie bites	957kJ	↑Fat	✓	Good

Tasty Joes

Product Name	Energy	Major Nutrients	Food Additives	Nutritious Rating
Burgers of beef	931kJ	↑Fat	HVP	Poor

Chicken

Mostly frozen chicken is a high salt, high fat, food additive storm. There are a few additive free varieties: *Steggles fairy snacks, Steggles tenders hot & spicy, Steggles mini roast spinach & cheese, IGA signature chicken Kiev and Ingham crumbed breast fillets.*

Barons Table

Product Name	Energy	Major Nutrients	Food Additives	Nutritious Rating
Chicken kiev	1012kJ	↑Fat	282, 200	Average

Bayview

Product Name	Energy	Major Nutrients	Food Additives	Nutritious Rating
Gluten free chicken nuggets	906kJ	↑Fat	319, 1520	Average
Gluten free chicken tenders	859kJ	✓	1520	Average

Chickadee

Product Name	Energy	Major Nutrients	Food Additives	Nutritious Rating
Chicken, sliced	563kJ	↑Fat ↑Salt	407	Average
Roast chicken sticks	864kJ	↑Fat ↑Salt	320	Average
Devil wing dings	1002kJ	↑Fat ↑Salt	124, HVP	Average
Tenders, sweet chilli		↑Fat ↑Salt	102, 124, 320,	Average

Coles

Product Name	Energy	Major Nutrients	Food Additives	Nutritious Rating
Chicken breast nuggets	998kJ	↑Fat	HVP, YE	Average
Chicken breast tenders	895kJ	↑Fat	YE	Average
Chicken kiev	1093kJ	↑Fat	200, 160b	Average
Chicken kiev, mini	1230kJ	↑Fat	HVP, 223, 320	Average
Smart buy chicken nuggets	1190kJ	↑Fat ↑Salt	HVP, 627, 631, 160b, YE	Poor

IGA/Franklins

Product Name	Energy	Major Nutrients	Food Additives	Nutritious Rating
Signature, chicken kiev	1460kJ	↑Fat	✓	Average
Signature, chicken poppers	794kJ	↑Fat	627, 631	Poor
Signature, sweet chilli chicken strips	950kJ	↑Fat ↑Salt	220, 282	Average
Signature, chicken snitzels	920kJ	↑Fat	635	Poor
Black & Gold, chicken nuggets	1000kJ	↑Fat ↑Salt	HVP	Poor

Ingham

Product Name	Energy	Major Nutrients	Food Additives	Nutritious Rating
Chicken breast chippies	1062kJ	↑Fat ↑Salt	HVP, 220, 319	Average
Chicken breast fillets, crumbed	732kJ	↑Fat ↑Salt	✓	Average
Chicken breast kiev	1093kJ	↑Fat	282, 200, 160b	Average
Chicken breast munchies	1088kJ	↑Fat ↑Salt	635 319, 223	Average
Chicken breast nuggets	1015kJ	↑Fat ↑Salt	223	Average
Chicken breast steaks	889kJ	↑Fat	282	Average
Chicken breast medallions, teriyaki	899kJ	↑Fat ↑Salt	200, HVP	Average

Chicken breast tenders	825kJ	↑Fat ↑Salt	282, 319	Average
Chicken breast tenders, sweet chilli	847kJ	↑Fat ↑Salt	102, 282, 160b	Average
Chicken breast tempura	688kJ	✓	YE, HVO	Average
Duets, broccoli & cheese	830kJ	↑Fat ↑Salt	282, 200	Average
Duets, creamy mushroom	890kJ	↑Fat ↑Salt	200, 319	Average
Duets, spinach & ricotta	927kJ	↑Fat ↑Salt	200, HVP	Average
Duets, garlic butter	1000kJ	↑Fat	200, 160b	Poor
Chicken, strips	845kJ	↑Fat ↑Salt	319	Poor
Chicken stackers, Italian herb	1090kJ	↑Fat ↑Salt	250, 160b	Poor
Chicken Stackers, ham & cheese	1003kJ	↑Fat ↑Salt	250	Poor
Asteroids, tempura	880kJ	↑Fat ↑Salt	YE, 319	Poor
Asteroids, cheese & bacon	975kJ	↑Fat ↑Salt	YE, 211, 250, 220, 223, 200, 160b	Poor
Asteroids, buffalo	840kJ	↑Fat ↑Salt	YE, 319	Poor
Family nuggets	1087kJ	↑Fat ↑Salt	319	Poor
Tempura nuggets	728kJ	↑Salt	YE	Poor
Chicken snitzel	1029kJ	↑Fat ↑Salt	282, 319	Poor
Chicken selections, sweet chilli	753kJ	↑Fat ↑Salt	HVP	Average
Thigh, traditional roast turkey	619kJ	↑Fat ↑Salt	HVP	Average
Breast, traditional roast turkey	454kJ	↑Salt	319	Average

Specialised Chicken

Product Name	Energy	Major Nutrients	Food Additives	Nutritious Rating
Garlic balls	1203kJ	↑Fat ↑Salt	621, 282, 160b, 102, 122	Average
Chicken breast nuggets	1207kJ	↑Fat ↑Salt	160b, HVP, 635	Average
Chicken chippies	1253kJ	↑Fat ↑Salt	160b, HVP, 635	Average
Chicken breast kiev	885kJ	↑Fat	631, 627, 621, 282, 320, 160b	Average

Steggles

Product Name	Energy	Major Nutrients	Food Additives	Nutritious Rating
Breast fingers, salt n pepper	894kJ	↑Fat ↑Salt	627, 631, YE, HVP	Average
Breast fingers, original	874kJ	✓	HVP	Average
Breast fingers, salt n vinegar	981kJ	↑Fat ↑Salt	HVP	Average
Breast fingers, salt n pepper	894kJ	↑Fat ↑Salt	YE, 627, 631, HVP	Average
Breast chunks, southern style	689kJ	↑Salt	YE, HVP, 631, 627	Average
Breast steaks	601kJ	✓	HVP, YE	Average
Fairy snacks	**735kJ**	**✓**	**✓**	**Average**
Dino snacks, tempura	752kJ	↑Fat	✓	Average
Fillets, roast garlic	609kJ	↑Salt	YE,	Average
Fillets, crumbed	969kJ	↑Fat	160b, 635	Average
Fillets, southern style	715kJ	↑Fat ↑Salt	HVP, YE	Average
Strips, crunchy southern style	850kJ	↑Fat ↑Salt	HVP, 631, 635, 627, YE	Poor
Crackles, tempura	742kJ	↑Fat ↑Salt	631, 627, HVP, VP, YE	Poor
Crackles, cheese	1001kJ	↑Fat	YE, 627,	Poor

		↑Salt	631, 200	
Crackles, garlic	875kJ	↑Fat ↑Salt	YE, 627, 631	Poor
Tenders, hot n spicy	**639kJ**	**↑Salt**	✓	**Average**
Tenders, crumbed breast	847kJ	↑Fat	160b, HVP, YE, 631, 627	Average
Tenders, sweet chilli	974kJ	↑Fat ↑Salt	102, 110, HVP	Average
Tenders, little	993kJ	↑Fat	YE, HVP, 631, 627	Average
Southern style burger	657kJ	↑Salt	HVP, VP	Poor
Skinless diced chicken	506kJ	↑Salt	407, YE, HVP	Poor
Chicken wings	1120kJ	↑Fat ↑Salt	HVP, 631, 635	Average
Mini roasts, spinach & cheese	**885kJ**	**↑Fat**	✓	**Average**
Mini roasts, sundried tomato	886kJ	↑Fat	220	Average
Skewers, honey soy	626kJ	✓	YE	Average
Skewers, satay	623kJ	✓	282	Average

Woolworths/Safeways

Product Name	Energy	Major Nutrients	Food Additives	Nutritious Rating
Homebrand chicken nuggets	1130kJ	↑Fat	HVP, YE, 160b	Poor

Fish

Most of the frozen fish range in high in fat and salt. There are select varieties that are additive free in *the Birdseye, I&J and Supermarket brands*. The best overall brand is *Ocean House*.

Bayview

Product Name	Energy	Major Nutrients	Food Additives	Nutritious Rating
Gluten free fish bites	798kJ	✓	319, 1520	Average
Gluten free flounder wild caught crumbed	843kJ	↑ Fat	319, 1520	Average
Whiting fillets	896kJ	↑ Fat	319, 1520, 160b	Average
Crumbed flathead	1000kJ	↑ Fat	319, 160b, 1520, HVP	Average

Birdseye

Product Name	Energy	Major Nutrients	Food Additives	Nutritious Rating
Oven bake, herb & garlic	955kJ	↑Fat	✓	Average
Oven bake, lemon	933kJ	↑Fat	✓	Average
Oven bake, lemon pepper	950kJ	↑Fat	631, 627	Average
Oven bake, lightly battered	952kJ	↑Fat	✓	Average
Oven bake, original	944kJ	↑Fat	✓	Average
Oven bake, salmon cakes	834kJ	↑Fat	✓	Average
Oven bake, fish cakes	972kJ	↑Fat	631, 627, HVP, YE	Average
Oven bake, tuna cakes	809kJ	✓	✓	Average
Natural fish fillets, Atlantic salmon lemon pepper	1070kJ	↑ Fat	✓	Good
Natural fish fillets,	768kJ	↑ Fat	✓	Good

Atlantic salmon provenvale				
Natural fish fillets, Atlantic salmon skinless	**1010kJ**	↑ Fat	✓	**Good**
Natural fish fillets, seasoned barramundi garlic & herb	758kJ	✓	YE	Average
Natural fish fillets, seasoned barramundi cracked pepper & lemon	753kJ	✓	YE	Average
Fish fillets, lemon & parsley	338kJ	✓	HVP	Average
Fish fillets, roasted garlic & spring onion	338kJ	✓	HVP, 160b	Average
Fish fillets, Thai coconut curry	339kJ	✓	HVP	Average
Crumbed fish, barramundi	934kJ	↑ Fat	VPE	Average
Crumbed fish, deep sea dory	884kJ	↑ Fat	VPE	Average
Crumbed fish, deep sea dory lemon	**956kJ**	↑ Fat	✓	Average
Crumbed fish, hoki	**924kJ**	↑ Fat	✓	Average
Crumbed fish, tropical snapper	**899kJ**	↑ Fat	✓	Average
Crumbed fish, southern blue whiting	**916kJ**	↑ Fat	✓	Average
Crumbed fish, spinach & feta	**673kJ**	↑ Fat	✓	Average
Crumbed fish, lightly seasoned garlic & parsley	661kJ	✓	160b, YE	Average
Crumbed fish, lemon pepper	659kJ	✓	160b	Average
Fish fillet fingers	**855kJ**	↑ Fat	✓	*Average*
Fish fingers	**869kJ**	↑ Fat	✓	*Average*

IGA/Franklins

Product Name	Energy	Major Nutrients	Food Additives	Nutritious Rating
Signature range, crumbed fish	911kJ	↑ Fat	319	Average
Signature range, crumbed fish with lemon	911kJ	↑ Fat	319	Average
Black & Gold fish fingers	787kJ	↑ Fat	160b	Average
Black & Gold fish portions	825kJ	↑ Fat	319	Average
Black & Gold fish potions. lemon	822kJ	↑ Fat	319	Average

Coles

Product Name	Energy	Major Nutrients	Food Additives	Nutritious Rating
Fish fillet, battered	883kJ	↑ Fat	✓	Average
Fish fillet, crumbed	882kJ	↑ Fat	160b, 319	Average
Gyoza prawns	930kJ	↑ Fat	VEP	Average
Fish fingers	846kJ	↑ Fat	160b	Average
Crumbed fish, herb & garlic	905kJ	↑ Fat	319	Average

I&J

Product Name	Energy	Major Nutrients	Food Additives	Nutritious Rating
Fish fillets, beer battered	787kJ	↑ Fat	✓	Average
Fish kievs	734kJ	✓	✓	Average
Fish flame grills, lemon pepper	370kJ	✓	YE	Average
Crispy fillets, lemon	890kJ	↑ Fat	✓	Average
Crispy fillets, original	884kJ	↑ Fat	✓	Average
Crispy fillets, tempura	842kJ	↑ Fat	✓	Average
Light n crispy lightly seasoned fillets	892kJ	↑ Fat	YE	Average
Seafood basket	1230kJ	↑ Fat	✓	Average
Fish fingers	870kJ	↑ Fat	HVP, 160b	Average

Salt n pepper calamari	996kJ	↑ Fat ↑ Salt	✓	Average

Pacific West

Product Name	Energy	Major Nutrients	Food Additives	Nutritious Rating
Fish fillets, beer battered	798kJ	↑ Fat ↑ Salt	621	Average
Tempura fillets	793kJ	↑ Fat ↑ Salt	621	Average
Salt n pepper squid	1005kJ	↑ Fat	621	Average
Squid chips	928kJ	↑ Fat ↑ Salt	621	Average
Lemon pepper squid	653kJ	✓	102, 621	Average
Barramundi, crumbed	**921kJ**	✓	✓	**Average**
Blue eyed cod, beer battered	672kJ	✓	621	Average
Flathead fillets	963kJ	↑ Fat	621	Average
Prawns, beer battered	1043kJ	↑ Fat	621	Average
Popcorn shrimp, jalapeno	1071kJ	↑ Fat	621	Average
Popcorn shrimp, traditional	1079kJ	↑ Fat	621	Average
Fish cocktails, beer battered	798kJ	↑ Fat ↑ Salt	621	Average

Ocean House

Product Name	Energy	Major Nutrients	Food Additives	Nutritious Rating
Thai fish cakes	1511kJ	✓	HVP	Average
Honey prawns	**1370kJ**	↑ Fat ↑ Sugar	✓	**Average**
Tempura prawn	**2550kJ**	↑ Fat ↑ Sugar	✓	**Average**
Prawn wraps	**2435kJ**	↑ Fat ↑ Sugar	✓	**Average**

Sealord

Product Name	Energy	Major Nutrients	Food Additives	Nutritious Rating
Fish tapas	874kJ	✓	✓	Average
Hoki tempura	891kJ	↑ Fat	YE, HVP	Average

Woolworths/Safeways

Product Name	Energy	Major Nutrients	Food Additives	Nutritious Rating
Homebrand Fish fingers	874kJ	↑ Fat	160b	Average
Homebrand crumbed fish	891kJ	↑ Fat	✓	Average
Homebrand crumbed fish, lemon	935kJ	↑ Fat	✓	Average

Vegetables

The frozen vegetables are generally the same; I would choose what is on special.

It might shock you to know that in many instances, frozen can have a higher nutrient density than fresh. Frozen vegetables are snap-frozen soon after harvest, whereas fresh vegetables can sit in cold storage or on the supermarket shelf continuing to respire, with the nutrient composition slowly deteriorating. Of course I'm a big advocate of growing your own vegetables and eating everything fresh!

Birds Eye

Product Name	Energy	Major Nutrients	Food Additives	Nutritious Rating
Create a meal, black bean	177kJ	✓	✓	Good
Create a meal, honey soy	244kJ	✓	✓	Good
Create a meal, teriyaki	221kJ	✓	YE	Good
Create a meal, korma	255kJ	✓	YE	Good
Country Harvest, baby beans, carrot & corn	135kJ	✓	✓	Good
Country Harvest, broccoli & cauliflower	108kJ	✓	✓	Good
Country Harvest, carrot, cauliflower & broccoli	122kJ	✓	✓	Good
Country Harvest, carrot, cauliflower, broccoli & sugar snap peas	133kJ	✓	✓	Good
Country Harvest, carrot, peas & corn	267kJ	✓	✓	Good
Country Harvest, mixed vegetables	195kJ	✓	✓	Good

Country Harvest, garden mix	119kJ	✓	✓	Good
Country Harvest, peas, corn & capsicum	346kJ	✓	✓	Good
Country Harvest, vegetables in cheese sauce	514kJ	✓	✓	Good
Country Harvest, spring greens	174kJ	✓	✓	Good
Country Harvest, peas & sweetcorn	366kJ	✓	✓	Good
Oven Roast potatoes. Rosemary & garlic	597kJ	✓	✓	Good
Singles, baby beans	111kJ	✓	✓	Good
Singles, baby peas	243kJ	✓	✓	Good
Singles, broccoli	118kJ	✓	✓	Good
Singles, brussels sprouts	kJ	✓	✓	Good
Singles, carrot rings	134kJ	✓	✓	Good
Singles, cauliflower	kJ	✓	✓	Good
Singles, chopped onion	129kJ	✓	✓	Good
Singles, chopped spinach	90kJ	✓	✓	Good
Singles, sliced bean	476kJ	✓	✓	Good
Singles, corn cobs	117kJ	✓	✓	Good
Steamfresh, broccoli, carrot & corn	202kJ	✓	✓	Good
Steamfresh, broccoli, cauliflower & carrot	116kJ	✓	✓	Good
Steamfresh, broccoli, corn, peas & greenbeans	242kJ	✓	✓	Good
Steamfresh, carrots, peas & corn	266kJ	✓	✓	Good
Stir fry vegetables, Chinese	127kJ	✓	✓	Good
Stir fry vegetables, Cantonese	147kJ	✓	✓	Good
Stir fry vegetables,	131kJ	✓	✓	Good

chow mein				
Stir fry vegetables, Japanese	kJ	✓	✓	Good
Stir fry vegetables, Malaysian	222kJ	✓	✓	Good
Stir fry vegetables, Shanghai	206kJ	✓	✓	Good
Flavour Infusion, basil & garlic	229kJ	✓	✓	Good
Flavour Infusion, garlic & ginger	158kJ	✓	✓	Good
Flavour Infusion, lemon grass & ginger	kJ	✓	✓	Good
Flavour Infusion, Thai style	141kJ	✓	✓	Good

Coles

Product Name	Energy	Major Nutrients	Food Additives	Nutritious Rating
Sliced beans	117kJ	✓	✓	Good
Broad beans	223kJ	✓	✓	Good
Broccoli florets	118kJ	✓	✓	Good
Brussels sprouts	kJ	✓	✓	Good
Baby carrots	131kJ	✓	✓	Good
Carrots, cauliflower & broccoli	116kJ	✓	✓	Good
Carrots, peas & corn	268kJ	✓	✓	Good
Cauliflower & broccoli	108kJ	✓	✓	Good
Cauliflower	97kJ	✓	✓	Good
Corn cobs	476kJ	✓	✓	Good
Corn kernels	476kJ	✓	✓	Good
Mixed vegetables	249kJ	✓	✓	Good
Chopped onions	129kJ	✓	✓	Good
Sliced onions	kJ	✓	✓	Good
Peas & corn	353kJ	✓	✓	Good
Peas	257kJ	✓	✓	Good
Minted peas	256kJ	✓	✓	Good
Peas, carrot &	163kJ	✓	✓	Good

		Major Nutrients	Food Additives	Nutritious Rating
cauliflower				
Potato, mashed	427kJ	✓	✓	Good
Smart buy green beans	74kJ	✓	✓	Good
Smart buy, corn kernels	504kJ	✓	✓	Good
Smart buy, peas	257kJ	✓	✓	Good
Smart buy, mixed vegetables	187kJ	✓	✓	Good
Stir fry, Thai style	141kJ	✓	✓	Good
Winter vegetable mix	119kJ	✓	✓	Good

Changs

Product Name	Energy	Major Nutrients	Food Additives	Nutritious Rating
Stir fry vegetables , bok choy	97kJ	✓	✓	Good
Stir fry vegetables, snow peas	103kJ	✓	✓	Good

Heinz

Product Name	Energy	Major Nutrients	Food Additives	Nutritious Rating
Steam fresh beans, carrots & broccoli	125kJ	✓	✓	Good
Steam fresh broccoli, carrots & cauliflower	120kJ	✓	✓	Good
Steam fresh broccoli, peas & carrot	140kJ	✓	✓	Good
Steam fresh broccoli, carrot & corn	215kJ	✓	✓	Good
Stir fry, Shanghai	120kJ	✓	✓	Good
Golden mix	290kJ	✓	✓	Good
Romano mix	135kJ	✓	✓	Good
Chunky mix	115kJ	✓	✓	Good
Classic mix	235kJ	✓	✓	Good
Cauliflower & broccoli	110kJ	✓	✓	Good
Peas & super sweet corn	340kJ	✓	✓	Good
Peas, corn & capsicum	370kJ	✓	✓	Good

		Major Nutrients	Food Additives	Nutritious Rating
Green beans	105kJ	✓	✓	Good
Baby beans	105kJ			Good
Baby peas	290kJ	✓	✓	Good
Super sweet corn	370kJ	✓	✓	Good
Minted peas	340kJ	✓	✓	Good
Chopped spinach	140kJ	✓	✓	Good

Home Country Organics

Product Name	Energy	Major Nutrients	Food Additives	Nutritious Rating
Green beans	100kJ	✓	✓	Good
Stir fry mix	177kJ	✓	✓	Good
Corn kernels	460kJ	✓	✓	Good
Peas, corn, carrots	256kJ	✓	✓	Good
Peas	255kJ	✓	✓	Good
Whole leaf spinach	150kJ	✓	✓	Good

IGA/Franklins

Product Name	Energy	Major Nutrients	Food Additives	Nutritious Rating
Black & Gold green beans	118kJ	✓	✓	Good
Black & Gold chow mein stir fry veggies	168kJ	✓	✓	Good
Black & Gold corn kernels	325kJ	✓	✓	Good
Black & Gold mixed vegetables	256kJ	✓	✓	Good
Black & Gold peas	257kJ	✓	✓	Good
Black & Gold cauliflower florets	94kJ	✓	✓	Good
Black & Gold broccoli florets	134kJ	✓	✓	Good

Logan Farm

Product Name	Energy	Major Nutrients	Food Additives	Nutritious Rating
Chopped spinach	102kJ	✓	✓	Good
Garden peas	273kJ	✓	✓	Good

Extra juicy corn	350kJ	✓	✓	Good

Macro Organic

Product Name	Energy	Major Nutrients	Food Additives	Nutritious Rating
Peas	340kJ	✓	✓	Good
Broad beans	298kJ	✓	✓	Good

Midwest

Product Name	Energy	Major Nutrients	Food Additives	Nutritious Rating
Peas	340kJ	✓	✓	Good
Sweet corn	128kJ	✓	✓	Good
Green beans	106kJ	✓	✓	Good

McCain

Product Name	Energy	Major Nutrients	Food Additives	Nutritious Rating
Green beans	151kJ	✓	✓	Good
Peas & super sweet corn	478kJ	✓	✓	Good
Baby peas	300kJ	✓	✓	Good
Peas, corn, carrots	334kJ	✓	✓	Good
Peas	373kJ	✓	✓	Good
Purely potato cubes	kJ	✓	✓	Good
Peas & corn	380kJ	✓	✓	Good
Baby beans premium	151kJ	✓	✓	Good
Winter mix	128kJ	✓	✓	Good
Stir fry supreme	136kJ	✓	✓	Good
Defence mix	225kJ	✓	✓	Good
Vision mix	307kJ	✓	✓	Good
Mixed vegetables	187kJ	✓	✓	Good
Carrots, cauliflower, broccoli & sugar snap peas	126kJ	✓	✓	Good
Garden peas	277kJ	✓	✓	Good
Super juicy corn	390kJ	✓	✓	Good
Corn cobettes	372kJ	✓	✓	Good

Super juicy corn cobettes	397kJ	✓	✓	Good

Woolworths/Safeways

Product Name	Energy	Major Nutrients	Food Additives	Nutritious Rating
Select baby peas	100kJ	✓	✓	Good
Select broccoli florets	177kJ	✓	✓	Good
Select julienne carrots	460kJ	✓	✓	Good
Select diced onion	256kJ	✓	✓	Good
Select cauliflower florets	255kJ	✓	✓	Good
Select sliced onion	150kJ	✓	✓	Good
Select cauliflower & broccoli	117kJ	✓	✓	Good
Select Brussels sprouts	197kJ	✓	✓	Good
Select chopped spinach	160kJ	✓	✓	Good
Homebrand peas	340kJ	✓	✓	Good
Homebrand corn kernels	326kJ	✓	✓	Good
Homebrand corn cobs	410kJ	✓	✓	Good
Homebrand green beans	118kJ	✓	✓	Good
Homebrand mixed vegetables	181kJ	✓	✓	Good

Fruit

Berry Fruits

Product Name	Energy	Major Nutrients	Food Additives	Nutritious Rating
Blackberries	320kJ	✓	✓	Excellent
Strawberries	189kJ	✓	✓	Excellent
Boysenberries	235kJ	✓	✓	Excellent

Coles

Product Name	Energy	Major Nutrients	Food Additives	Nutritious Rating
Mixed berries	180kJ	✓	✓	Excellent
Raspberries	220kJ	✓	✓	Excellent
Blueberries	215kJ	✓	✓	Excellent

Creative

Product Name	Energy	Major Nutrients	Food Additives	Nutritious Rating
Fruit blueberries	220kJ	✓	✓	Excellent
Mixed berries	200kJ	✓	✓	Excellent
Raspberries	230kJ	✓	✓	Excellent
Strawberries	90kJ	✓	✓	Excellent
Forrest berries	190kJ	✓	✓	Excellent
Blackberries	210kJ	✓	✓	Excellent
Pitted cherries	250kJ	✓	✓	Excellent
High antioxidant mix	165kJ	✓	✓	Excellent
Smoothie cubes, breakfast	637kJ	↑ Sugar	✓	Excellent
Smoothie cubes, tropical	367kJ	↑ Sugar	✓	Excellent
Smoothie cubes, strawberry	380kJ	↑ Sugar	✓	Excellent
Smoothie cubes, berry	554kJ	↑ Sugar	✓	Excellent

Garden Supreme

Product Name	Energy	Major Nutrients	Food Additives	Nutritious Rating
Boysenberries	196kJ	✓	✓	Excellent

Harvest Time

Product Name	Energy	Major Nutrients	Food Additives	Nutritious Rating
Strawberries	96kJ	✓	✓	Excellent
Mixed berries	177kJ	✓	✓	Excellent
Raspberries	110kJ	✓	✓	Excellent
Mango cheeks	275kJ	✓	✓	Excellent

IGA/Franklins

Product Name	Energy	Major Nutrients	Food Additives	Nutritious Rating
Signature blueberries	220kJ	✓	✓	Excellent
Signature mixed berries	225kJ	✓	✓	Excellent
Signature raspberries	220kJ	✓	✓	Excellent

McCain

Product Name	Energy	Major Nutrients	Food Additives	Nutritious Rating
Blueberries	184kJ	✓	✓	Excellent
Four berry mix	211kJ	✓	✓	Excellent
Raspberries	202kJ	✓	✓	Excellent
Three berry mix	233kJ	✓	✓	Excellent
Baby strawberry berry mix	210kJ	✓	✓	Excellent

Nannas

Product Name	Energy	Major Nutrients	Food Additives	Nutritious Rating
Raspberries	225kJ	✓	✓	Excellent
Mixed berries	198kJ	✓	✓	Excellent

Organics

Product Name	Energy	Major Nutrients	Food Additives	Nutritious Rating
Goji berries	220kJ	✓	✓	Excellent

Sara Lee

Product Name	Energy	Major Nutrients	Food Additives	Nutritious Rating
Raspberries	192kJ	✓	✓	Excellent
Mixed berries	208kJ	✓	✓	Excellent

Fridge Section

Flavoured Milk and Custard

The best bands for flavoured milk are *Bannister downs and Dare.*

Ambrosia

Product Name	Energy	Major Nutrients	Food Additives	Nutritious Rating
Devon custard pots	429kJ	↑ Sugar	160b	Average
Ready made custard	672kJ	↑ Sugar	160b	Average

Bannister Downs

Product Name	Energy	Major Nutrients	Food Additives	Nutritious Rating
Café au late	210kJ	✓	✓	Average
Chocolate milk	270kJ	✓	✓	Average
Mango smoothie	240kJ	✓	✓	Average

Brownes

Product Name	Energy	Major Nutrients	Food Additives	Nutritious Rating
Custard	498kJ	↑ Sugar	160b, 220	Average
Choc chill milk	281kJ	✓	407	Average
Chocolate mint chill milk	292kJ	↑ Sugar	407	Average
Coffee chill	**250kJ**	✓	✓	**Average**
Coffee Chill lite	183kJ	✓	407, 951	Average
Mocha chill milk	289kJ	✓	407	Average
Perc coffee chill milk	**241kJ**	✓	✓	**Average**
Strawberry chill milk	272kJ	✓	122	Average
Vanilla chill milk	258kJ	✓	407, 202	Average
Supershake, chocolate	336kJ	↑ Sugar	220, 407	Average
Kick, cappuccino	**362kJ**	✓	✓	**Average**
Kick, double esspresso	**397kJ**	↑ Sugar	✓	**Average**
Supershake, chocolate	336kJ	↑ Sugar	220, 407	Average

honeycomb				
Supershake, cookies & cream	390kJ	↑ Sugar	220, 407	Average
Supershake, vanilla malt	337kJ	↑ Sugar	220, 407	Average

Coles

Product Name	Energy	Major Nutrients	Food Additives	Nutritious Rating
Custard, lite	324kJ	✓	407, 160b	Average
Custard, pouring	399kJ	↑ Sugar	407, 160b	Average

Dare

Product Name	Energy	Major Nutrients	Food Additives	Nutritious Rating
Double Expresso	369kJ	✓	✓	Average
Expresso	356kJ	✓	✓	Average

Harvey Fresh

Product Name	Energy	Major Nutrients	Food Additives	Nutritious Rating
Affogato, reduced fat milk	270kJ	✓	✓	Average
Cappuccino iced coffee	240kJ	✓	✓	Average
Chocolate milk	270kJ	✓	407	Average
Country custard	400kJ	↑ Sugar	407	Average

Masters

Product Name	Energy	Major Nutrients	Food Additives	Nutritious Rating
Choc berry chilled milk	285kJ	✓	407	Average
Chocolate milk	263kJ	✓	407	Average
Custard	442kJ	↑ Sugar	102, 110, 407	
Iced coffee milk	255kJ	✓	407	Average
Iced coffee milk, light	230kJ	✓	407	Average
Mocha milk	366kJ	✓	133, 155, 407	Average
Spearmint milk	254kJ	✓	102, 133	Average
Strawberry milk	286kJ	✓	122, 124, 102	Average

Pauls

Product Name	Energy	Major Nutrients	Food Additives	Nutritious Rating
Custard	421kJ	↑ Sugar	407	Average
Custard, double thick	490kJ	↑ Sugar	407	Average
Custard, 99% fat free	324kJ	✓	407	Average
Custard, premium	574kJ	↑ Sugar	407	Average
Good to go smoothie, mango passion	338kJ	↑ Sugar	✓	Average
Good to go smoothie, mixed berry	338kJ	↑ Sugar	✓	Average

Yoghurt and Dairy Snacks

Personally I make my own yoghurt, it is so easy and much cheaper, but if I were to buy it would be *Jalna or Mundella*. In the kids ranges I would choose *Brownes kids or Paul's characters.*

Ambrosia

Product Name	Energy	Major Nutrients	Food Additives	Nutritious Rating
Apple crumble pudding	660kJ	↑ Sugar	160b, 422, 220	Average
Raspberry jelly pudding	377kJ	↑ Sugar	160b, 122, 220	Average
Rice pudding	417kJ	✓	✓	Average
Strawberry jelly pudding	364kJ	↑ Sugar	160b, 122, 220	Average

Brownes

Product Name	Energy	Major Nutrients	Food Additives	Nutritious Rating
Deluxe, mango passion	434kJ	↑ Sugar	160b	Good
Deluxe, peaches & cream	456kJ	↑ Sugar	✓	Good
Deluxe, vanilla	429kJ	↑ Sugar	✓	Good
Deluxe, strawberry	476kJ	↑ Sugar	163	Good
Deluxe, mixed berry	444kJ	↑ Sugar	✓	Good
Deluxe, mango	443kJ	↑ Sugar	✓	Good
Diet, strawberry shortcake	194kJ	✓	950, 951, 957	Good
Diet, tropical cheesecake	198kJ	✓	950, 951, 957	Good
Diet, vanilla crème	196kJ	✓	950, 951, 957	Good
Light, blueberry	330kJ	↑ Sugar	163	Good
Light, mango	307kJ	↑ Sugar	440	Good
Light, mixed berry	337kJ	↑ Sugar	✓	Good
Light, peach, banana,	363kJ	↑ Sugar	440	Good

passion				
Light, peach mango	**339kJ**	**↑ Sugar**	✓	**Good**
Light, strawberry	340kJ	↑ Sugar	440	Good
Light, traditional	210kJ	↑ Sugar	440	Good
Light, vanilla	335kJ	↑ Sugar	440	Good
Traditional, apricot	412kJ	↑ Sugar	407, 440	Good
Traditional, fruit salad	466kJ	↑ Sugar	160b	Good
Traditional, mango	**416kJ**	**↑ Sugar**	✓	**Good**
Traditional, muesli munch	438kJ	↑ Sugar ↑ Fat	202, 440	Good
Traditional, natural	**315kJ**	✓	✓	**Good**
Traditional, passionfruit	439kJ	↑ Sugar	440, 160b	Good
Traditional, strawberry	379kJ	↑ Sugar	163	Good
Kids, banana	**443kJ**	**↑ Sugar**	✓	**Good**
Kids, strawberry	**441kJ**	**↑ Sugar**	✓	**Good**
Kids, vanilla	**396kJ**	**↑ Sugar**	✓	**Good**

Coles

Product Name	Energy	Major Nutrients	Food Additives	Nutritious Rating
Peach, mango & passionfruit yoghurt	475kJ	↑ Sugar	160b	Good
Strawberry yoghurt	470kJ	↑ Sugar	120	Good
Strawberry lite yoghurt	358kJ	↑ Sugar	120	Good
Vanilla yoghurt	**487kJ**	**↑ Sugar**	✓	**Good**

Dairy Farmers

Product Name	Energy	Major Nutrients	Food Additives	Nutritious Rating
Chocolate custard	528kJ	↑ Sugar	✓	Average
Yoghurt, blueberry field	420kJ	↑ Sugar	✓	Good
Yoghurt, citrus cheesecake	464kJ	↑ Sugar	✓	Good
Yoghurt, orchard	413kJ	↑ Sugar	160b	Good

peaches & mango				
Yoghurt, strawberries & cream	448kJ	↑ Sugar	120, 160b	Good
Yoghurt, vanilla cream	**423kJ**	**↑ Sugar**	✓	**Good**
Yoghurt, vanilla light	226kJ	✓	160b	Good
Yoghurt, vine passionfruit	410kJ	↑ Sugar	160b	Good

Fruche

Product Name	Energy	Major Nutrients	Food Additives	Nutritious Rating
Yoghurt, strawberry fields	424kJ	↑ Sugar	120, 202	Good
Yoghurt, tropical mango	427kJ	↑ Sugar	202, 160b	Good
Yoghurt, vanilla bean	427kJ	↑ Sugar	202, 160b	Good
Yoghurt, vanilla berry	416kJ	↑ Sugar	202, 160b, 120	Good

Jalna

Product Name	Energy	Major Nutrients	Food Additives	Nutritious Rating
A2 natural yoghurt	322kJ	✓	✓	Good
Biodynamic natural yoghurt	350kJ	✓	✓	Good
Strawberry yoghurt	528kJ	↑ Sugar	✓	Good
Vanilla low fat yoghurt	441kJ	✓	✓	Good

Mundella

Product Name	Energy	Major Nutrients	Food Additives	Nutritious Rating
Greek yoghurt, honey	552kJ	↑ Sugar	✓	Good
Greek yoghurt, natural	498kJ	✓	✓	Good
Greek yoghurt, vanilla	549kJ	↑ Sugar	✓	Good

Sunkissed fruits yoghurt	412kJ	↑ Sugar	✓	Good
Vanilla yoghurt, reduced fat	403kJ	↑ Sugar	✓	Good
Woodlands fruit yoghurt	497kJ	↑ Sugar	223	Good

Nestle

Product Name	Energy	Major Nutrients	Food Additives	Nutritious Rating
Chocolate desserts	526kJ	↑ Sugar	407	Good
Milo dairy snacks	539kJ	↑ Sugar	407, 202	Good

Pauls

Product Name	Energy	Major Nutrients	Food Additives	Nutritious Rating
Character yoghurt, banana	361kJ	✓	✓	Good
Character yoghurt, peach	339kJ	✓	✓	Good
Character yoghurt, strawberry	361kJ	✓	✓	Good

Ski

Product Name	Energy	Major Nutrients	Food Additives	Nutritious Rating
D'lite yoghurt, berry basket	384kJ	↑ Sugar	✓	Good
D'lite yoghurt, honey buzz	411kJ	↑ Sugar	✓	Good
D'lite yoghurt, island escape	375kJ	↑ Sugar	✓	Good
D'lite yoghurt, peach & mango	374kJ	↑ Sugar	160b	Good
D'lite yoghurt, peach, mango & passionfruit	367kJ	↑ Sugar	160b	Good
D'lite yoghurt,	375kJ	↑ Sugar	120	Good

strawberry & boysenberry				
D'lite yoghurt, summer passion	371kJ	↑ Sugar	160b	Good
D'lite yoghurt, vanilla crème	379kJ	↑ Sugar	✓	Good
D'lite yoghurt, wild blueberry	376kJ	↑ Sugar	✓	Good
D'lite yoghurt, wild strawberry	369kJ	↑ Sugar	120	Good
Divine yoghurt, berry heaven	437kJ	↑ Sugar	✓	Good
Divine yoghurt, mango	437kJ	↑ Sugar	160b	Good
Divine yoghurt, passionfruit	415kJ	↑ Sugar	160b	Good
Divine yoghurt, tropical fruit salad	428kJ	↑ Sugar	✓	Good
Divine yoghurt, wild strawberry	422kJ	↑ Sugar	120	Good

Soylife

Product Name	Energy	Major Nutrients	Food Additives	Nutritious Rating
Apricot & mango yoghurt	331kJ	✓	160b, 202	Good
Lemon crème	375kJ	↑ Sugar	160b	Good

Yoplait

Product Name	Energy	Major Nutrients	Food Additives	Nutritious Rating
Le rice, apple & cinnamon	455kJ	↑ Sugar	160b	Average
Le rice, choc coconut rough	481kJ	↑ Sugar	220	Average
Le rice, raspberry & white chocolate	452kJ	↑ Sugar	120	Average
Le rice, smooth caramel	461kJ	↑ Sugar	160b	Average

Le rice, vanilla	**454kJ**	↑ Sugar	✓	Average
For Me yoghurt, banana & honey	175kJ	✓	160b, 951, 950	Good
For Me yoghurt, field berries	170kJ	✓	160b, 200, 120	Good
For Me yoghurt, French vanilla	164kJ	✓	200, 951, 950, 160b	Good
For Me yoghurt, mango	167kJ	✓	160b, 951, 950	Good
For Me yoghurt, sticky date	162kJ	✓	200, 951, 950, 160b	Good
For Me yoghurt, strawberry	150kJ	✓	200, 951, 950, 160b, 120	Good
Original yoghurt, blueberry	353kJ	↑ Sugar	120, 200	Good
Original yoghurt, berry bliss	353kJ	↑ Sugar	120, 200	Good
Original yoghurt, natural	**306kJ**	✓	✓	**Good**
Original yoghurt, rhubarb custard	369kJ	↑ Sugar	200	Good
Original yoghurt, strawberry	426kJ	↑ Sugar	160b, 120, 200	Good
Original yoghurt, vanilla	372kJ	↑ Sugar	200	Good
Petite Miams, berry	480kJ	↑ Sugar	120	Good
Petite Miams, strawberry	476kJ	↑ Sugar	120	Good
Petite Miams, vanilla	**486kJ**	**↑ Sugar**	✓	**Good**
Gogurts	356kJ	↑ Sugar	120	Good
Smackers, strawberry	357kJ	↑ Sugar	120	Good

Vaalia

Product Name	Energy	Major Nutrients	Food Additives	Nutritious Rating
Yoghurt, apricot, mango & peach	380kJ	↑ Sugar	160b	Good
Yoghurt, French vanilla	425kJ	↑ Sugar	160b	Good
Yoghurt, Greek style	624kJ	✓	✓	**Good**
Yoghurt, lemon crème	449kJ	↑ Sugar	160b	Good
Yoghurt, luscious berries	403kJ	↑ Sugar	120	Good
Yoghurt, strawberry	413kJ	↑ Sugar	120	Good

Dips

Brands that have a few additive free varieties are Black Swan (pea, mint & zest lemon, roasted garlic hommus, sweet corn, bell pepper & coriander, Zucchini, pumpkin & feta), Coles (classic guacamole, classic guacamole spicy) and Chris' (spring onion, tzatziki).

Black Swan

Product Name	Energy	Major Nutrients	Food Additives	Nutritious Rating
Baby spinach & feta	1310kJ	↑ Fat	220	Average
Beetroot & tzatziki	590kJ	↑ Fat	220	Average
Capsicum & feta	1200kJ	↑ Salt ↑ Fat	220	Average
Caramelised French onion	1090kJ	↑ Fat	220	Average
Fresh guacamole	518kJ	↑ Fat	220	Average
Pea, mint & zesty lemon	**613kJ**	✓	✓	**Average**
Roasted garlic hommus	801kJ	↑ Fat	220, 223	Average
Roasted garlic tzatziki	**501kJ**	✓	✓	**Average**
Skinny hommus	826kJ	↑ Fat	220, 223	Average
Skinny roasted capsicum	840kJ	↑ Salt ↑ Fat	220	Average
Smoked salmon	1220kJ	↑ Salt ↑ Fat	223, 160b, 320, 120, 220	Average
Sweet corn, bell pepper & coriander	**603kJ**	↑ Fat	✓	**Average**
Zucchini, pumpkin & feta	**517kJ**	↑ Fat	✓	**Average**

Coles

Product Name	Energy	Major Nutrients	Food Additives	Nutritious Rating
Avocado	996kJ	↑ Fat	223	Average
Beetroot & mint	532kJ	↑ Salt	202, 223	Average
Capsicum, light	256kJ	✓	202, 220	Average
Classic guacamole	**795kJ**	**↑ Fat**	✓	**Average**
Classic guacamole, spicy	**795kJ**	**↑ Fat**	✓	**Average**
French onion	276kJ	↑ Fat	220, 223	Average
Hommus	837kJ	↑ Fat	220, 223	Average
Hommus, light	398kJ	✓	220, 223	Average
Sundried tomato	773kJ	↑ Salt ↑ Fat	220	Average
Tzatziki	356kJ	✓	220, 223	Average
Tzatziki, light	286kJ	✓	220, 223	Average

Copperpot

Product Name	Energy	Major Nutrients	Food Additives	Nutritious Rating
Cheese & chive	935kJ	↑ Fat	320, 202	Average
French onion	941kJ	↑ Fat	320, 202, 220	Average
Greeky tzatziki	627kJ	↑ Fat	320, 202	Average
Heavenly hommus	1130kJ	↑ Fat	320, 202, 211, 223	Average
Razzle dazzle basil	2180kJ	↑ Fat	320, 202, 220	Average
Roasted capsicum	1020kJ	↑ Fat	320, 202, YE	Average
Spinach, feta & cashews	1070kJ	↑ Fat	202, 320, 220	Average
Layered, basil, capsicum & cream cheese	1160kJ	↑ Fat	320, 202, 220	Average
Layered, guacamole	810kJ	↑ Fat	202, 122, 211, 223	Average
Layered, spicy salsa	996kJ	↑ Fat	202, 122, 211, 223	Average
Layered, sundrieds & cream cheese	1210kJ	↑ Fat	320, 202, 220	Average

Chris'

Product Name	Energy	Major Nutrients	Food Additives	Nutritious Rating
Caviar	1341kJ	↑ Fat	124, 223, 220	Average
Cheese & chives	1148kJ	↑ Fat	220, 223	Average
Corn relish	1015kJ	↑ Fat	223, 320	Average
Creamy basil	1344kJ	↑ Fat	202, 211, 320, 220	Average
Hommus	821kJ	↑ Fat	220	Average
Hommus, light & fresh	732kJ	↑ Fat	320	Average
Roasted capsicum	562kJ	↑ Salt ↑ Fat	220, 202, 211	Average
Spicy capsicum	1003kJ	↑ Salt ↑ Fat	110, 220, 124	Average
Spicy yellow pepper	1150kJ	↑ Salt ↑ Fat	223, 211, 202	Average
Spinach, pinenut, pecorino & chilli	1292kJ	↑ Fat	223, 320, 202, 211	Average
Spring onion	1200kJ	↑ Fat	✓	Average
Three olives	1633kJ	↑ Salt ↑ Fat	202, 211, 223, 320	Average
Tzatziki	417kJ	✓	✓	Average
White caviar & almond	1619kJ	↑ Salt ↑ Fat	223, 211, 202	Average

Kraft

Product Name	Energy	Major Nutrients	Food Additives	Nutritious Rating
French onion	933kJ	↑ Salt ↑ Fat	200	Average
French onion, light	869kJ	↑ Salt ↑ Fat	200	Average
Gherkin	884kJ	↑ Salt ↑ Fat	200	Average
Onion & bacon	970kJ	↑ Salt ↑ Fat	200	Average
Prawn & crab	985kJ	↑ Salt ↑ Fat	200, 223	Average
Smoked salmon	1002kJ	↑ Salt	200, 129, 223	Average

		↑ Fat		
Philadelphia, mango chutney	821kJ	↑ Salt ↑ Fat	200	Average
Philadelphia, three olives	847kJ	↑ Fat	200	Average
Philadelphia, tomato chutney	788kJ	↑ Fat	200, 220	Average
Philadelphia, sweet chilli	758kJ	↑ Fat	200	Average

Red Rock

Product Name	Energy	Major Nutrients	Food Additives	Nutritious Rating
Balsamic, beetroot, feta & cashew	1350kJ	↑ Fat	320, 223, 202	Average
Hommus, pinenut & caramelised onion	1440kJ	↑ Fat	320, 223, 202, 211	Average
Moroccan sweet potato, sesame & pistachio	1240kJ kJ	↑ Fat	320, 223, 202	Average
Red capsicum, percorino & cashew	1450kJ	↑ Fat	320, 220, 202	Average
Red capsicum, white bean, rosemary & pistachio	1120kJ	↑ Fat	320, 211, 202	Average
Thai sweet chilli, lemongrass & cashews	1700kJ	↑ Fat ↑ Sugar	320, 223, 202	Average
Yoghurt, cucumber, feta & dill	644kJ	↑ Fat	202, 320	Average

Wattle Farm

Product Name	Energy	Major Nutrients	Food Additives	Nutritious Rating
Chunky, basil	2130kJ	↑ Fat	220	Average
Chunky, beetroot	1850kJ	↑ Salt ↑ Fat	211, 223, 220	Average
Chunky, baby spinach	2460kJ	↑ Fat	223, 220	Average
Chunky, chilli red	2120kJ	↑ Salt ↑ Fat	220, 202	Average
Chunky, exotic Thai	2430kJ	↑ Fat	211, 223, 220	Average

Chunky, roasted pumpkin	2220kJ	↑ Salt ↑ Fat	211, 220	Average
Chunky, rocket	2140kJ	↑ Fat	220	Average
Chunky, spicy tomato & basil	1940kJ	↑ Salt ↑ Fat	220, 202	Average
Chunky, sweet chilli	1940kJ	↑ Salt ↑ Fat	220, 202	Average

Willow Farm

Product Name	Energy	Major Nutrients	Food Additives	Nutritious Rating
French onion	885kJ	↑ Fat	320, 223, 220	Average
Semi dried tomato	656kJ	↑ Salt ↑ Fat	220	Average

Fresh Juice

Commercial fresh juice isn't any healthier than the long life varieties, but in my opinion they do taste better. Orange juice contains the least amount of sugar, while apple contains the highest amount. The best brands are: *Cole, Charlies, Berri, Nudie and Golden circle.*

Berri

Product Name	Energy	Major Nutrients	Food Additives	Nutritious Rating
Apple & pineapple juice	207kJ	↑ Sugar	✓	Good
Apple & mango juice	221kJ	↑ Sugar	✓	Good
Breakfast juice	204kJ	↑ Sugar	✓	Good
Orange juice	**187kJ**	✓	✓	**Good**
Orange juice, pulp free	**187kJ**	✓	✓	**Good**
Super juice, immune	202kJ	↑ Sugar	✓	Good

Brownes

Product Name	Energy	Major Nutrients	Food Additives	Nutritious Rating
Orange C juice	200kJ	↑ Sugar	202	Average
Orange & mango juice	191kJ	↑ Sugar	202	Average

Coles

Product Name	Energy	Major Nutrients	Food Additives	Nutritious Rating
Apple juice	225kJ	↑ Sugar	✓	Good
Apple juice, cloudy	198kJ	↑ Sugar	✓	Good

Product Name	Energy	Major Nutrients	Food Additives	Nutritious Rating
Apple & mango juice	203kJ	↑ Sugar	✓	Good
Apple, pineapple & guava juice	193kJ	↑ Sugar	✓	Good
Orange juice	160kJ	✓	✓	Good
Orange juice, pulp free	160kJ	✓	✓	Good
Orange juice, preservative free	174kJ	✓	✓	Good
Tropical juice	200kJ	✓	✓	Good

Charlies

Product Name	Energy	Major Nutrients	Food Additives	Nutritious Rating
Lemonade	190kJ	↑ Sugar	✓	Average
Orange lemonade	192kJ	↑ Sugar	✓	Average
Orange & mango lemonade	190kJ	↑ Sugar	✓	Average
Peach & passionfruit lemonade	192kJ	↑ Sugar	✓	Average
Raspberry lemonade	193kJ	↑ Sugar	✓	Average

Daily Juice Co

Product Name	Energy	Major Nutrients	Food Additives	Nutritious Rating
Apple juice	187kJ	✓	202	Good
Breakfast juice	204kJ	↑ Sugar	202	Good
Classic orange juice	196kJ	✓	202	Good
Orange juice, pulp free	170kJ	✓	202	Good
Orange & mango juice	197kJ	✓	202	Good

Golden Circle

Product Name	Energy	Major Nutrients	Food Additives	Nutritious Rating
Finest, Apple, cranberry &	200kJ	↑ Sugar	✓	Good

pomegranate juice				
Finest, orange juice	170kJ	✓	✓	Good
Finest, orange juice pulp free	170kJ	✓	✓	Good
Finest, pineapple juice	215kJ	↑ Sugar	✓	Good
Raw, berry burst juice	180kJ	✓	✓	Good
Raw, citrus crush	200kJ	✓	✓	Good

Harvey Fresh

Product Name	Energy	Major Nutrients	Food Additives	Nutritious Rating
100% orange juice	180kJ	✓	202	Good
100%orange & passionfruit juice	200kJ	✓	202	Good
Tempt, apple	200kJ	↑ Sugar	202	Average
Tempt, orange	190kJ	✓	202	Average
Tempt, orange & mango	190kJ	↑ Sugar	202	Average
Tempt, orange & passionfruit	190kJ	✓	202	Average

Mildura

Product Name	Energy	Major Nutrients	Food Additives	Nutritious Rating
Sunrise, apple & guava	172kJ	✓	202, 211	Average
Sunrise, orange & mango	180kJ	✓	160b, 202, 211	Average
Sunrise, orange & passionfruit	170kJ	✓	160b, 202, 211	Average
Sunrise, tropical	168kJ	✓	160b, 202, 211	Average

Nudie

Product Name	Energy	Major Nutrients	Food Additives	Nutritious Rating
Apple juice	191kJ	↑ Sugar	✓	Good
Breakfast juice	368kJ	✓	✓	Good
Coconut water	130kJ	✓	✓	Good
Cranberry & raspberry	203kJ	✓	✓	Good

juice				
Mango & passionfruit juice	226kJ	✓	✓	Good
Orange juice	170kJ	✓	✓	Good
Orange juice, pulp free	170kJ	✓	✓	Good
Orange, mango & pineapple juice	183kJ	✓	✓	Good

Original Juice Co

Product Name	Energy	Major Nutrients	Food Additives	Nutritious Rating
Apple & mango juice	215kJ	↑ Sugar	✓	Good
Breakfast juice	210kJ	✓	✓	Good
Orange juice	170kJ	✓	✓	Good
Orange juice, pulp free	170kJ	✓	✓	Good
Black label, apple & forest fruit juice	199kJ	✓	✓	Good
Black label, apple, lime & mint juice	200kJ	✓	✓	Good
Black label, Apple, peach & apricot	202kJ	↑ Sugar	✓	Good
Black label, grapefruit	177kJ	✓	✓	Good

Tofu & Vegetarian

I really wish pre-packaged vegetarian food was done a lot better; unfortunately they often contain preservatives and/or flavour enhancers. Tofu is reliably additive free.

Australian Eat Well

Product Name	Energy	Major Nutrients	Food Additives	Nutritious Rating
Chickpea & spinach sausages	411kJ	↑ Salt	HVP, 202, 407	Good
Tomato, basil & onion sausages	463kJ	↑ Salt	HVP, 202, 407	Good

Joyce Tofu

Product Name	Energy	Major Nutrients	Food Additives	Nutritious Rating
Firm	255kJ	✓	✓	Good
Silken	190kJ	✓	✓	Good
Stir-fry	665kJ	✓	✓	Good

Nutri Soy Organic

Product Name	Energy	Major Nutrients	Food Additives	Nutritious Rating
Tofu	440kJ	✓	✓	Good

Sanitarium

Product Name	Energy	Major Nutrients	Food Additives	Nutritious Rating
Bacon style rashes	980kJ	↑ Salt ↑ Fat	YE	Good
BBQ sausages	851kJ	↑ Salt ↑ Fat	407, YE, 635	Good
Hot dogs	840kJ	↑ Salt ↑ Fat	407, 160b	Good
Rosemary, sage &	1070kJ	↑ Salt	407, YE, HVP	Good

parsley sausages		↑ Fat		
Smoked deli slices	720kJ	↑ Salt ↑ Fat	407, YE, 635	Good
Sundried tomato & olive sausages	880kJ	↑ Salt	407, YE, HVP	Good
Thai sweet chilli lime burgers	730kJ	↑ Salt ↑ Fat	407, YE, 220	Good
Vegie sausages	911kJ	↑ Salt ↑ Fat	635, YE	Good

Soyco Tofu

Product Name	Energy	Major Nutrients	Food Additives	Nutritious Rating
Chinese	714kJ	↑ Fat	✓	Good
Japanese	732kJ	↑ Fat	✓	Good
Malaysian	732kJ	↑ Fat	✓	Good
Thai	714kJ	↑ Fat	✓	Good

Fruit and Vegetable Composition

Product Name	Energy	Nutrients
Apple	207kJ	Calcium, folate, potassium, vitamin C, vitamin K
Apricot	156kJ	Calcium, folate, iron, potassium, vitamin C, vitamin B5
Asparagus	79kJ	Calcium, folate, iron, magnesium, niacin, potassium, vitamin C, zinc
Avocado	879kJ	Calcium, folate, iron, magnesium, niacin, potassium, vitamin C, zinc
Banana	358kJ	Calcium, folate, iron, magnesium, niacin, potassium, vitamin C, vitamin B6
Beans	69kJ	Calcium, folate, iron, magnesium, potassium, vitamin C, vitamin K, zinc
Broccoli	101kJ	Calcium, folate, iron, magnesium, niacin, potassium, vitamin C, zinc
Brussels' sprout	103kJ	Calcium, folate, iron, magnesium, niacin, potassium, vitamin C, zinc
Cabbage	65kJ	Calcium, folate, iron, magnesium, potassium, vitamin C, vitamin K
Capsicum	79kJ	Calcium, folate, iron, magnesium, potassium, vitamin A, vitamin C
Carrot	103kJ	Calcium, folate, iron, magnesium, potassium, vitamin A, vitamin C
Cauliflower	80kJ	Calcium, folate, iron, magnesium, potassium, vitamin C
Celery	51kJ	Calcium, folate, magnesium, potassium, vitamin C
Cherry	224kJ	Calcium, folate, magnesium, potassium, vitamin C
Cucumber	48kJ	Calcium, folate, magnesium, vitamin C
Grape	267kJ	Calcium, folate, magnesium, potassium, vitamin C
Grapefruit	111kJ	Calcium, folate, magnesium, niacin, potassium, vitamin C
Honey dew melon	132kJ	Calcium, folate, iron, magnesium, potassium, vitamin C

Kiwifruit	204kJ	Calcium, folate, iron, magnesium, potassium, vitamin C
Leek	101kJ	Calcium, folate, iron, magnesium, potassium, vitamin C, zinc
Lettuce	27kJ	Calcium, folate, magnesium, potassium, vitamin C
Mandarin	162kJ	Calcium, folate, magnesium, potassium, vitamin C
Mango	236kJ	Calcium, folate, iron, magnesium, niacin, potassium, vitamin C, zinc
Mushroom	98kJ	Folate, magnesium, potassium, vitamin B12
Nectarine	156kJ	Calcium, folate, magnesium, potassium, vitamin C
Orange	156kJ	Calcium, folate, iron, magnesium, potassium, vitamin C, vitamin K
Onion	111kJ	Calcium, folate, iron, magnesium, niacin, potassium, vitamin C
Passionfruit	193kJ	Calcium, iron, magnesium, niacin, potassium, vitamin C, zinc
Pea	249kJ	Calcium, folate, iron, magnesium, niacin, potassium, vitamin C, zinc
Peach	132kJ	Calcium, folate, magnesium, potassium, vitamin C
Pear	218kJ	Calcium, folate, magnesium, potassium, vitamin C, vitamin B5
Persimmon	278kJ	Calcium, folate, iron, magnesium, potassium, vitamin C
Pineapple	158kJ	Calcium, folate, iron, magnesium, potassium, vitamin C
Plum	146kJ	Calcium, folate, magnesium, potassium, vitamin C
Potato	272kJ	Calcium, folate, iron, magnesium, niacin, potassium, vitamin C, vitamin B6zinc
Pumpkin	176kJ	Calcium, folate, iron, magnesium, niacin, potassium, vitamin C, zinc
Rockmelon	91kJ	Calcium, folate, iron, magnesium, potassium, vitamin C
Silverbeet	62kJ	Calcium, folate, iron, magnesium,

		potassium, vitamin A, vitamin C, vitamin K
Squash	112kJ	Calcium, folate, magnesium, potassium, vitamin C
Strawberry	81kJ	Calcium, folate, iron, magnesium, potassium, vitamin C
Swede	112kJ	Calcium, folate, iron, magnesium, niacin, potassium, vitamin C
Sweet potato	311kJ	Calcium, folate, iron, magnesium, niacin, potassium, vitamin C, zinc
Sweetcorn	426kJ	Calcium, folate, iron, magnesium, niacin, potassium, vitamin C, zinc
Tomato	56kJ	Calcium, folate, iron, magnesium, niacin, potassium, vitamin C
Watermelon	96kJ	Calcium, folate, iron, magnesium, potassium, vitamin C
Zucchini	66kJ	Calcium, folate, iron, magnesium, niacin, potassium, vitamin C, zinc

Source: Nutritional value of Australian foods (ANZFA) & Serve nutrition software (AUSNUT)

Glossary

HF	Hydrolysed fat
HO	Hydrolysed oil
HVO	Hydrolysed vegetable oil
HVP	Hydrolysed vegetable protein
VE	Vegetable extract
VP	Vegetable powder
VPE	Vegetable protein extract
YE	Yeast extract

For more information and updates visit my website www.asnatureintended.biz and find me on facebook at my page the undeniable truth about FOOD.

Other Titles

The Undeniable Truth About Food: A phases approach to making changes that make a real difference to you and the planet. (2012) Published by SBPRA

The Additive Free Cookbook. (2012) Published by Amazon

References

Allen, D.H., Van Nunens, S., Loblay, R., Clark, L. & Swain, A. (1984). Adverse reactions to foods, *Medical Journal Australia,* 141(S37-S42)

Aranitoyyannis, I.S. & Bosnea, L. (2004). Migration of substances from food packaging materials to food. *Critical Review Food Science Nutrition. 44(2): 63-76.*

Ashraf-Ur-Rahman, F.R.Chowdhury, & B. Alam. (2008). Artificial ripening: what are we eating. *Journal of Medicine,* (9): 42-44.

Barker, A. (1975). Organic vs inorganic nutrition and horticultural crop quality. *Horticultural Science,* 10: pp. 50-53.

Bateman, B., Warner, J., Hutchinson, E. et al. (2004). The effects of double blind, placebo controlled artificial food colourings and benzoate preservative challenge on hyperactivity on the general population: sample of preschool children. *Archives of Disabled Children,* 89: 506-11.

Barnard, N.D., Cohen, J., Jenkins, D.J., Turner-McGrievy, G., Gloede, L., Green, A. Ferdowsian, H. (2009). A low-fat diet elicits greater macronutrient changes, but is comparable in adherence and acceptability, compared with a more conventional diabetes diet among individuals with type 2 diabetes. *The American journal of clinical nutrition.* Feb; 109(2): pp. 263-273.

Briggs, D.R. (1997). Food additives. Wahlqvist, M.L. (Ed.), *Allen & Unwin, Australia.*

Briggs, D.R. (1997). Naturally occurring toxicants and food contaminants. Wahlqvist, M.L. (Ed.), *Allen & Unwin, Australia.*

Briggs, D.R. & Lennard, L.B. (1997). Recent developments in food technologies. (In). Food and Nutrition. Wahlqvist, M.L. (Ed.), *Allen & Unwin, Australia.*

Carlson, E., Chva, J. & Belcher, S. (2008). Bisphenol A found in polycarbonate plastics and epoxy resins.

Castle, L., Jickells, S.M., Gilbert, J. & Harrisons, W. (1990). Migration testing of plastics and microwave-active materials for high temperature food applications. *Food Additive Contamination. Nov-Dec,* 7(6): 779-796.

Castle, L., Mercer, A.J., Startin, J.R. & Gilbert, J. (1987). Migration from plasticized films into foods: migration of di-(2-ethylhexyl)adipate from PVC film used for retail food packaging. *Food Additive Contamination. Oct-Dec,* 4(4): 399-406.

Chan, E., Griffiths, S., & Chan, C. (2008). Public health risks of melamine in milk products. *Lancet;* *372.*

Cobiac, L. (1994). Lactose: A review of intakes and of importance of health of Australians and New Zealanders. *Supplement to Food Australia,* 46(1-28)

Cooper, J.E., Kendig, E.L. Belcher, S.M. (2011). Assessment of bisphenol A released from reusable, aluminium and stainless steel water bottles. *Chemosphere, Dept. of Pharmalogy and cell biophysics; University of Cincinnati College of Medicine.*

Craig, W.J., Mangels, A.R., American Dietetic Association. (2009). Position of the American Dietetic Association: vegetarian diets. *Journal of the American Dietetic Association,* July; 109(7): pp. 1266-1282.

Cwiek-Ludwicka, K., Jurkiewicz, M., Slelmach, A. & Polterak, H. (2010). Part A chemical analysis control: exposure risk assessment. *Food Additive Contamination. Oct; 27(10): 1478-1486.*

David, T.J. (1993). *Food additive intolerance in childhood.* Blackwell Scientific Publications, London.

Davis, D.R. (2009). Declining fruit and vegetable nutrient composition: what is the evidence? *Horticultural Science,* 44(1) pp.15-19.

Dengate, S. (2008). *Fed up.* Random House, NSW.

Dobias, J., Chudackova, K., Voldrich, M. & Marek, M. (2000). Properties of polyethylene films with incorporated benzoic anhydride and 4-hydroxybenzoic acid and their suitability for food packaging. *Food Additive Contamination. Dec;17(12):1047-1053.*

Editorial. (2007). Food safety reforms in the USA. *The Lancet;* 369: 12/05/07.

Eady, J. (2008). *Additive alert.* Additive Alert, WA.

Epstein, S. (2002). *Unreasonable risk.* Environmental toxicology, Illinois.

Fauconnier, M.L., Panahaleux, V., Vanzereren, E., Marlier, M. & Wathelet, J.P. (2001). Modelling migration from high-density polyethylene containers into concentrated solutions used as food flavourings. *Food Additive Contamination. Nov; 18(11): 1040-1045.*

Fieldhouse, P. (2002). Food and nutrition. *Nelson Thornes, UK.*

Feingold, B.F. (1975). Hyperkinesis and learning disabilities linked to artificial food colours and flavours. *American Journal of Nursing; 75;* pp.797-803.

Fergusson, J. *The vitamin murders.* Portebello Books, London.

Foster, E., Mathers J.C. & Adamson, A.J. (2010). Part A Chemical analysis control exposure risk assessment: Packaged food intake by British children aged 0-6 years. *Food Additive Contamination. Mar; 27(3): 380-388.*

Franz, R. (2002). Programme on the recyclability of food-packaging materials with respect to food safety considerations: polyethylene terephthalate (PET), paper and board, plastics covered by functional barriers. *Food Additive Contamination. 19 Suppl.: 93-110.*

Garde, J.A., Catala, R., Gavara, R. & Hernandez, R.J. (2001). Characterizing the migration of antioxidants from polypropylene into fatty food stimulants. *Food Additive Contamination. Aug; 18(8): 750-762.*

Gilbert, J., Castle, L., Jickells, S.M. & Sharman, M. (1994). Current research of food contact materials undertaken by the ministry of agriculture, fisheries and food. *Food Additive Contamination. Mar-Apr; 11(2): 231-240.*

Gilbert, J., Startin, J.R. & McGuinness, J.D. (1986). Compositional analysis of commercial PVC bottles and studies of aspects of specific and overall migration in foods and stimulants. *Food Additive Contamination. Apr-Jun; 3(2): 133-143.*

Goddard, J.M., Talbert, J.N. & Hotchkiss, J.H. (2007). Covalent attachment of lactase to low-density polyethylene. *Journal of Food Science. Jan; 72(1): E036-041.*

Heath, J.L. & Reilly, M. (1981). Migration of actyl-tribylcitrate from plastic film into poultry during microwave cooking. *Poultry Science. Oct; 60(10): 2258-2264.*

Jenke, D. & Couch, T. (2006). A consideration of the impact of solution on the accumulation of organic substances leached from plastic used in container/closure systems. *Journal of Pharmacological Science Technology. Jan-Feb; 60(1): 60-71.*

Jones, G.P. (1997). Food processing. (In). Wahlqvist, M.L. (Ed.), *Allen & Unwin, Australia.*

Jones, G.P. (1997). Minerals. (In). Wahlqvist, M.L. (Ed.), *Allen & Unwin, Australia.*

Kennedy, E.T., Bowman, S.A., Spence, J.T., Freedmen, M., King, J. (2001) Popular diets: correlation to health, nutrition and obesity. *Journal of American Dietetic Association.* April; 101(4): pp. 411- 420.

Lau, K. (2005). Synergistic interactions between commonly used food additives in a developmental neurotoxicity test. *Toxicology Science (12)*

Layo-Rosales, J.E., Rosales-Riveria, G.C., Lynch, A.M., Rice, C.P. & Torrents, A. (2004). Migration of nonylphenol from plastic containers to water and milk. *Journal of Agriculture & Food Chemistry. (2004). Apr; 52(7):*

2258-2264.

Le, H.H., Carson, E.M., Chva, J.P. & Belcher, S.M. (2008). Bisphenol A is released from polycarbonate drinking bottles and mimics the neurotoxic actions of estrogen in developing cerebellar neurons. *Toxicology Letters. Jan 30; 176(2): 149-156.*

Lehr, K.M., Welsh, G.C., Bell, C.D. & Lickly, T.D. (1993). The 'vapour phase' migration of styrene from general purpose polystyrene and high impact polystyrene. *Food Chemical Contamination. Nov; 31(11): 793-798*

Lickly, T.D., Lehr, K.M. & Walsh, G.C. (1995). Migration of styrene from polystyrene foam food-contact articles. *Food Chemical Toxicology. Jun; 33(6): 475-481.*

Loblay, R. & Swain, A.R. (1996). Food intolerance. In *Recent Advances in Clinical Nutrition 2.* Wahlqvist, M.L. & Truswell, A.S. (eds). John Libbey, London.

Loewenberg, S. (2008). US to debate tightening legislation on safety of chemicals. *Lancet;* 372: 23-24.

Mayer, A.M. (1997). Historical changes in mineral content of fruits and vegetables: a cause for concern. *British Food Journal;* 99: pp.207-11.

McCann, D., & Barrett, A. et al. (2007). Food additives and hyperactive behaviour in 3 year olds and 8/9 year old children in the community: a randomised, double blinded placebo controlled trial. *Lancet; 370* pp.1560-67.

Millstone, E. Lang, T. (2008). Risking regulatory capture at the UK's Food Standards Agency. *The Lancet; 372:* 12/07.08

Moors, S., Diel, P. & Degen, G.H. (2006). Toxicokinetics of bisphenol A inpregnant DA/Han rats after single IV applications. *Archives Toxicology. Oct; 80 (10): 647-655.*

N.a. (2009). Evidence on declining fruit and vegetable nutrient composition. *U.S. Food Policy.* 3/2/09.

Na. (2009). Food safety, food additives. *Centre for science in the public interest.*

Palanza, P.,Gloiosa, L., Vom Saal, F. S. & Parmigaiani, S. (2008). Effects of developmental exposure to bisphenol A on brain and behaviour in mice. *Environmental Research. Oct; 108(8): 150-157.*

Papaspyrides, C.D. & Tingas, S.G. (1998). Comparison of isopropanol and isooctane as food stimulants in plasticizer migration tests. *Food Additive Contamination. Aug-Sept; 15(6): 681-689.*

Perry, J. (2008). China's tainted infant formula sickens nearly 13,000 babies. *British Medical Journal; 337.*

Petersen, J.H., Lillemark, L. & Lund, L. (1997). Migration from PVC cling films compared with their field of application. . *Food Additive Contamination. May-Jun; 14(4): 345-353.*

Petersen, J.H., Naamansen, E.T & Nielsen, P.A. (1995). PVC cling film in contact with cheese: health aspects related to global migration and specific migration of DEHA. *Food Additive Contamination. Mar-Apr; 12(2): 245-253.*

Rijk, R. & deKruijk, N. (1993). Migration testing with olive oils in a microwave oven. *Food Additive Contamination. Nov-Dec;10(6):631-645.*

Read, R.S.D. Jones, G.P. (1997). Food energy and energy expenditure. (In). Wahlqvist, M.L. (Ed.), *Allen & Unwin, Australia.*

Schab, D. & Trihn, N. (2004). Do artificial food colours promote hyperactivity in children with hyperactive syndromes? A meta-analysis of double blind placebo controlled trials. *Journal of Developmental behaviour paediatrics;* 25: pp 423-34.

Shibko, S. & Bumenthal, H. (). Pthalic acid esters used in food packaging materials.

Slimak, K.M. (2003). Reduction of autistic traits following dietary intervention and elimination of exposure to environmental substances. *In Proceedings of 2003 International Symposium on indoor air quality and health hazards, National Institute of Environmental Health Science, USA, and Architectural Institute of Japan, January8-11, 2003, Tokyo, Japan, vol 2 pp206-216.*

Smith, B. (1993). Organic foods vs supermarket foods: element levels. *Journal of Applied Nutrition;* 45: pp.35-39.

Song, Y.S., Begley, T., Paquette, K. & Komolprasert, V. (2003). Effectiveness of polypropylene film as a barrier to migration from recycled paperboard packaging to fatty and high moisture food. *Food Additive Contamination. Sept; 20(9): 875-883.*

Swanson, J.M., Sergeant, J., Taylor, E. et al. (1998). Attention deficit hyperactivity disorder and hyperkinetic disorder. *Lancet;* 351: 429-33.

Tapsell, L.C., Hemphill, I., Cobiac, L., Patch, C.S., Sullivan, D.R., Fenech, M., Roodenrys, S., Keogh, J.B., Cliffton, P.M., Williams, P.G., Fazio, V.A., Inge, K.E. (2006). Health benefits of herbs and spices: the past, present and future. *The medical journal of Australia.* Aug; 185(4 Suppl): pp. S4-24.

Tehrany, E.A. & Desobry, S. (2004). Partition co-efficient in food/packaging systems: a review. *Dec; 21(12): 1186-1202.*

Till, D., Schwope, A.D., Ehnthoit, D.J.,Sidman, K.R., Whelan, R.H., Schwartz, P.S & Reid, R.C. (2003). Indirect food additive migration from polymeric food packaging materials. *Critical Review Toxocology; 18(3): 215-243.*

Vandenberg, L.N., Hauser, R., Marcus, M. Olea, N. & Welshons, W. (2007). Human exposure to bisphenol A (BPA). *Reproductive Toxicolgy. Aug-Sept; 24(2): 139-177.*

Vitrac, O. & Leblanc, J.C. (2007). Consumer exposure to substances in plastic packaging. Assessment of the contribution of styrene from yogurt pots. *Food Additive Contamination; 24(2): 194-215.*

Vogtmann, H. (1988). From healthy soil to healthy food: an analysis of the quality of food produced under contrasting agricultural systems. *Nutrition Health;* 6: 21-35.

Wagner, M. & Oehlmann, J. (2009). Endrocrine disruptors in bottled mineral water: total estrogenic burden and migration from plastic bottles. *Environmental Science Pollution Research Institute. May; (16): 278-286.*

Wahlqvist, M.L. (1997). Vitamins and vitamin-like compounds. *Allen & Unwin, Australia.*

Walker-Smith, J.A. (1984). Cow's milk protein intolerance in infancy. In *Food intolerance.* Chandra, R.K., (ed). Elsevier, New York.

Wikipedia. (2011). The free encyclopedia. *en.wikipedia.org*

Williams, D. (2008). Living with autism. In *Everyday Health;* 18(3).

Wilson, B. (2008). *Swindled: from poison sweets to counterfeit coffee, the dark history of food cheats.* John Murray, London.

Worthington, V. (2001). Nutritional quality of organic versus conventional fruits, vegetables and grains. *Journal of Alternative and Complementary Medicine;* 7(2): pp. 161-173.

www.ingramcontent.com/pod-product-compliance
Lightning Source LLC
Chambersburg PA
CBHW082128290526

45794CB00008B/2969